# Statistical Methodologies with
# Medical Applications

# Statistical Methodologies with Medical Applications

**Poduri S.R.S. Rao**

*Professor of Statistics*
*University of Rochester*
*Rochester, New York, USA*

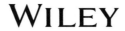

*Library of Congress Cataloging-in-Publication Data*

Names: Rao, Poduri S.R.S., author.
Title: Statistical methodologies with medical applications / Poduri S.R.S. Rao.
Description: Chichester, West Sussex, United Kingdom ; Hoboken : John Wiley & Sons Inc., 2016. |
  Includes bibliographical references and index.
Identifiers: LCCN 2016022669| ISBN 9781119258490 (cloth) | ISBN 9781119258483 (Adobe PDF) |
  ISBN 9781119258520 (epub)
Subjects: | MESH: Statistics as Topic
Classification: LCC RA409 | NLM WA 950 | DDC 610.2/1–dc23
LC record available at https://lccn.loc.gov/2016022669

A catalogue record for this book is available from the British Library.

Cover Image: Gun2becontinued/Gettyimages

Set in 10/12pt Times by SPi Global, Pondicherry, India
Printed and bound in Malaysia by Vivar Printing Sdn Bhd

10  9  8  7  6  5  4  3  2  1

*To my grandchildren*
*Asha, Sita,*
*Maya and Wyatt*

# Contents

# Topics for illustrations, examples and exercises

Heights, weights and BMI (Body Mass Index) of sixteen and twenty-year-old boys from growth charts

Immunization coverage of one-year-olds: Measles, DTP3 and HEP B3 from WHO reports

Medical insurance for children

Sudden Infant Syndrome (SIDS)

Population growth rates and fertility

Age, family size, income and health insurance

Healthcare expenditure in Africa, Asia and Europe

Vaccination for flu for different age groups

Emergency department visits for cold symptoms, injuries and other reasons.

Overweight and obesity

Trends of adult obesity

BMI and mortality

Smoking, heart disease and cancer risk

Air pollution and cancer risk

Hypertension, systolic and diastolic blood pressures (SBP, DBP) of males and females.

Cholesterol levels: LDL and HDL

Effects of overweight on LDL

Low-dose aspirin and reduction of certain types of cancer

Celiac disease and the benefits of gluten-free diet

Statins and the reduction of LDL

Exercise and its benefits for blood pressure levels

Weight loss with diets of combinations of low and high levels of fatty acids and protein

Medical rehabilitation of stroke patients

Functional independence measures of stroke patients from medical rehabilitation

*Sources*: Reports of WHO, CDC, U.S. Health Statistics; *Journal of the American Medical Association* (*JAMA*); *New England Journal of Medicine* (*NEJM*), *Lancet* and other published literature.

# Preface

Statistical analysis, evaluation and inference are essential for every type of medical study and clinical experiment. Physicians and medical clinics and laboratories routinely record the blood pressures, cholesterol levels and other relevant diagnostic measurements of patients. Clinical experiments evaluate and compare the effects of medical treatments and procedures. Medical journals report the research findings on the relative risks and odds ratios related to hypertension, abnormal cholesterol levels, obesity, harmful effects of smoking habits and excessive alcohol consumption and similar topics.

Estimation of the means, standard deviations, proportions, odds ratios, relative risks and related statistical measures of health-related characteristics are of importance for the above types of medical studies. Evaluation of the errors of estimation, ascertaining the confidence limits for the population characteristics of interest, tests of hypotheses and statistical inference, and Chisquare tests for independence and association of categorical variables are important aspects of many medical studies and clinical experiments. Statistical inference is employed, for instance, to assess the relationship between obesity and hypertension and the association between air pollution and bronchial problems. A variety of similar problems require statistical investigations and inference. Regression analysis is widely used to determine the relationship of clinical outcomes and physical attributes. In several clinical investigations, correlations between diagnostic observations are examined to search for the causal factors. Analysis of Variance and Covariance procedures are extensively employed to examine the differences between the effects of medical treatments. All the above types of statistical methods, procedures and techniques required for medical studies, research and evaluations are presented in the following chapters. Topics such as the Meta-analysis, Survival Analysis and Hazard Ratios, and nonparametric statistics are also included.

Following the descriptive statistical measures in the first chapter, definitions of probability, odds ratios and relative risk appear in Chapters 2 and 3. Binomial, normal, Chisquare and related probability distributions essential for the statistical methods and applications are presented in Chapter 4. Estimation of the means, variances, proportions and percentages, odds ratios and relative risks, Standard Errors (S.E.) of the estimators and confidence intervals appear in Chapters 5 and 6. Tests of hypotheses of means, proportions and variances, p-values, power of a test, sample size required for a specified power are the topics for Chapters 7 and 8. The Chisquare tests for goodness of fit and independence are presented in Chapter 9. Linear, multiple and logistic regressions and correlation are the topics for Chapter 10. Chapter 11 presents the Analysis of Variance (ANOVA) and Covariance procedures, Randomized bocks,

Latin square designs, fixed and random effects models, and two-way cross-classification with and without interaction. Meta-analysis and Survival Analysis in Chapters 12 and 13 are followed by the nonparametric statistics in Chapter 14. The final chapter contains topics in ANOVA and tests of hypotheses including the Simultaneous Confidence Intervals and Bootstrap Confidence Intervals.

Examples, illustrations and exercises with solutions are presented in each chapter. They are constructed from the observations of practical situations, research studies appearing in *The New England Journal of Medicine* (*NEJM*), *Journal of the American Medical Association* (*JAMA*), *Lancet* and other medical journals, and the summaries presented in the *Health Statistics* of the *Center for Disease Control* (CDC) in the United States and the *World Health Organization* (WHO). They are related to a variety of medical topics of general interest including the following: (a) heights, weights and Body Mass Index (BMI) of ten-to-twenty-year-old boys and girls; (b) immunization of children; (c) overweight, obesity, hypertension and high cholesterol levels of adults; (d) benefits of fat-free and gluten-free diets and exercise, and (e) healthcare expenditures and medical insurance.

BMI is the ratio of the weight in kilograms to the square of the height in meters. A person is considered to be of normal weight if the BMI is 18.5–24, overweight if it is 25–29, and obese if it is 30 or more. For the blood cholesterol levels of adults, LDL less than 100 mg/dL and HDL higher than 40 mg/dL are considered optimal. Systolic and diastolic blood pressures, SBP and DBP of 120/80 mmHg are considered desirable. Illustrations and examples and exercises throughout the chapters are related to these medical measurements and other health-related topics. Readily available software programs in *Excel, Minitab* and R are utilized for the solutions of the illustrations, examples and exercises.

The various topics in these chapters are presented at the level of comprehension of the students pursuing statistics, biostatistics, medicine, biological, physical and natural sciences and epidemiological studies. Each topic is illustrated through examples. More than one hundred exercises with solutions are included. This book can be recommended for a one-semester or two-quarter course for the above types of students, and also for self-study. One or two semesters of training in the principles and applications of statistical methods provides adequate preparation to pursue the different topics. The various statistical methods for medical studies presented in this manuscript can also be of interest to clinicians, physicians, and medical students and residents.

I would like to thank the editor, Ms. Kathryn Sharples, for her interest in this project. Thanks to Charles Heckler, Kevin Rader and Nicholas Zaino for their expert reviews of the manuscript. Thanks also to Sarah Briscoe, Isabelle Weir and Patricia Digiorgio for their assistance in assembling the manuscript on the word processor. Special thanks to my wife and daughter, Drs. K. R. Poduri M.D, FAAPMR, and Ann Poduri Hug M.D, MPH for sharing their medical expertise in selecting the various topics and illustrations throughout the chapters.

**Poduri S.R.S. Rao**
Professor of Statistics
University of Rochester

# List of abbreviations

WHO: World Health Organization
CDC: Center for Disease Control
LDL: Low Density Lipoprotein
HDL: High Density Lipoprotein
LDL and HDL are measures of cholesterol levels in units of milligrams for Deciliter (mg/dl)
SBP : Systolic Blood Pressure
DBP: Diastolic Blood Pressure
SBP and DBP are measures of pressure in the blood vessels in units of millimeters of mercury (mmHg)
BMI: Body Mass Index

# 1

# Statistical measures

## 1.1 Introduction

Medical professionals, hospitals and healthcare centers record heights, weights and other relevant physical measurements of patients along with their blood pressures cholesterol levels and similar diagnostic measurements. National organizations such as the Center for Disease Control (CDC) in the United States, the World Health Organization (WHO) and several national and international organizations record and analyze various aspects of the healthcare status of the citizens of all age groups. Epidemiological studies and surveys collect and analyze health-related information of the people around the globe. Clinical trials and experiments are conducted for the development of effective and improved medical treatments.

Statistical measures are utilized to analyze the various diagnostic measurements as well as the outcomes of clinical experiments. The mean, mode and median described in the following sections locate the centers of the distributions of the above types of observations. The variance, standard deviation (S.D.) and the related coefficient of variation (C.V.) are the measures of dispersion of a set of observations. The quartiles, deciles and percentiles divide the data respectively into four, ten and one hundred equal parts. The skewness coefficient exhibits the departure of the data from its symmetry, and the kurtosis coefficient its peakedness. The measurements on the heights, weights and Body Mass Indexes (BMIs) of a sample of twenty-year-old boys obtained from the Chart Tables of the CDC (2008) are presented in Table 1.1. These measurements for the ten and sixteen- year old boys and girls are presented in Appendix Tables T1.1–T1.4.

*Statistical Methodologies with Medical Applications*, First Edition. Poduri S.R.S. Rao.
© 2017 John Wiley & Sons, Ltd. Published 2017 by John Wiley & Sons, Ltd.

Table 1.1    Heights (cm), weights (kg) and BMIs of twenty-year old boys.

| Height | Weight | BMI |
|--------|--------|-------|
| 162 | 54 | 20.58 |
| 163 | 55 | 20.70 |
| 167 | 58 | 20.80 |
| 168 | 59 | 20.90 |
| 170 | 60 | 20.76 |
| 172 | 62 | 20.96 |
| 172 | 63 | 21.30 |
| 173 | 66 | 22.05 |
| 174 | 68 | 22.46 |
| 176 | 72 | 23.24 |
| 176 | 75 | 24.21 |
| 176 | 75 | 24.21 |
| 177 | 78 | 24.90 |
| 178 | 80 | 25.25 |
| 178 | 82 | 25.88 |
| 180 | 84 | 25.93 |
| 184 | 86 | 25.40 |
| 184 | 88 | 25.99 |
| 186 | 95 | 27.46 |
| 188 | 102 | 28.86 |

$BMI = Weight/(Height)^2$.

## 1.2    Mean, mode and median

The diagnostic measurements of a sample of $n$ individuals can be represented by $x_i, i = (1,2,\ldots,n)$. Their mean or average is

$$\bar{x} = \sum_{i=1}^{n} x_i/n = (x_1 + x_2 + \ldots + x_n)/n. \tag{1.1}$$

For the heights of the boys in Table 1.1, the mean becomes $\bar{x} = (162 + 163 + \ldots + 188)/20 = 175.2$ cm. Similarly, the mean of their weights is 73.1 kg. For the BMI, which is (Weight/Height$^2$), the mean becomes 23.59.

The mode is the observation occurring more frequently than the remaining observations. For the heights of the boys, it is 176 cm. The median is the middle value of the observations. If the number of observations $n$ is odd, it is the $(n + 1)$th observation. If $n$ is an even number, it is the average of the $(n/2)$th and the next observation. Both the mode and median of the twenty heights of the boys in Table 1.1 are equal to 176 cm, which is slightly larger than the mean of 175.2 cm.

| 2 | 16 23 |
| 4 | 16 78 |
| 9 | 17 02234 |
| (6) | 17 666788 |
| 5 | 18 044 |
| 2 | 18 68 |

*Figure 1.1 Stem and leaf display of the heights of the twenty boys. Leaf unit = 1.0. The median class has (6) observations. The cumulative number of observations below and above the median class are (2, 4, 9) and (5, 2).*

The mean, mode and median locate the center of the observations. The mean is also known as the first moment $m_1$ of the observations. For the healthcare policies, for instance, it is of importance to examine the average amount of the medical expenditures incurred by families of different sizes or specified ranges of income. At the same time, useful information is provided by the median and modal values of their expenditures. Figure 1.1 is the Stem and Leaf display of the heights in Table 1.1. The cumulative number of observations below and above the median appear in the first column. The second and third columns are the stems, with the attached leaves.

## 1.3   Variance and standard deviation

The variance is a measure of the dispersion among the observations, and it is given by

$$s^2 = \sum_{i=1}^{n}(x_i-\bar{x})^2/(n-1)$$
$$= \left[(x_i-\bar{x})^2 + (x_2-\bar{x})^2 + ...(x_n-\bar{x})^2\right]/(n-1). \tag{1.2}$$

The divisor $(n-1)$ in this expression represents the *degrees of freedom* (d.f.). If $(n-1)$ of the observations and the sum or mean of the $n$ observations are known, the remaining observation is automatically determined. The expression in (1.2) can also be expressed as $\sum_{i\neq j}(x_i-x_j)^2/n(n-1)$, which is the average of the squared differences of the $n(n-1)$ pairs of the observations. The standard deviation (S.D.) is given by $s$, the positive square root of the variance. The second central moment of the observations $m_2 = \sum(x_i-\bar{x})^2/n$ is the same as $(n-1)s^2/n$. For the twenty heights of boys in

Table 1.2    Summary figures for the heights, weights and BMIs of the 20 boys in Table 1.1.

|  | Height | Weight | BMI |
|---|---|---|---|
| Mean ($\bar{x}$) | 175.2 | 73.1 | 23.59 |
| Variance ($s^2$) | 51.33 | 188.09 | 6.53 |
| $m_2$ | 48.76 | 178.69 | 6.21 |
| S.D.(s) | 7.16 | 13.71 | 2.56 |
| C.V.(%) | 4.09 | 18.76 | 10.85 |
| $m_3$ | −18.86 | 913.69 | 5.24 |
| $K_1$ | −0.055 | 0.383 | 0.341 |
| $m_4$ | 5690 | 70901 | 75.93 |
| $K_2$ | 2.39 | 2.22 | 1.97 |

Table 1.1, $s^2 = \left[(162-175.2)^2 + (163-175.2)^2 + \ldots + (188-175.2)^2\right]/19 = 51.33$ and $m_2 = (19/20)(51.33) = 48.76$. The standard deviation becomes $s = 7.16$ cm.

The unit of measurement is attached to both the mean and standard deviation; kg for weight and cm for height. It is kg/(meter-squared) for the BMI. The coefficient of variation (C.V.), is the ratio of the standard deviation to the mean ($s/\bar{x}$) and is devoid of the unit of measurement of the observations. The mean, variance, standard deviation and C.V. for the above three characteristics for the 20 boys in Table 1.1 are presented Table 1.2.

## 1.4    Quartiles, deciles and percentiles

Any set of data can be arranged in an ascending order and divided into four parts with one quarter of the observations in each part. Twenty-five percent of the observations are below the first quartile $Q_1$ and 75 percent above. Similarly, half the number of observations are below the median, which is the second quartile $Q_2$, and half above. Three-quarters of the observations are below the third quartile $Q_3$ and one-fourth above. As seen in Section 1.2, the median of the heights in Table 1.1 is 176 cm. The average of the fifth and sixth observations is 171 cm, which is the first quartile. Similarly, the third quartile is 179 cm, which is the average of the fifteenth and sixteenth observations. The box and whiskers plot in Figure 1.2 presents the positions of these quartiles.

Ten percent of the observations are below the first decile and 90 percent above. Ninety percent of the observations are below the ninth decile and 10 percent above. One percent of the observations are below the first percentile and 99 percent above. Similarly, 99 percent of the observations are below the ninety-ninth percentile and 1 percent above.

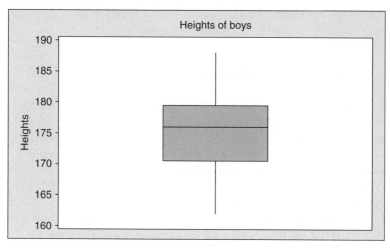

*Figure 1.2 Box and whiskers plot of the heights of boys in Table 1.1, obtained from Minitab. The middle line of the box is the median $Q_2$. The bottom and top lines are the first and third quartiles $Q_1$ and $Q_3$. The tips of the vertical line, whiskers, are the upper and lower limits $Q_1 + 1.5(Q_3 - Q_1)$ and $Q_1 - 1.5(Q_3 - Q_1)$.*

## 1.5 Skewness and kurtosis

Physical or diagnostic measurements $x_i, i = (1, 2, \ldots, n)$, of a group of individuals may not be symmetrically distributed about their mean. The third central moment, $m_3 = \sum_1^n (x_i - \bar{x})^3 / n$ will be zero if the observations are symmetrically distributed about the mean. It will be positive if the observations are skewed to the right and negative if they are skewed to the left. For the symmetrically distributed observations, the third, fifth, seventh and all the odd central moments will be zero. The *Pearsonian coefficient of skewness* is given by $K_1 = m_3 / m_2^{3/2}$, which does not depend on the unit of measurement of the observations unlike $m_2$ and $m_3$. For any set of observations symmetrically distributed about its mean, $m_3 = 0$ and hence $K_1 = 0$. For the positively skewed observations, $m_3$ and $K_1$ are positive. For the negatively skewed observations, they are negative. For the heights of the boys in Table 1.1, $m_3 = -18.86$ and $K_1 = -18.86 / (48.76)^{3/2} = -0.055$. These heights are slightly negatively skewed.

The fourth central moment of the observations, $m_4 = \sum_1 (x_i - \bar{x})^4 / n$, becomes large as the distribution of the observations becomes peaked and small as it becomes flat. The *Pearsonian coefficient of kurtosis* is given by $K_2 = m_4 / m_2^2$, which does not depend on the unit of measurement. For the normal distribution, which is extensively employed for statistical analysis and inference, $K_1 = 0$ and $K_2 = 3$. For the observations on all the three characteristics in Table 1.1, the fourth moments are large, as seen from Table 1.2, but $K_2$ is smaller than three.

## 1.6   Frequency distributions

Any set of clinical measurements or medical observations can be classified into a convenient number of groups and presented as the *frequency distribution*. The CDC, National Center for Health Statistics (NCHS) and other organizations present various health-related measurements on the U.S. population in the form of summary tables. These measurements are obtained from periodic or continual surveys of the population in the country and also from the administrative medical records of the population. They are arranged according to age groups, education, income levels, male-female classification and other characteristics of interest. Similar summary figures are presented by the WHO and healthcare organizations throughout the world. For the sake of illustration, the twenty heights of the boys in Table 1.1 are arranged in Table 1.3 into seven classes of the same width of five, and displayed as the histogram in Figure 1.3.

In general, the n observations can be divided into $k$ classes with $n_i$ observations in the $i$th class, $n = \sum_1^k n_i$. The mid-values of the classes can be denoted by $(x_1, x_2, \ldots, x_k)$. With the above notation, the mean of the $n$ observations becomes

$$\bar{x} = \sum_1^k f_i x_i = (n_1 x_1 + n_2 x_2 + \ldots + n_k x_k)/n, \tag{1.3}$$

where $f_i = n_i/n$ is the relative frequency in the $i$th class and $\sum_1^k f_i = 1$. From the above table and (1.3), the mean of the heights is

$$\bar{x} = (1 \times 160 + 2 \times 165 + \ldots + 1 \times 190)/20 = 175.25.$$

Since the 20 observations are grouped, this mean differs slightly from the actual value of 175.2 cm.

Table 1.3   Frequency distribution of the heights of the 20 boys in Table 1.1.

| Class | Mid-$x_i$ | Frequency ($n_i$) | Relative frequency ($f_i$) |
|---|---|---|---|
| 157.5–162.5 | 160 | 1 | 0.05 |
| 162.5–167.5 | 165 | 2 | 0.10 |
| 167.5–172.5 | 170 | 4 | 0.20 |
| 172.5–177.5 | 175 | 6 | 0.30 |
| 177.5–182.5 | 180 | 3 | 0.15 |
| 182.5–187.5 | 185 | 3 | 0.15 |
| 187.5–192.5 | 190 | 1 | 0.05 |
| | | $n = 20$ | $\Sigma f_i = 1$ |

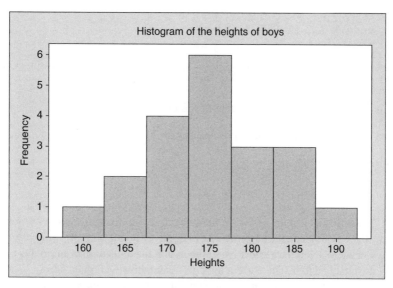

*Figure 1.3   Histogram of the distribution of the heights of the boys in Table 1.3 obtained from* Minitab.

For the grouped data, the second moment becomes

$$m_2 = \sum_{i=1}^{k} f_i(x_i - \bar{x})^2 = \left[ n_1(x_1 - \bar{x})^2 + n_2(x_2 - \bar{x})^2 + \ldots + n_k(x_k - \bar{x})^2 \right]/n. \qquad (1.4)$$

Now, $s^2 = \sum_{1}^{k} n_i(x_i - \bar{x})^2 / (n-1) = nm_2/(n-1)$. From (1.4), for the heights of the boys, $m_2 = 56.19$ and $s^2 = 59.14$, which differ from the actual values 48.76 and 51.33 as a result of the grouping. From the grouped data, the third and fourth central moments are obtained from $m_3 = \sum_{1}^{k} f_i(x_i - \bar{x})^3$ and $m_4 = \sum_{1}^{k} f_i(x_i - \bar{x})^4$. In general, the $r$th central moment for the grouped data is given by $m_r = \sum_{1}^{k} f_i(x_i - \bar{x})^r$.

## 1.7   Covariance and correlation

The heights and weights of the 20 boys in Table 1.1 can be denoted by $(x_i, y_i), i = (1, 2, \ldots, n)$. With the subscripts $(x, y)$ for these characteristics, as presented in Table 1.2, the standard deviations of these characteristics are $s_x = 7.16$ and $s_y = 13.71$. Their covariance is given by

$$s_{xy} = \sum_1^n (x_i - \bar{x})(y_i - \bar{y})/(n-1)$$

$$= [(x_1 - \bar{x})(y_1 - \bar{y}) + (x_2 - \bar{x})(y_2 - \bar{y}) + \ldots + (x_n - \bar{x})(y_n - \bar{y})]/(n-1). \quad (1.5)$$

It is the sum of the cross-products of the deviations of $(x_i, y_i)$ from their means divided by $(n-1)$. It can also be expressed as $s_{xy} = \left( \sum_1^n x_i y_i - n\bar{x}\bar{y} \right)/(n-1)$. The sample correlation coefficient of $(x, y)$ is

$$r = s_{xy}/s_x s_y. \quad (1.6)$$

It will be positive as $y$ increases with $x$ and negative if it decreases, and vice versa. In general, the covariance can be positive or negative. It can range from a very small negative value to a very large positive number, and the units of measurements of both $x$ and $y$ are attached to it. The correlation coefficient, however, ranges from $-1$ to $+1$, and it is devoid of the units of measurements of the two characteristics. If $x$ increases as $y$ increases, or $x$ decreases as $y$ decreases, their covariance and correlation will be positive; negative otherwise. If $x$ and $y$ are not related, $s_{xy}$ and $r$ will be zero. For the heights and weights of the twenty-year-old boys in Table 1.1, from (1.5), (1.6) and Table 1.2, $s_{xy} = (1814.61/19) = 95.51$ and $r = 95.51/(7.16 \times 13.71) = 0.97$. In this case, these two characteristics are highly positively correlated as expected. Figure 1.4 displays the relationship of the weights and heights of the twenty boys in Table 1.1.

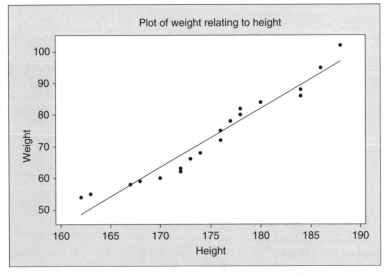

*Figure 1.4   Plot of the weights of the twenty-year-old boys on their heights from the observations in Table 1.1.*

# 1.8   Joint frequency distribution

When the number of observations on two variables $(x, y)$ is not small, they can be grouped into the joint frequency distribution. National and international organizations present the health-related characteristics in this form. For the sake of illustration, age $(x)$ and weight $(y)$ of a sample of $n = 200$ adults classified into $r = 3$ rows and $c = 3$ columns are presented in Table 1.4.

With the first and second subscripts $i = (1, 2, ...,r)$ and $j = (1, 2,...,c)$ representing the rows and columns respectively, the $i$th row and $j$th column consists of $n_{ij}$ adults. The total number of observations in the $i$th row and $j$th column respectively

are   $n_{i.} = \sum_{j=1}^{c} n_{ij}$ and $n_{.j} = \sum_{j=1}^{r} n_{ij}$.   The   overall   sample   size   becomes   $n = \sum_{i=1}^{r}$

$\sum_{j=1}^{c} n_{ij} = \sum_{i=1}^{r} n_{i.} = \sum_{j=1}^{c} n_{.j}$.   The row and column totals are the marginal totals. They

provide the frequency distributions of the age and weight respectively. The means, variances and standard deviations for the row and column classifications are obtained from these distributions as described in Section 1.6. With the mid-values $(x_1, x_2, ..., x_r)$ of the row classification and $(y_1, y_2, ..., y_c)$ of the column classification, the covariance of $(x, y)$ is obtained from

$$s_{xy} = \sum_{i=1}^{r} \sum_{j=1}^{c} n_{ij}(x_i - \bar{x})(y_i - \bar{y})/(n-1). \tag{1.7}$$

The correlation coefficient is found from $r = s_{xy}/s_x s_y$.

From Table 1.4, the mean, variance and standard deviation of the age are

$$\bar{x} = (35 \times 70 + 45 \times 90 + 55 \times 40)/200 = 43.5,$$

$$s_x^2 = \left[70(35 - 43.5)^2 + 90(45 - 43.5)^2 + 40(55 - 43.5)^2\right]/199 = 53.02,$$

and $s_x = 7.28$.

Table 1.4    Age $(x)$ and weight $(y)$ of $n = 200$ adults.

| | | Weight (lbs) | | | |
|---|---|---|---|---|---|
| | | 140–150 | 150–160 | 160–170 | Total |
| | 30–40 | 20 | 30 | 20 | 70 |
| Age (years) | 40–50 | 15 | 35 | 40 | 90 |
| | 50–60 | 5 | 15 | 20 | 40 |
| | Total | 40 | 80 | 80 | 200 |

Similarly, for the weight, $\bar{y} = 157$, $s_y^2 = 56.28$ and $s_y = 7.50$. From (1.7),

$$s_{xy} = [20(35-43.5)(145-157) + \ldots + 20(55-43.5)(165-157)]/199 = 10.55.$$

The correlation of age and weight now becomes $r_{xy} = 10.55/(7.28 \times 7.50) = 0.19$, which is not very high.

## 1.9     Linear transformation of the observations

For computations, it may become convenient to transform the data first. For instance, we may subtract 170 from each of the heights in Table 1.1, and divide the result by 10. The new observations now become $u_i = (x_i - 170)/10 = (1/10)x_i - 17$. We may also first divide each height by 100 and then subtract 5. Now, $u_i = (1/100)x_i - 5$. In either case, the new observations take the form of $u_i = ax_i + b$, where $(a, b)$ are positive or negative constants. The mean of the transformed observations becomes

$$\bar{u} = \sum u_i/n = \sum (ax_i + b)/n = a \sum x_i/n + b = a\bar{x} + b. \qquad (1.8)$$

Their variance becomes

$$\begin{aligned} s_u^2 &= \sum (u_i - \bar{u})^2/(n-1) \\ &= \sum [(ax_i + b) - (a\bar{x} + b)]^2/(n-1) \\ &= a^2 \sum (x_i - \bar{x})^2/(n-1) = a^2 s_x^2. \end{aligned} \qquad (1.9)$$

With the above type of transformation, computations for $\bar{u}$ and $s_u^2$ become simple. Now, $\bar{x}$ is obtained from $(\bar{u} - b)/a$ and $s_x^2$ from $s_u^2/a^2$. Note that adding or subtracting a constant displaces the mean, but it has no effect on the variance. Multiplying $x_i$ by the constant $a$ results in multiplying its variance by $a^2$, and the standard deviation by $a$.

As found earlier, the average of the heights of the twenty boys is 175.2 cm. To convert $x_i$ in cm to $y_i$ in inches, $y_i = 0.3937 x_i$. Now, the average height is $\bar{y} = (0.3937)\bar{x} = (0.3937)(175.2) = 68.98$ inches or close to 5 feet 9 inches. The variance becomes $s_y^2 = (0.3937)^2 s_x^2 = (0.3937)^2 (51.33) = 7.9561$ and $s_y = (0,3937)s_x = 2.82$ inches.

## 1.10     Linear combinations of two sets of observations

Consider the gains in weights $(x_i, y_i), i = (1,2,\ldots,n)$ of a sample of $n$ adults on two occasions. The total $t_i = (x_i + y_i)$, difference $d_i = (y_i - x_i)$, a weighted combination $u_i = (ax_i + by_i)$, with specified constants $(a, b)$ may be of interest. The mean and variance of $t_i$ are

$$\bar{t}=\sum_1^n t_i/n=\sum_1^n (x_i+y_i)/n=\bar{x}+\bar{y} \qquad (1.10)$$

and

$$V(t_i)=\sum_1^n (t_i-\bar{t})^2/(n-1)=\sum_1^n \left[(x_i-\bar{x})^2+(y_i-\bar{y})^2+2(x_i-\bar{x})(y_i-\bar{y})\right]/(n-1)$$

$$=s_x^2+s_y^2+2s_{xy}, \qquad (1.11)$$

where $\left(s_x^2,s_y^2\right)$ are the variances and $s_{xy}$ the covariance of $x$ and $y$. The standard deviations of $x$ and $y$ are $s_x$ and $s_y$, and the sample correlation is $r=s_{xy}/s_x s_y$, $(-1<r<1)$. The standard deviation $s_t$ of $t_i$ is the positive square root of $V(t_i)$.

Similarly, the mean, variance, and standard deviation of $d_i$ are $\bar{d}=\bar{y}-\bar{x}$, $V(d_i)=s_y^2+s_x^2-2s_{xy}$ and the standard deviation $s_d$ of $d_i$ is the positive square root of $V(d_i)$. If $u_i=ax_i+by_i+c$, where $(a, b, c)$ are constants, $\bar{u}=a\bar{x}+b\bar{y}+c$ and $V(u_i)=V(ax_i+by_i)=a^2 s_x^2+b^2 s_y^2+2abs_{xy}$. The standard deviation $s_u$ of $u_i$ is obtained from the square root of $V(u_i)$.

For an illustration, consider the gains in weights (lbs) $(x_i, y_i)$ of $n=5$ adults on two occasions: (5, 10), (10, 5), (10, 10), (5, –5), and (5, 10); the fourth candidate lost 5 lbs.

From these observations, the mean, variance and standard deviation of $x_i$ are (7, 7.5, 2.74). Corresponding figures for $y_i$ are (6, 42.5, 6.52). The covariance and correlation are $s_{xy}=3.75$ and $r=0.21$. The mean, variance and standard deviation of $t_i$ and $d_i$ respectively become (13, 57.5, 7.58) and (–1, 42.5, 6.52). With $a=(1/4)$, $b=(3/4)$ and $c=-5$, the mean, variance, and standard deviation of $u_i$ become (1.25, 57.78, 5.08).

# Exercises

**1.1.** Find the summary figures for the 20 ten-year old boys and girls in Tables T1.1 and T1.2.

**1.2.** (a) Find the means and standard deviations of the three characteristics for the sixteen-year-old boys and girls in Tables T1.3 and T1.4. (b) Find the means and S.D.s for the heights with grouping.

**1.3.** The mid-values of weights (lbs.) along with the systolic blood pressures, SBPs, of 200 adults are presented below. Find the means and standard deviations of the weights and blood pressures and their correlation.

|  | | SBP (y) | | |
|---|---|---|---|---|
|  | | 130 | 150 | Total |
| Weight (x) | 145 | 32 | 44 | 76 |
|  | 155 | 28 | 40 | 68 |
|  | 165 | 20 | 36 | 56 |
|  | Total | 80 | 120 | 200 |

**1.4.** Fertility rates per woman ($x$ in %) and the corresponding annual population growth rates ($y$ in %) in 192 countries of the world in 2006 are available from the tables of the WHO (2008). The fertility rates ranged from 1.2 to 7.3 percent. The population growth rate was negative in 18 countries and ranged from 0 to 4 percent in 188 countries. Combining the very small values of ($x, y$) with the adjacent cells, the mid-values of the percentages and the frequencies are presented below. Find the means, standard deviations and the correlation of these two characteristics.

|  | | Population growth rate (y %) | | | | |
|---|---|---|---|---|---|---|
|  | | 0.5 | 1.5 | 2.5 | 3.5 | Total |
| Fertility rate (x %) | 2 | 71 | 40 | 2 | 2 | 115 |
|  | 3.5 | 8 | 13 | 8 | 1 | 30 |
|  | 5.5 | 1 | 8 | 26 | 12 | 47 |
|  | Total | 80 | 61 | 36 | 15 | 192 |

**1.5.** Ross et al. (2006) analyzed the use of healthcare services by the lower- and higher-income insured and uninsured adults in the United States. The data were obtained from a nationally representative survey of a sample of 194,943 adults conducted by the CDC in 2002. The responding size ($n$) of the sample and the percentages of the insured (I) and uninsured (U) for the age, income and household classifications were presented as follows. Estimate the means, medians and standard deviations of age, income and household size for the insured and uninsured.

| Age | I | U | Income ($ 1,000) | I | U | Household size | I | U |
|---|---|---|---|---|---|---|---|---|
| 18–29 | 24 | 38 | < 15 | 8 | 23 | 1 | 11 | 10 |
| 30–39 | 24 | 24 | 15–25 | 12 | 34 | 2 | 29 | 24 |
| 40–49 | 25 | 21 | 25–35 | 13 | 18 | 3 | 21 | 21 |
| 50–64 | 27 | 18 | 35–50 | 19 | 13 | 4 | 22 | 20 |
|  |  |  | 50-75 | 21 | 7 | 5 | 17 | 25 |
|  |  |  | ≥ 75 | 27 | 5 |  |  |  |
| $n = 194,943$ | | | $n = 172,778$ | | | $n = 194,695$ | | |

**1.6.** Immunization coverage of the one-year-olds in the countries of the world for measles, DTP3 and HepB3 are presented in Table T1.5. Find the means and standard deviations for each of these types of coverage.

**1.7.** Convert the average and standard deviation of the weights in Table 1.2 into pounds from kilograms.

**1.8.** With the observations in Section (1.10), find the means, variances and standard deviations of (a) $u_i = (1/2)x_i + (1/2)y_i - 10$ and (b) $v_i = (1/3)x_i + (2/3)y_i + 5$.

**1.9.** Find the covariance and correlation of $u_i$ and $v_i$ of Exercise 1.8.

# 2

# Probability, random variable, expected value and variance

## 2.1 Introduction

The basic principles of probability are essential for the development of statistical theory, inference and applications. Probabilities of mutually exclusive, independent and dependent events are described in the following sections. *Bayes' theorem* is illustrated through an example. General definitions of a probability distribution, expected value, variance and moments of a random variable are presented.

## 2.2 Events and probabilities

Clinically examining the difference between the effects of two or more medical treatments and evaluating the benefits of different diets for weight reduction or hypertension control are two illustrations of *experiments*. The outcome of an experiment can be a success or failure, *Event A* and its complement *Event B*. For instance, an exercise program may increase the HDL of a person by less than 10, or by more than 10 mg/dL. These two events can be denoted by A and its complement B. In a random sample of 100 persons participating in the exercise program, HDL may increase by less than 10 mg/dL for 40 persons and more than 10 mg/dL for the remaining. Thus (*4/10*)th or 40 percent of the outcomes are in favor of the event A and (*6/10*)th or 60 percent in favor of its complement B. If we repeat the experiment, a large number of times with 100 persons each time, the fractions in favor of A can be (4/10, 3/10, 4/10, 7/10,…,) and their average may become 0.45. This long-run average of the fraction, the *relative frequency*, is the probability P(A) of the event A. The probability of the event

*Statistical Methodologies with Medical Applications*, First Edition. Poduri S.R.S. Rao.
© 2017 John Wiley & Sons, Ltd. Published 2017 by John Wiley & Sons, Ltd.

B becomes $P(B) = 0.65 = 1 - P(B)$. The *long-run relative frequency* of an event is defined as its probability.

The number of cases favorable to an event relative to the number of all possible cases provides another definition for its probability. For instance, consider a group of 10 physicians consisting of 6 pediatricians and 4 of another specialty. If one physician is selected randomly from the 10, the probability that a pediatrician appears is 6/10.

For both the above definitions of probability, an event A and its complement B are considered. In general, there can be more than two events. For instance, an exercise program may increase the HDL by less than 5, 5–10, 10–20 and more than 20 mg/dL. These events can be denoted by A, B, C, and D. Their probabilities are defined as above, and in this case $P(A) + P(B) + P(C) + P(D) = 1$.

## 2.3   Mutually exclusive events

Consider the event of success A and of failure B, its complement. These two events are *mutually exclusive*, and $P(A) + P(B) = 1$. Similarly, if A, B, and C are the only three mutually exclusive events of the outcome of an experiment, $P(A) + P(B) + P(C) = 1$. A medical treatment may result, for instance, in the three events of success, failure and indeterminate, which are mutually exclusive.

## 2.4   Independent and dependent events

The events A, B, C,… are *independent* if the outcome of one does not depend on the outcome of the remaining. Denote by A and B respectively, the events of a person being overweight and having elevated systolic blood pressure (SBP). If these two events are *independent* with $P(A) = 0.40$ and $P(B) = 0.20$, the probability of a person being overweight and having elevated SBP becomes $P(A \text{ and } B) = (0.40)(0.20) = 0.08$. In general, this probability is expressed as

$$P(AB) = P(A)P(B). \tag{2.1}$$

On the other hand, the above events can be *dependent*. If 30 percent of the persons with elevated SBP are overweight, this *conditional probability* is expressed as $P(A|B) = 0.30$. Now, the probability of a person in the above group to be overweight and to have high SBP becomes

$$P(AB) = P(A|B)\, P(B). \tag{2.2}$$

The probability in this case is $(0.30)(0.20) = 0.06$. Note that $P(AB) = P(A|B)P(B)$, which is the same as $P(BA) = P(B|A)P(A)$. It should also be noted that mutually exclusive events are necessarily dependent.

## 2.5    Addition of probabilities

A person can be overweight (A) or have elevated SBP (B), or have both these attributes. The probability of this event is

$$P(A \text{ or } B) = P(A) + P(B) - P(AB). \tag{2.3}$$

The joint probability $P(AB)$ is subtracted since it is added twice when the probabilities of A and B are added. If A and B are independent, $P(A \text{ or } B) = 0.40 + 0.20 - (0.40)(0.20) = 0.52$. On the other hand, if $P(A|B) = 0.30$, $P(A \text{ or } B) = 0.40 + 0.20 - (0.30)(0.20) = 0.54$.

## 2.6    Bayes' theorem

Consider the probabilities for an adult in a large population to be a cigarette smoker (S) and a smoker of cigar-type tobacco products (T) to be 0.6 and 0.4 respectively. It may be known that the probabilities for a smoker to be hypertensive (H) and normotensive (N) respectively are 0.8 and 0.2. Similarly, these probabilities for a cigar type of products may be known to be 0.4 and 0.6. Bayes' theorem combines the *prior* probabilities of cigarette or cigar smoking of the adults and their *conditional* probabilities of being hypertensive or normotensive. This procedure results in the *posterior* probabilities of a hypertensive or normotensive adult to be a smoker of cigarettes or cigars.

For the above population, the prior probabilities of an adult's being a smoker of cigarettes or cigars respectively are $P(S) = 0.6$ and $P(T) = 0.4$. The probabilities of a cigarette smoker becoming hypertensive or normotensive respectively are $P(H|S) = 0.8$ and $P(N|S) = 0.2$. Now, the probability for an adult to be a cigarette smoker and hypertensive is $P(HS) = P(SH) = (0.8)(0.6) = 0.48$. The probability for being a cigarette smoker and normotensive is $P(NS) = P(SN) = (0.2)(0.6) = 0.12$.

The probabilities of a cigar smoker becoming hypertensive or normotensive are $P(H|T) = 0.4$ and $P(N|T) = 0.6$. Now, the probability of an adult's being a cigar smoker and hypertensive is $P(HT) = P(TH) = (0.4)(0.4) = 0.16$. The probability of being a cigar smoker and normotensive is $P(NT) = P(TN) = (0.4)(0.6) = 0.24$.

Since a hypertensive adult can be a cigarette or cigar smoker, the probability of being hypertensive is $P(H) = P(HS) + P(HT) = 0.48 + 0.16 = 0.64$. Since a normotensive adult can be a cigarette or cigar smoker, the probability of being a normotensive adult is $P(N) = P(NS) + P(NT) = 0.12 + 0.24 = 0.36$.

The above probabilities can be summarized as follows:

| Prior Probability | Conditional Probability | Joint Probability |
|---|---|---|
| $P(S) = 0.60$ | $P(H|S) = 0.80$ | $P(HS) = (0.80)(0.60) = 0.48$ |
| | $P(N|S) = 0.20$ | $P(NS) = (0.20)(0.60) = 0.12$ |
| $P(T) = 0.40$ | $P(H|T) = 0.40$ | $P(HT) = (0.40)(0.40) = 0.16$ |
| | $P(N|T) = 0.60$ | $P(NT) = (0.40)(0.60) = 0.24$ |
| | | $P(H) = P(HS) + P(HT) = 0.64$ |
| | | $P(N) = P(NS) + P(NT) = 0.36$ |

Now, the *posterior probability* of a hypertensive adult to be a cigarette smoker is $P(S|H) = P(SH)/P(H) = (0.48/0.64) = 3/4$ or 75 percent, and to be a cigar smoker it is $P(T|H) = P(TH)/P(H) = (0.16/0.64) = (1/4)$ or 25 percent. The probability of a normotensive adult to be a cigarette smoker is $P(S|N) = P(SN)/P(N) = (0.12/0.36) = 1/3$ or 33.3 percent, and to be a cigar smoker, it is $P(T|N) = P(TN)/P(N) = (0.24/0.36) = 2/3$ or 67.7 percent.

## 2.7    Random variables and probability distributions

Random variables are associated with the events of the outcomes of the experiments. For instance, the decrease of weights as a result of an exercise program for a large group of adults can be considered to be a random variable. If the weights of a proportion p of the adults decrease, this outcome can be represented by the random variable $X$ taking the value one with probability $p$, and it can be expressed as $P(X = 1) = p$. The probability for the complementary event of the weight not decreasing is expressed as $P(X = 0) = (1 - p) = q$. These events of decrease and its complement are mutually exclusive; they are also dependent.

If a treatment for hypertension reduces SBP by $x_1$ mmHg for a proportion $p_1$ of the participating adults of a clinic and by $x_2$ mmHg for the remaining proportion $p_2 = 1 - p_1$, the probabilities for theses outcomes can be expressed as $P(X = x_1) = p_1$ and $P(X = x_2) = p_2$. As an illustration, $x_1 = 10$ mmHg with $p_1 = 0.70$ and $x_2 = 30$ mmHg with $p_2 = 0.30$. The probability distribution function or the probability mass function (p.m.f.) of $X$ is specified through this description. In general, the p.m.f. of $X$ may consist of $k$ values $(x_1, x_2 ..., x_k)$ with corresponding probabilities $(p_1, p_2, ..., p_k)$, $0 \leq p_i \leq 1$ and $\sum_1^k p_i = 1$.

## 2.8    Expected value, variance and standard deviation

With the complete specification of the p.m.f. as in the above section, the expected value of $X$ is defined as

$$\mu = E(X) = x_1 p_1 + x_2 p_2 + ... + x_k p_k = \Sigma x_i p_i. \tag{2.4}$$

This expected value, also referred to as the mean, is the *weighted average* of the values of the random variable, with the probabilities $p_i$ as the weights. The variance is defined as

$$\sigma^2 = E(X - \mu)^2 = \sum_1^k (x_i - \mu)^2 p_i$$
$$= (x_1 - \mu)^2 p_1 + (x_2 - \mu)^2 p_2 + ... + (x_k - \mu)^2 p_k. \tag{2.5}$$

It is the weighted average of the squared deviations of the observations from the expected value, with $p_i$ as the weights, and it becomes the same as $\sum_{1}^{k} x_i^2 p_i - \mu^2$.

To illustrate the expected value and variance, consider two examples of weight reduction: (1) $(x_1, x_2) = (1, 0)$ with $(p_1, p_2) = (0.6, 0.4)$ and (2) $(x_1, x_2) = (6, 10)$ with $(p_1, p_2) = (0.5, 0.5)$. The first case represents the decrease of weight, without any specification of the amount, with a probability of 0.6, and not decreasing with a probability of 0.4. The expected value now is $E(X) = 1(0.6) + 0(0.4) = 0.6$. The second case refers to decreases of 6 and 10 lbs with a 50 percent chance for each outcome. For these outcomes, $E(X) = 6(0.5) + (10)(0.5) = 8$, that is, on the average there is a decrease of 8 lbs. The variance for the first case is $\sigma^2 = (1 - 0.6)^2 (0.6) + (0 - 0.6)^2 (0.4) = 0.24$. For the second case, $\sigma^2 = (6 - 8)^2 (0.5) + (10 - 8)^2 (0.5) = 4$.

For another characteristic $X$, consider the three values $(x_1, x_2, x_3) = (-2, 0, 10)$ with probabilities $(p_1, p_2, p_3) = (0.2, 0.3, 0.5)$. Now, $E(X) = (-2)(0.2) + (0)(0.3) + (10)(0.5) = 4.6$, and $\sigma^2 = (-2 - 4.6)^2 (0.2) + (0 - 4.6)^2 (0.3) + (10 - 4.6)^2 (0.5) = 29.64$.

## 2.9   Moments of a distribution

The mean of a random variable $E(X)$ is the first moment, denoted by $\mu$. The second, third, fourth, ..., moments of $X$ are $\mu_2' = E(X^2), \mu_3' = E(X^3), \mu_4' = E(X^4), ....$ The second third, fourth *central moments* are $\mu_2 = E(X - \mu)^2, \mu_3 = E(X - \mu)^3, \mu_4 = E(X - \mu)^4, ....$ The second moment is the same as $\sigma^2 = V(X)$.

## Exercises

**2.1.** Eighty percent of the employees of a university received the flu vaccine and 20 percent did not. For those who receive the vaccine, there is a 10 percent chance of being affected by flu and 90 percent chance of not being affected. For those who do not receive the vaccine, the chances of getting affected and not affected by flu respectively are 60 and 40 percent. For the persons affected and not affected by flu, find the probabilities of their receiving or not receiving the vaccine.

**2.2.** Sixty percent of the adults over seventy years are overweight and 50 percent have low HDL. Find the chances for an adult to be overweight or to have low HDL if (a) weight and HDL are independent and (b) if there is 40 percent chance for the HDL of an overweight adult to be low.

**2.3.** From Tables 64 and 65, *Health United States* (2012), during 2007–2010, 30.6 and 27.4 percent of the adults twenty years or older respectively were hypertensive (A) and had cholesterol levels exceeding 240 mg/dL (B). These two events can be considered to be independent. Find the probabilities for the following events: An adult is (a) hypertensive with cholesterol exceeding 240 mg/dL and (b) either hypertensive or the cholesterol exceeds 240 mg/dL. In a random sample of two adults, find the probability for at least one adult to be (c) hypertensive, and (d) have cholesterol of 240 mg/dL or higher.

# 3

# Odds ratios, relative risk, sensitivity, specificity and the ROC curve

## 3.1 Introduction

The *odds ratio* is a measure of the effect of, for instance, overweight or smoking of persons on medical complications such as diabetes and hypertension. *Relative risk*, for instance, of exposure to air pollution for longer and shorter periods of time, is the ratio of the probabilities of their effects on complications like respiratory problems.

Physical examinations and laboratory tests are conducted to diagnose the medical complications of patients. *Sensitivity* and *specificity* are the probabilities of a diagnostic test correctly classifying the presence or absence of a medical complication. The *ROC curve* is a plot of the sensitivity against (1 – specificity) for a range of the classifications.

## 3.2 Odds ratio

Odds ratios (OR) are obtained from observational, retrospective, epidemiological and case-control studies. In the latter type, case and control refer respectively to having and not having a medical complication. A sample of 200 persons are classified in Table 3.1.

From these observations, the odds of a hypertensive to be a smoker *versus* non-smoker are $(a/c) = 45/35 = 9/7$. Similarly, the odds for a nonhypertensive person to

*Statistical Methodologies with Medical Applications*, First Edition. Poduri S.R.S. Rao.

Table 3.1    Smoking and hypertension.

|  | Hypertension | Nonhypertension | Total |
|---|---|---|---|
| Smokers | $a = 45$ | $b = 15$ | $(a + b) = 60$ |
| Nonsmokers | $c = 35$ | $d = 105$ | $(c + d) = 140$ |
| Total | $(a + c) = 80$ | $(b + d) = 120$ | $(a + b + c + d) = 200$ |

be a smoker versus nonsmoker are $b/d = 15/105 = 1/7$, which are much smaller than 9/7 for the hypertensive persons. The relative odds or the odds ratio for these two groups is

$$OR = \frac{a/c}{b/d} = \frac{ad}{bc}. \qquad (3.1)$$

These are the odds of smoking for a hypertensive person relative to that of a nonhypertensive person. For the above 200 persons, estimate of (3.1) becomes $\widehat{OR} = 9$.

The odds of a smoker to be hypertensive versus nonhypertensive are $(a/b)$. The odds of a nonsmoker to be hypertensive versus nonhypertensive are $(c/d)$. The odds that a smoker is a hypertensive person relative to that of a nonhypertensive person again becomes $(a/b)/(c/d) = (ad/bc)$. If the proportions $p_1 = a/(a+c)$ and $p_2 = b/(b+d)$ are available, the OR in (3.1) can be obtained from $[p_1(1-p_2)]/[p_2(1-p_1)]$.

As an illustration, from the survey of 194,943 U.S. adults conducted by the CDC in 2002, Ross et al. (2006) presented the percentages and the ORs for the insured and uninsured adults of different income levels receiving services for cardiovascular risk reduction and other health related characteristics. For another illustration, Muhm et al. (2007) presented the odds ratios of passenger problems like muscular discomfort, exertion and fatigue for attributes like altitude, oxygen saturation, age and male-female classification. The observations were obtained from a simulated commercial flight on volunteers.

## 3.3    Relative risk

From Table 3.1, the *risk* of hypertension for the smokers is $a/(a+b) = 45/60$ or 75 percent. This risk for the nonsmokers is $c/(c+d) = 35/140$ or 25 percent. The relative risk of hypertension for the two groups becomes

$$RR = \frac{a/(a+b)}{c/(c+d)}, \qquad (3.2)$$

which is the ratio of their probabilities. For the 200 persons in the above table, the estimate of RR of hypertension becomes $\widehat{RR} = (45/60)/(35/140) = 3$.

Table 3.2     Heights (feet), weights (pounds) and relative risks for the (25–59) years-old-persons.

| Relative risk | | 1.38 Underweight | 1 Healthy weight | 0.83 Healthy weight | 1.20 Overweight | 1.83 Obese |
|---|---|---|---|---|---|---|
| Height | 5.0 | <95 | 95–128 | 129–154 | 155–179 | >180 |
| | 5.5 | <115 | 115–155 | 156–186 | 187–217 | >218 |
| | 6.0 | <136 | 136–184 | 185–221 | 222–258 | >258 |

Relative risk is commonly used in cohort studies and randomized controlled experiments. If $a$ and $c$ are small relative to $b$ and $d$ respectively, the numerator and denominator of (3.2) become close to $(a/b)$ and $(c/d)$, and the RR does not differ much from the OR in (3.1).

The Body Mass Index (BMI) is a measure relating body fat to weight and height of a person. As illustrated in Chapter 1 for the twenty-year-old boys, it is computed from (weight in kilograms)/(square of the height in centimeters). From the National Health and Nutrition Examination Survey (NHANES), 1999–2002, (32.8, 23.8, 31.8) percent of the U.S. population of age (25–59, 60–69, ≥ 70) years respectively were estimated to have BMI of (18.5–25.0). Flegal et al. (2005) estimated the risk of mortality for ranges of the BMI from the data of three of the above surveys between 1971 and 1994. Relative to the persons with BMI of (18.5–25.0), the risk was higher for the underweight persons with BMIs less than 18.5 and obese persons with BMI of 30 or higher, but not for the overweight persons with BMI of (25–30). Converting the BMI (B) from the metric system, with height ($x$ in feet) and weight ($y$ in pounds) the BMI becomes $B = (y/2.2046)/(x/3.28)^2$. The results in Table 3.2 for the heights, weights and relative risks for the (25–59) year-old persons are obtained from the summary figures presented by the above authors. For the (60–69) and 70 year-old persons, the relative risk was found to be more than 1.38 for the underweight persons and less than 1.83 for the obese persons.

For another illustration, foods prepared with partially hydrogenated vegetable oils contain transfats which have been found to be associated with Coronary Heart Disease (CHD) and similar complications. For four large-scale studies Mozaffarian et al. (2006) present the relative risks of CHD for the substitution of 2 percent of the total energy intake of carbohydrates with transfatty acids. They were 1.33, 1.26, 1.14 and 1.28.

## 3.4   Sensitivity and specificity

Consider the outcomes of 100 diagnostic tests presented in Table 3.3. *Sensitivity* is the proportion of the persons with the disease identified by the test as having the disease. In this illustration, the estimate of this proportion $a/(a+c)$ becomes $40/60 = 2/3$ or

Table 3.3    Results of a diagnostic test.

|  | Disease | No disease | Total |
|---|---|---|---|
| Test + | $a = 40$ | $b = 15$ | $(a + b) = 55$ |
| Test − | $c = 20$ | $d = 25$ | $(c + d) = 45$ |
| Total | $(a + c) = 60$ | $(b + d) = 40$ | $(a + b + c + d) = 100$ |

66.7 percent. *Specificity* is the proportion of the persons without the disease identified by the test as not having the disease. In this case, the estimate of this proportion $d/(b+d)$ becomes 25/40 or 62.5 percent. It is desirable that both these measures for a test should be high.

## 3.5    The receiver operating characteristic (ROC) curve

From Table 3.3, the proportion of the *true positive* cases is $a/(a+c)$, which is the same as the sensitivity, and its estimate is $(40/60) = 2/3$. The proportion of the *true negative* cases is $d/(b+d)$, which is the specificity, and its estimate becomes $= (25/40) = (5/8)$. The proportion of the *false positive* cases is $b/(b+d)$, which is same as (1 − specificity), and its estimate becomes $= (15/40) = (3/8)$. For the ROC curve, sensitivity is plotted against (1 − specificity). The probability of *false negatives* is $c/(a+c)$ with its estimate of (1/3). Both the false positives and false negatives can have serious consequences.

In several types of clinical diagnosis, the test classifies the disease as present (positive) or not present (negative) based on specific ranges or demarcations of a continuous characteristic such as weight or age of the patients. The ROC curve is a plot of the sensitivity, true positive, against (1 − specificity), false positive, at the classification ranges. It originated during World War II for signal detection and is employed for assessing the accuracy of medical diagnostic tests.

## Exercises

**3.1.** The LDL of 400 persons consuming high and low fat diets are as follows. Find the odds for a (1) high and (2) normal LDL persons to be on a high fat diet, and (3) the odds ratio.

|  | LDL High | LDL Normal | Total |
|---|---|---|---|
| High fat | $a = 150$ | $b = 100$ | $(a + b) = 250$ |
| Low fat | $c = 70$ | $d = 80$ | $(c + d) = 150$ |
| Total | $(a + c) = 220$ | $(b + d) = 180$ | $(a + b + c + d) = 400$ |

**3.2.** From the observations in Exercise 3.1, find the risk of high LDL from the fat and nonfat diets and their relative risks.

**3.3.** The complaint of pain in the ribs of 150 athletes could be due to physical exertion or bronchial complications. The results of a test for bronchial infection of the athletes are as follows. Find (1) the sensitivity and (2) specificity of the test.

|  | Infection | No infection | Total |
|---|---|---|---|
| Test positive | $a = 30$ | $b = 20$ | $(a+b) = 50$ |
| Test negative | $c = 40$ | $d = 60$ | $(c+d) = 100$ |
| Total | $(a+c) = 70$ | $(b+d) = 80$ | $(a+b+c+d) = 150$ |

**3.4.** The number of hypertensive and normotensives among 150 adult males of different weights are given below. Find the sensitivity and specificity of the test classifying an adult male as hypertensive if his weight is above (a) 190, and (b) 200.

| Weight (lbs) | Hypertensive | Normotensive |
|---|---|---|
| 180 | 8 | 80 |
| 190 | 10 | 25 |
| 200 | 12 | 15 |
| Total | 30 | 120 |

# 4

# Probability distributions, expectations, variances and correlation

## 4.1  Introduction

As in any application, the random variables corresponding to medical experiments and observations can be discontinuous or continuous type. They can also be categorical, ordered or ranked. The numbers of clinics, hospitals, physicians and patients are examples of discrete or discontinuous random variables.

The random variables related to a number of diagnostic variables, for instance, blood pressure and cholesterol levels, dosages of drugs and lengths of medical treatments, take continuous values. For such cases, the p.d.f. (probability density function) of a random variable is denoted by $f(x)$ along with its range $(a < x < b)$ and can be depicted as a curve. The area under this curve over its entire range becomes equal to one. The c.d.f., $F(x)$, is the area under f(x) from **a** to **x**. Note that $F(a) = 0$ and $F(b) = 1$. The expected values, variances and higher order moments for these distributions are found through integral calculus.

The distributions of some of the discontinuous and continuous random variables commonly used in medical studies and research along with their expected values are presented in the following sections. Further topics in this chapter include (a) the joint and conditional distributions of two discrete random variables, (b) conditional and unconditional means and variances and (c) the bivariate normal distribution with its properties.

---

*Statistical Methodologies with Medical Applications*, First Edition. Poduri S.R.S. Rao.
© 2017 John Wiley & Sons, Ltd. Published 2017 by John Wiley & Sons, Ltd.

## 4.2    Probability distribution of a discrete random variable

Consider a random variable $X$ taking values $(x_1, x_2, ..., x_k)$ with probabilities $(p_1, p_2, ..., p_k)$, $\sum_1^k p_i = 1$. The expected value $E(X)$ of $X$ is

$$\mu_X = E(X) = \sum_1^k x_i p_i,  \tag{4.1}$$

which is the weighted average of $X$ with the probabilities $p_i$ as the weights. The variance $V(X)$ of $X$ is

$$\sigma_X^2 = E(X - \mu_X)^2 = \sum_1^k \left( x_i^2 - 2\mu_X x_i + \mu_X^2 \right) p_i$$

$$= \sum_1^k x_i^2 p_i - \mu_X^2 = E\left(X^2\right) - \mu_X^2.  \tag{4.2}$$

As an illustration, if $X$ takes values $(-5, 10, 15)$ with probabilities $(0.2, 0.3, 0.5)$, $\mu_X = (-5)(0.2) + 10(0.3) + 15(0.5) = 9.5$. Its variance becomes $\sigma_X^2 = (-5 - 9.5)^2 (0.2) + (10 - 9.5)^2 (0.3) + (15 - 9.5)^2 (0.5) = 57.25$. The standard deviation of $X$ is $\sigma_X = 7.57$.

For a linear transformation $Y = aX + b$ with constants $(a, b)$, $\mu_Y = E(aX + b) = a\mu_X + b$ and $\sigma_Y^2 = E(Y - \mu_Y)^2 = E[(aX + b) - (a\mu_X + b)]^2 = a^2 E(X - \mu_X)^2 = a^2 \sigma_X^2$.

## 4.3    Discrete distributions

### 4.3.1    Uniform distribution

In the simplest form of this distribution, which is also known as the rectangular distribution, the random variable $X$ takes the values $(1, 2, ..., n)$ with the probability of $(1/n)$ at each value. This distribution can be formally expressed as

$$P(X = i) = 1/n, \quad i = (1, 2, ..., n),  \tag{4.3}$$

with $\sum_{i=1}^n P(X = i) = 1$. From these probabilities

$$E(X) = 1(1/n) + 2(1/n) + ... + n(1/n) = [n(n+1)/2]/n = (n+1)/2  \tag{4.4a}$$

and

$$E\left(X^2\right) = \left(1^2 + 2^2 + ... + n^2\right)/n = [n(n+1)(2n+1)/6]/n = (n+1)(2n+1)/6.  \tag{4.4b}$$

The variance of $X$ is given by $V(X) = E\left[(X - E(X))^2\right] = \left\{E(X^2) - 2[E(X)]^2 + [E(X)]^2\right\} = E(X^2) - [E(X)]^2$. From (4.4a) and (4.4b),

$$V(X) = (n+1)(2n+1)/6 - (n+1)^2/4 = \left(n^2 - 1\right)/12. \tag{4.5}$$

As an illustration, if $X$ takes values $(1, 2,..., 10)$ with probability of $1/10$ for each value, $E(X) = 5.5$ and $V(X) = (99/12) = (33/4) = 8.25$. The standard deviation of $X$, S.D.$(X)$, is the positive square root of its variance. For this illustration, S.D.$(X) = \sqrt{8.25} = 2.87$ approximately.

If $X$ takes $b$ values $(a, a+1, a+2,..., a+b-1)$ each with probability $(1/b)$, $E(X) = [a + a + (b-1)]/2 = a + (b-1)/2$. In this case, $E(X^2) = \left[a^2 + (a+1)^2 + ... + (a+b-1)^2\right]/b$, and $V(X)$ can be obtained from $E(X^2) - [E(X)]^2$.

## 4.3.2  Binomial distribution

For an illustration of this distribution, consider 28 per cent of a large adult male population to be obese. For practical purposes, the probability for any adult in this population to be obese can be considered to be 0.28 and the chances of these adults being obese is *independent* of each other. Given this probability, the chances, for instance, of two adult males randomly selected from a list of six to be obese are obtained as follows. There are $_6C_2 = 6!/(2!4!) = 15$ possible combinations of two adults being selected from the six. The chances of the two selected adults to be obese is $(0.28)^2$ and the chances of the remaining four adults to be not obese is $(1 - 0.28)^4 = (0.72)^4$. Thus, the probability for two of the six adults selected to be obese is $15(0.28)^2(0.72)^4 = 0.316$ or close to 32 percent. Similarly, there are $_6C_3 = 6!/(3!3!) = 20$ combinations of three adults being selected from the six. In this case, the probability of three adults selected from the six to be obese is $20(.28)^3(.72)^3 = 0.1639$ or about 16.4 percent.

In general, the binomial distribution refers to n independent *trials* or selections, with the probability of the outcome, success or failure, remaining the same at each trial. The number of successes $X$ can be expressed as $\sum\limits_{i=1}^{n} X_i$, where $X_i$ is the *Bernoulli* random variable with $P(X_i = 1) = p$ and $P(X_i = 0) = (1 - p) = q$. The probabilities of $X$ taking different values are given by the binomial distribution,

$$P(x) = P(X = x) = {}_nC_x p^x q^{n-x} \quad x = (0, 1, 2, ..., n) \tag{4.6}$$

These probabilities are the same as the $(n+1)$ terms in the expansion of $(p+q)^n$.

As shown in Appendix A4, the expected value and variance of $X$ are $E(X) = np$ and $V(X) = npq$. Further, the variance of the number of failures $V(n - X)$ is the same as $V(X)$, and the covariance, Cov $(X, n - X)$, becomes equal to $(-npq)$. The correlation of the number of successes $X$ and the number of failures $(n - X)$ becomes equal to $(-1)$. As can be expected, one unit increase in the number of successes $X$ results in one unit decrease in the number of failures $(n - X)$ and *vice versa*.

An estimator of $p$ is given by the sample proportion of successes $\hat{p} = X/n$. The expected value $E(\hat{p})$ and variance $V(\hat{p})$ of this estimator are equal to $p$ and $pq/n$. Similarly, the estimator of $q$ is $\hat{q} = (n-X)/n = (1-\hat{p})$. The expected value $E(\hat{q})$ and variance $V(\hat{q})$ of this estimator become equal to $q$ and $pq/n$. Further, $Cov(\hat{p},\hat{q}) = -pq/n$ and the correlation of these estimators becomes $(-1)$.

Note that for the *Bernoulli* random variable $E(X_i) = 1(p) + 0(q) = p$, and $V(X_i) = (1-p)^2 p + (0-1)^2 q = pq$. The above results for the binomial random variable $X$ also follow from these results.

### 4.3.3 Multinomial distribution

As seen in the above section, the binomial distribution refers to two classes or categories. For the *multinomial* distribution, the population is considered to be consisting of $k \geq 3$ classes. The probabilities of the outcomes for these classes $(p_1, p_2, ..., p_k)$, $\sum_{i=1}^{k} p_i = 1$, remain the same at each trial or selection. In a random sample of size $n$, the probability of observing $(n_1, n_2, ..., n_k)$ units from the $k$ classes becomes

$$P(n_1, n_2, ...n_k) = \frac{n!}{n_i! n_2! ... n_k!} p_1^{n_2} p_2^{n_2} ... p_k^{n_k} \qquad (4.7)$$

Note that $(n_1, n_2, ..., n_k)$ are the random variables. From (4.7), the expected value and variance of the number observed in the $i$th class become $E(n_i) = np_i$ and $V(n_i) = np_i(1-p_i)$. The covariance of the number observed in the $i$th and $j$th classes becomes $(-np_i p_j)$.

As an illustration, consider (25, 30, 25 and 20) percent of the adults in the age groups (25–35, 35–45, 45–55 and 55–65) years respectively in a large population to be obese. From (4.7), the probability of selecting three from each of these four groups in a random sample of $n = 12$ from this population becomes $[12!/3!3!3!3!](0.25)^3 (0.30)^3$ $(0.25)^3 (0.20)^3 = 369600(5.27344)10^{-8} = 0.0195$ or close to 2 percent. In a random sample of $n = 100$ adults from this population, the expected value, variance and standard deviation of the number of adults observed, for instance, from the first age group are $100(0.25) = 25$, $100(0.25)(0.75) = 18.75$ and 4.33.

### 4.3.4 Poisson distribution

Some types of allergies, failures of medical treatments and mistakes in surgical procedures may occur very infrequently. In such cases, the outcome of the event follows the *Poisson* distribution. As an illustration, if one in 10 million of the 110 million adult male population in Table T4.1 is allergic to an antibiotic, the probability for any of these adults to be allergic can be considered to be $p = 1/10^7$ and on the average $\lambda = (110 \times 10^6)(1/10^7) = 11$ persons of this population will be allergic to that antibiotic. The probabilities of the Poisson distribution are given by

$$P(X=x) = e^{-\lambda}\lambda^x/x! \quad x = (0, 1, 2, \ldots) \tag{4.8}$$

The random variable $X$ for this discrete distribution can take values from zero to an infinitely large number. The probabilities for the binomial distribution in (4.6) approach the probabilities in (4.8) as $n$ becomes large and $p$ becomes small. As shown in Appendix A4, from (4.8), $E(X) = \lambda$ and $V(X) = \lambda$. The probabilities for different ranges of $X$ can be found from (4.8), from published tables of this distribution or software programs. When $\lambda = 11$, for instance, we find that $P(X \le 5) = 0.0375$, $P(5 \le X \le 10) = 0.4448$, and $P(X \ge 11) = 0.5401$.

### 4.3.5    Hypergeometric distribution

The binomial and multinomial distributions refer to sampling units *with* replacement from infinite populations. For several statistical estimations and analyses, the sample units are selected randomly *without* replacement from populations of finite sizes. Consider a finite population of $N$ units, consisting of two groups of sizes $N_1$ and $N_2 = (N - N_1)$, that is, in the proportions $P_1 = (N_1/N)$ and $P_2 = (N_2/N) = (1 - P_1)$. In a sample of n units selected randomly without replacement from the N units, the probability of observing $n_1$ and $n_2 = (n - n_1)$ units from the two groups is given by the *hypergeometric* distribution

$$P(n_1, n_2) = \frac{{}_{N_1}C_{n_1}\,{}_{N_2}C_{n_2}}{{}_{N}C_{n}} \quad (0 \le n_1 \le N_1, 0 \le n_2 \le N_2) \tag{4.9}$$

The numerator of this expression is the number of selections of $n_1$ units from the first group of size $N_1$ and $n_2$ units from the second group of size $N_2$. The denominator is the number of selections of n units from the population of size $N$. For this distribution, $E(n_1) = nP_1$ and $E(n_2) = nP_2$. Further,

$$V(n_1) = V(n_2) = n[(N-n)/(N-1)]P_1P_2 \tag{4.10a}$$

and

$$\text{Cov}(n_1, n_2) = -V(n_1). \tag{4.10b}$$

For large $N$, the variance in (4.10a) becomes the same as the variance $nP_1P_2$ of the binomial random variable with $n$ trials and probability of success $P_1$.

For an example, according to the World Health Organization (WHO) report for 2006, $N = 27$ countries had the highest per capita government expenditure for health; $N_1 = 19$ above \$2000 and $N_2 = 8$ below that figure. For a sample of size $n = 10$ selected randomly *without* replacement from the 27 countries, the expected values are $E(n_1) = 10(19/27) = 7.04$ and $E(n_2) = 10(8/27) = 2.96$, close to 7 and 3. From (4.10a), $V(n_1) = V(n_2) = 1.3633$.

Consider a sample of size 10 units selected randomly with replacement from an infinitely large population following the binomial distribution in (4.6) with probability of success of (19/27). The expected value now is $10(19/27) = 7.04$, same as above.

However, the variance of the number of successes becomes $10(19/27)(8/27) = 2.09$. The variance has increased from 1.3633 since a unit can appear in the sample more than once.

## 4.4    Continuous distributions

### 4.4.1    Uniform distribution of a continuous variable

The p.d.f (probability density function) of this random variable is given by

$$f(x) = 1/(b-a)  \quad a < x < b \tag{4.11}$$

This distribution is symmetric. Its mean and variance are given by $E(X) = (a+b)/2$ and $V(X) = (b-a)^2/12$. As an illustration, the total, male and female populations in the U.S. in 2008 from five to fifty-four years of age, presented in Table T4.1, can be represented by the uniform distributions with $a = 5$ and $b = 54$. The mean, variance and S.D. for the male population in this age range become 29.5, 200.08 and 14.15 respectively.

### 4.4.2    Normal distribution

The p.d.f of the *standard normal* variable $Z$ with mean $\mu = E(Z) = 0$ and variance $\sigma^2 = E(Z^2) = 1$ is given by

$$f(z) = \frac{1}{\sqrt{2\Pi}} e^{-\frac{1}{2}z^2}  \quad -\infty < z < \infty \tag{4.12}$$

This symmetric distribution, also known as the Gaussian distribution, has become essential for statistical analysis, applications and inference. This distribution with its probability (area) of $(1-\alpha)$ between $(-\alpha/2)$ and $(\alpha/2)$ is presented in Figure 4.1. Typical probabilities of this distribution are $P(-1.645 < Z < 1.645) = 0.90$ and $P(-1.96 < Z < 1.96) = 0.95$.

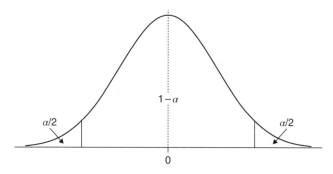

*Figure 4.1    Probabilities under the standard normal distribution; $(1-\alpha)$ percent of the area is between $-Z_{\alpha/2}$ and $Z_{\alpha/2}$, and $(\alpha/2)$ percent above $Z_{\alpha/2}$ and below $-Z_{\alpha/2}$.*

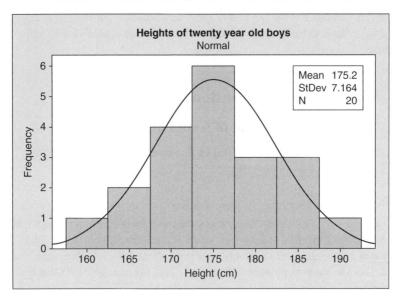

*Figure 4.2   Normal distribution fitted to the heights in Table 1.1 of the 20 twenty-year old boys.*

For this symmetric distribution, all the odd moments, $E(Z^3), E(Z^5), \ldots$ vanish. The skewness coefficient $E(Z^3)/\sigma^3$ becomes zero. The fourth moment is $E(Z^4) = 3$, and hence the coefficient of kurtosis becomes $E(Z^4)/\sigma^4 = 3$. The skewness and kurtosis of other distributions are assessed by comparing with these values of the standard normal distribution.

The p.d.f of a random variable $X$ following the normal distribution with mean $E(X) = \mu$ and variance $V(X) = E(X-\mu)^2 = \sigma^2$ is given by

$$f(x) = \frac{1}{\sigma\sqrt{2\Pi}} e^{-(x-\mu)^2/2\sigma^2}. \quad -\infty < x < \infty \qquad (4.13)$$

For this symmetric distribution, the third and fourth central moments become $\mu_3 = E(X-\mu)^3 = 0$ and $\mu_4 = E(X-\mu)^4 = 3\sigma^4$. Thus, the skewness and kurtosis coefficients become $K_1 = 0$ and $K_2 = 3$. This distribution fitted to the data of the heights of the 20 boys in Table 1.1 is presented in Figure 4.2. The straight line of the normal probability plot in Figure 4.3 refers to the cumulative probabilities of the standard normal distribution $Z$, and the percentages correspond to the observed heights. For instance, 10 percent, two of the 20, of the heights are below 163 inches.

## 4.4.3   Normal approximation to the binomial distribution

The probabilities for the binomial distribution can be obtained from (4.6). They are also available in the software programs and published tables. If the sample size $n$ is large, these probabilities can be obtained through the normal approximation with

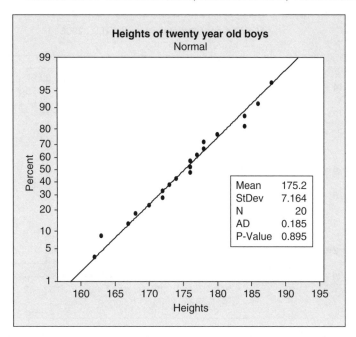

*Figure 4.3    Normal probability plot of the heights of the twenty boys in Table 1.1.*

mean $\mu = np$ and variance $\sigma^2 = npq$. As an illustration, when $n = 20$ and $p = 0.6$ for the binomial, $P(X \geq 10) = 0.8725$. For this distribution, the mean, variance and standard deviation are $\mu = 20(0.6) = 12$, $\sigma^2 = 20(0.6)(0.4) = 4.8$ and $\sigma = 2.19$. For the normal approximation, $P(X \geq 10) = P[(X-\mu)/\sigma] > (9.5-12)/2.19$, that is, $P(Z > -1.14) = 0.8729$, which is close to the exact value of 0.8723. To include 10 for $X$, the *continuity correction* 0.5 is subtracted.

For another illustration, $P(8 \leq X \leq 10) = 0.2236$ from (4.6). With the normal approximation, this probability becomes $P[(7.5 - 12)2.19 < Z < (10.5 - 12)/2.19] = P(-2.05 < Z < -0.68) = 0.228$. The normal approximation becomes closer to the actual probability as $n$ is large and $p$ is not too far from 0.5. Note that 0.5 is subtracted to include 8 and it is added to include 10.

### 4.4.4    Gamma distribution

Several nonnegative variables with positive skewness follow this distribution. The p.d.f of this random variable is

$$f(x) = \frac{1}{\Gamma(\alpha)\beta^\alpha} e^{-x/\beta} x^{\alpha-1} \quad x > 0 \tag{4.14}$$

where $\alpha > 0$ and $\beta > 0$ are the shape and scale parameters respectively. If $\alpha$ is an integer, $\Gamma(\alpha) = (\alpha-1)!$. For this random variable, $E(X) = \alpha\beta$ and $V(X) = \alpha\beta^2$. Both the

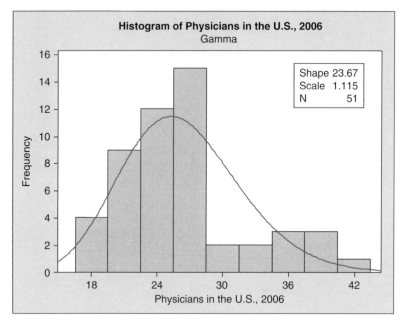

*Figure 4.4    Number of physicians per 10,000 civilian population in the U.S. in 2006 as presented in Table T4.2.*

skewness and peakedness of this distribution increase as $\alpha$ becomes small. The number of physicians per 10,000 civilian population in the 50 States of the U.S. in 2006, presented in Table T4.2, can be approximated through this distribution as shown in Figure 4.4. For this data, $E(X) = 26.41$, $V(X) = 33.89$, $\mu_3 = 178.78$ and $\mu_4 = 3765.72$.

### 4.4.5    Exponential distribution

The probability of this nonnegative random variable decreases as it increases. Its p.d.f is given by

$$f(x) = \frac{1}{\beta}e^{-x/\beta} \quad x > 0 \tag{4.15}$$

where $\beta > 0$ is the scale parameter. For this random variable, $E(X) = \beta$ and $V(X) = \beta^2$.

In 2006, the per capita healthcare expenditures in 191 countries of the world ranged from as low as four dollars to \$6,714 at the average exchange rate. For 135 of these countries, they ranged from four to 500 dollars, for 21 from 500 to 1000 dollars, and for the remaining from 1000 to 6,714 dollars. They are presented for the 135 countries in Table T4.3 and Figure 4.5. Averages and standard deviations for the three groups appear below the table.

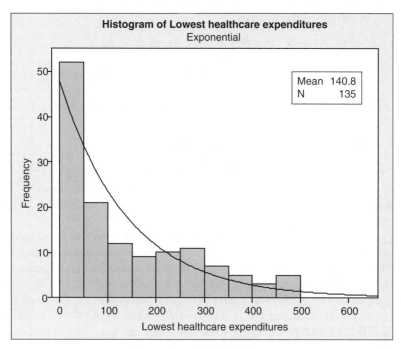

*Figure 4.5    Lowest per capita healthcare expenditure at the average exchange rate (US$); 135 countries; 2006. Source: WHO.*

An interesting property of this distribution is that it is "*memoryless.*" From (4.15),

$$P[X > (x+y)|(X > x)] = P[X > (x+y) \text{ and } (X > x)]/P(X > x)$$

$$= e^{-(x+y)/\beta}/e^{-x/\beta} = e^{-y/\beta} = P(X > y). \qquad (4.16)$$

The probability of $X$ exceeding $(x+y)$ does not depend on the probability of its exceeding $x$. For instance, $P(X > 50|X > 40) = P(X > 10)$. It is the same as $P(X > 30|X > 20)$, $P(X > 15|X > 5)$, and so on.

### 4.4.6    Chisquare distribution

This distribution has a very important role in a wide variety of statistical applications and inference. The p.d.f. of this random variable $X$ with $r$ *degrees of freedom* (d.f.) is

$$f(x)\frac{1}{2^{r/2}\Gamma(r/2)}e^{-x/2}x^{(r/2)-1}. \qquad (4.17)$$

It is the same as the Gamma distribution in (4.14) with $\alpha = r/2$ and $\beta = 2$. Its expected value and variance are $E(X) = r$ and $V(X) = 2r$.

### 4.4.7  Weibull distribution

The p.d.f., of the random variable $X$ in this case takes the form

$$f(x) = (\lambda/\beta)(x/\beta)^{\lambda-1} e^{-(x/\beta)^{\lambda}} \qquad x>0, \lambda>0, \beta>0 \qquad (4.18)$$

If $\lambda = 1$, the p.d.f of $Y = (X/\beta)$ becomes the exponential distribution $f(y) = e^{-y}$.

### 4.4.8  Student's $t$, and $F$ distributions

When $Z$ follows the standard normal distribution and $U$ follows the chisquare distribution with $f$ degrees of freedom, $t = Z/\sqrt{U/f}$ follows the $t$-distribution with $f$ degrees of freedom. For large $f$, the probabilities for this distribution differ very little from that of the standard normal distribution.

When $U_1$ and $U_2$ follow independent chisquare distributions with $f_1$ and $f_2$ degrees of freedom respectively, $F = (U_1/f_1)/(U_2/f_2)$ follows the $F$-distribution with $f_1$ and $f_2$ d.f. The upper percentiles of the $F$-distribution are tabulated. The lower percentile of $F(f_1, f_2)$ is given by the reciprocal of the upper percentile of $F(f_2, f_1)$. For instance, $P(F_{8,4} < 6.04) = 0.95$. To find the ninety-fifth lower percentile of $F$-distribution with eight and four d.f, note that $P(F_{4,8} < 3.84) = 0.95$. Since $(1/3.84) = 0.26$, $P(F_{8,4} > 0.26) = 0.95$, that is, $P(F_{8,4} < 0.26) < 0.05$. The lower and upper percentiles of these distributions are also available in the software programs.

## 4.5  Joint distribution of two discrete random variables

For many clinical and medical investigations and research, it is frequently important to study two variables $(X, Y)$ such as (age, weight) and (weight, SBP); more than two variables in several cases. Consider the mid-values ($x_1 = 35$, $x_2 = 45$, $x_3 = 55$) of age and ($y_1 = 145$, $y_2 = 155$, $y_3 = 165$) of weight of the 200 adults in Table 1.4 as the discrete values of $X$ and $Y$ respectively. The joint probability distribution of $(X, Y)$ in Table 4.1 is obtained from these 200 observations. The estimates of the proportions of the nine combinations are considered for the probabilities.

Table 4.1   Joint probability distribution of age $(X)$ and weight $(Y)$ of the 200 adults in Table 1.4

|  |  | Weight $(Y)$ | | | |
|---|---|---|---|---|---|
|  |  | $y_1 = 145$ | $y_2 = 155$ | $y_3 = 165$ | $P(X = xi)$ |
|  | $x_1 = 35$ | 0.10 | 0.15 | 0.10 | 0.35 |
| Age $(X)$ | $x_2 = 45$ | 0. 075 | 0.175 | 0.20 | 0.45 |
|  | $x_3 = 55$ | 0. 025 | 0.75 | 0.10 | 0.20 |

The joint probabilities $P(X = x_i, Y = y_j) = P(x_i, y_j)$, for the $i = (1, 2, \ldots, k)$ rows and $j = (1, 2, \ldots, l)$ columns appear in this table. For this illustration $k = 3$ and $l = 3$ for the age and weight classifications. The probability for each value of the age is obtained by adding over the columns. Similarly, the probability for each value of the weight is obtained by adding over the rows. The probability distributions for age and weight, $P(X = x_i) = P(x_i)$ and $P(Y = y_j) = P(y_j)$, are presented in the right-hand side column and the bottom row respectively.

From the above table, $P(x_1, y_1) = 0.10$, $P(x_1, y_2) = 0.15$, $P(x_1, y_3) = 0.10$ and $P(x_1) = (0.10 + 0.15 + 0.10) = 0.35$. The probabilities $P(x_2)$ and $P(x_3)$ for age and the probabilities for $Y$ on the bottom row are obtained similarly. From the probability distribution of $X$, its expected value, variance and standard deviation are

$$\mu_X = E(X) = \sum_{i=1}^{k} x_i P(x_i) = (35)(0.35) + (45)(0.45) + (55)(0.20) = 43.5,$$

$$\sigma_X^2 = V(X) = E(X - \mu_X)^2 = \sum_{1}^{k} (x_i - \mu_X)^2 P(x_i)$$

$$= (35 - 43.5)^2 (0.35) + (45 - 43.5)^2 (0.45) + (55 - 43.5)^2 (0.20) = 52.75$$

and $\sigma_X = 7.26$. Similarly, the expected value variance and standard deviation of $Y$ become 157, 56 and 7.48.

The Covariance of $(X, Y)$ is given by

$$\sigma_{XY} = Cov(X, Y) = E(X - \mu_X)(Y - \mu_Y) = \sum_{i=1}^{k} \sum_{j=1}^{l} (x_i - \mu_X)(y_j - \mu_Y) P(x_i, y_j), \quad (4.19)$$

which becomes the same as $E(XY) - \mu_X \mu_Y$. The correlation coefficient of $(X, Y)$ is $\rho_{XY} = \sigma_{XY} / \sigma_X \sigma_Y$, $-1 \leq \rho_{XY} \leq 1$. It may be positive or negative and does not depend on the unit of measurements of $(X, Y)$. From the probability distribution in Table 4.1, $\sigma_{XY} = 10.5$ and $\rho_{XY} = 10.5 / (7.26 \times 7.48) = 0.193$.

The estimates for the variances, standard deviations and covariance of age and weight found in Section 1.8 are slightly larger than the above exact values.

For a linear combination $U = aX + bY + c$, where $(a, b, c)$ are constants, $E(U) = a\mu_X + b\mu_Y + c$ and $V(U) = a^2 \sigma_X^2 + b^2 \sigma_Y^2 + 2ab\sigma_{XY}$. For two linear combinations $U_1 = a_1 X + b_1 Y + c_1$ and $U_2 = a_2 X + b_2 Y + c_2$, where $(a_1, b_1, c_1)$ and $(a_2, b_2, c_2)$ are constants, $Cov(U_1, U_2) = a_1 a_2 \sigma_X^2 + (a_1 b_2 + b_1 a_2)\sigma_{XY} + b_1 b_2 \sigma_Y^2$.

### 4.5.1  Conditional distributions, means and variances

In the case of variables such as height $(X)$ and weight $(Y)$, the probability distributions, expectations and variances of weight for given values of age would be of interest. From Table 4.1, the conditional probabilities of the three values of weight at age $X = x_1$ are

$$P(Y = y_1 | X = x_1) = P(y_1, x_1) / P(x_1) = (0.10) / (0.35) = 10/35,$$

$$P(Y = y_2 | X = x_1) = P(y_2, x_1) / P(x_1) = (0.15) / (0.35) = 15/35$$

and

$$P(Y = y_3 | X = x_1) = P(y_3, x_1)/P(x_1) = (0.10)/(0.35) = 10/35.$$

The probability distribution of $Y$ at $X = x_i$ is given by these three probabilities. The expected value of $Y$ at $X = x_i$ is

$$\mu_{Y.x_1} = E(Y | X = x_1) = \sum_{j=1}^{3} y_j P(Y = y_j | X = x_1). \qquad (4.20)$$

The variance of $Y$ at $X = x_1$ is given by

$$V(Y | X = x_1) = E(Y - \mu_{Y.x_1})^2 = \sum_{j=1}^{3} (y_j - \mu_{Y.x_1})^2 P(Y = y_j | X = x_1) \qquad (4.21)$$

The conditional means and variances of $Y$ at $x_2$ and $x_3$ are found similarly. From Table 4.1, the expected value, variance and standard deviation of the weights at age 35 become (155, 57.14 and 7.56). At age 45 and 55, they are (157.78, 53.40, 7.31) and (158.75, 48.44, 6.96) respectively.

## 4.5.2    Unconditional expectations and variances

The expectations and variances of random variables can be obtained from their marginal distributions. They can also be obtained from the conditional means and variances. Following the notation in Section (4.5.1),

$$E(Y) = \sum_i \sum_j y_j P(x_i, y_j) = \sum_i \sum_j y_j P(x_i) \frac{P(x_i, y_j)}{P(x_i)}$$

$$= \sum_i P(x_i) \left[ \sum_j y_j \frac{P(x_i, y_j)}{P(x_i)} \right] = \sum_i P(x_i) \left[ \sum_j y_j P(y_j | x_i) \right]$$

$$= \sum_i P(x_i) E(Y | x_i) = EE(Y | X). \qquad (4.22)$$

The unconditional mean of $Y$ is the expectation of its mean conditional on $X$. In the above section, the expectations of weight ($Y$) at age levels $(x_1, x_2, x_3) = (35, 45, 55)$ were found to be (155, 157.78, 158.75). Multiplying these conditional expectations with the probabilities (0.35, 0.45, 0.20) of $X$ and adding, $E(Y) = 155(0.35) + 157.78(0.45) + 158.75(0.20) = 157$. As seen in the above section, from the marginal distribution of $Y$, $E(Y) = 145(0.2) + 155(0.4) + 165(0.4) = 157$.

To find the unconditional variance $V(Y)$, note that, $E(Y^2) = EE(Y^2 | X)$. Now,

$$V(Y) = E(Y^2) - [E(Y)]^2 = EE(Y^2|X) - [EE(Y|X)]^2$$
$$= \left\{ EE(Y^2|X) - E[E(Y|X)]^2 \right\} + \left\{ E[E(Y|X)]^2 - [EE(Y|X)]^2 \right\}$$
$$= E[V(Y|X)] + V[E(Y|X)]. \tag{4.23}$$

The utility of the results in (4.22) and (4.23) is that the unconditional mean $E(Y)$ and variance $V(Y)$ of $Y$ can be found from its conditional mean and variance.

From the conditional variances of the weight found in the above section, $E[V(Y|X)] = 57.14(0.35) + (53.40)(0.45) + (48.44)(0.20) = 53.72$, rounding-off to two decimals. Further,

$$V[E(Y|X)] = (155 - 157)^2(0.35) + (157.78 - 157)^2(0.45)$$
$$+ (158.75 - 157)^2(0.20) = 2.28,$$

rounding-off to two decimals. Combining these two results, $V(Y) = 56$ as found from Table 4.1.

## 4.6  Bivariate normal distribution

This distribution has been of importance to study the relationship between two correlated normal variables $(x_1, x_2)$. Their joint density is given by

$$f(x_1, x_2) = \frac{e^{-q(x_1, x_2)/2}}{2\Pi(1 - \rho^2)^{1/2}}. \qquad (-\infty < x_1 < \infty), (-\infty < x_2 < \infty) \tag{4.24}$$

In this expression,

$$q(x_1, x_2) = \left[ \frac{(x_1 - \mu_1)^2}{\sigma_1^2} - 2\rho \frac{(x_1 - \mu_1)(x_2 - \mu_2)}{\sigma_1 \quad \sigma_2} + \frac{(x_2 - \mu_2)^2}{\sigma_2^2} \right] / (1 - \rho^2), \tag{4.25}$$

where $\rho = \sigma_{12}/\sigma_1\sigma_2$ is the correlation of $(x_1, x_2)$; $Cov(x_1, x_2) = \sigma_{12} = \sigma_{21}$ is the covariance of $(x_1, x_2)$. The marginal distributions $f(x_1)$ and $f(x_2)$ of $f(x_1, x_2)$ are normal with means $(\mu_1, \mu_2)$ and variances $(\sigma_1^2, \sigma_2^2)$. This joint density can be expressed as

$$f(x_1, x_2) = f(x_1)f(x_2|x_1) = f(x_2)f(x_1|x_2). \tag{4.26}$$

In this expression, $f(x_1|x_2)$ is the distribution of $x_1$ conditional on $x_2$ with mean $\mu_{1.2} = \mu_1 + \beta_{1.2}(x_2 - \mu_2)$ and variance $\sigma_{1.2}^2 = \sigma_1^2(1 - \rho^2)$, where $\beta_{1.2} = \sigma_{12}/\sigma_2^2$, and it is independent of $f(x_1)$. Similarly, $f(x_2|x_1)$ is the distribution of $x_2$ conditional on $x_1$ with mean $\mu_{2.1} = \mu_2 + \beta_{2.1}(x_1 - \mu_1)$ and variance $\sigma_{2.1}^2 = \sigma_2^2(1 - \rho^2)$, where $\beta_{2.1} = \sigma_{21}/\sigma_1^2$, and it is independent of $f(x_1)$. Note that $Cov(x_1, x_2) = \sigma_{12} = \sigma_{21}$.

# Exercises

**4.1.** Forty percent of the adults in a community are known to be hypertensive. In a sample of 15 adults selected from the community, find the probabilities of (a) exactly 5, (b) less than 5, (c) more than 10, and (d) (5–10) of the adults to be hypertensive.

**4.2.** Find the probabilities in Exercise 4.1 through the normal approximation.

**4.3.** The allergic reaction to an antibiotic was known to be mild, moderate and severe for (50, 40, 10) percent of a large group of patients. For a random sample of $n = 100$ patients, find the following : (a) Difference of the expected numbers for the mild and moderate and the standard deviation of the difference, and (b) Difference of the expected numbers for the mild and moderate from the difference of the expected numbers for the moderate to severe, and its standard deviation.

**4.4.** The number of individuals in a large population requiring gluten-free diet is known to follow the Poisson distribution with mean $\lambda = 10$. In a sample of these individuals, find the probabilities of (a) 5, (b) at most 5 and (b) (10–15) of these individuals requiring this diet.

**4.5.** Find the (a) upper and (b) lower ninety-fifth percentiles of the F-distribution with (6, 12) d.f.

# Appendix A4

## A4.1   Expected values and standard deviations of the distributions

*Bernoulli*:

$$P(X = 1) = p \text{ and } P(X = 0) = q = 1 - p.$$

$$E(X) = 1(p) + 0(q) = p. E(X^2) = 1(p) + 0(q) = p, \text{ and } V(X) = p - p^2 = pq.$$

Alternatively, $V(X) = (1-p)^2 p + (0-p)^2 q = q^2 p + p^2 q = pq.$

*Binomial*:

$$E(X) = \sum_{x=0}^{n} x(_nC_x p^x q^{n-x}) = np \sum_{x=1}^{n-1} C_{x-1} p^{x-1} q^{(n-1)-(x-1)} = np.$$

Similarly, $E[X(X-1)] = n(n-1)p^2$. Hence, $E(X^2) = n(n-1)p^2 + (np)$ and $V(X) = npq$.

Alternatively, $X = (X_1 + X_2 + \ldots + Xn)$, where $X_i$, $i = (1, 2, \ldots, n)$ are Bernoulli random variables with probability of success $p$ and failure $q$. Hence $E(X) = (p + p + \ldots + p) = np$ and $V(X) = V(X_1) + (X_2) + \ldots + V(X_3) = (pq + pq + \ldots + pq) = npq.$

*Multinomial*:

As in the case of the Binomial distribution, from (4.7), $E(n_i) = np_i$, $E[n_i(n_i-1)] = n(n-1)p_i^2$ and $V(n_i) = np_i(1-p_i)$. Further, $E(n_in_j) = n(n-1)p_ip_j$ and $Cov(n_i, n_j) = E(n_in_j) - E(n_i)E(n_j) = -np_ip_j$.

*Poisson*:

From (4.8), $E(X) = \sum_{x=0} x\left(e^{-\lambda}\dfrac{\lambda^x}{x!}\right) = \lambda\sum_{x=1} e^{-\lambda}\dfrac{\lambda^{x-1}}{(x-1)!} = \lambda$.

Similarly, $E[X(X-1)] = \lambda^2$. Hence, $E(X^2) = (\lambda^2 + \lambda)$ and $V(X) = \lambda$.

*Hypergeometric*:

From (4.9), $E(n_1) = n(N_1/N)$, $E[n_1(n_1-1)] = [n(n-1)/N(N-1)]N_1(N_1-1)$. Hence, $V(n_1) = n[(N-n)/(N-1)](N_1/N)(N_2/N)$. Since $n_2 = n-n_1$, $E(n_2) = n(N_2/N)$ and $V(n_2)$ is the same as $V(n_1)$.

## A4.2   Covariance and correlation of the numbers of successes x and failures (n – x) of the binomial random variable

As defined in (4.19), the covariance of two random variables can be expressed as

$$\sigma_{XY} = E(XY) - \mu_X\mu_Y.$$

From (4.6),

$$E[X(n-X)] = \sum_{x=0}^{n} x(n-x)(_nC_x p^x q^{n-x}) = n(n-1)pq\sum_{x=1}^{n-1} {}_{n-1}C_{x-1}p^{x-1}q^{(n-1)-(x-1)}$$

$$= n(n-1)pq.$$

Now, $Cov[X,(n-X)] = E[X(n-X)] - E(X)E(n-X) = n(n-1)pq - (np)(nq) = -npq$. This result can also be obtained from noting that $V[X+(n-X)] = V(n) = 0$.

# 5

# Means, standard errors and confidence limits

## 5.1 Introduction

For the statistical evaluation of a treatment for hypertension, for instance, means and standard deviations of the SBPs and DBPs of samples of patients are obtained before and after administering the treatment. Several types of statistical analyses of the physical and diagnostic characteristics of the patients in the healthcare clinics or the individuals participating in an experiment utilize the sample means, standard deviations and similar summary figures. Clinical experiments provide the means, standard deviations and other summary figures of the observations for estimating the effects of medical treatments and their comparisons.

The *Standard Error (S.E.)* of an estimator for a population parameter such as the mean or proportion is the standard deviation of its sampling distribution. The conceptually possible repetitions of the random sample results in this distribution. The *Confidence limits* for a parameter provide its upper and lower bounds. They are derived from the probability distribution of its estimator.

Estimation of the means, difference of two means, proportions and their differences, variance, ratio of two variances along with the confidence limits for these quantities are presented in the following sections.

*Statistical Methodologies with Medical Applications*, First Edition. Poduri S.R.S. Rao.
© 2017 John Wiley & Sons, Ltd. Published 2017 by John Wiley & Sons, Ltd.

## 5.2    Expectation, variance and standard error (S.E.) of the sample mean

Consider the SBPs of a population following a probability distribution with expected value $E(X) = \mu$ and variance $\sigma^2 = E(X-\mu)^2$. The observations of the SBPs of a random sample of size $n$ selected independently from this population can be represented by $(X_1, X_2, ..., X_n)$, or simply as $X_i, i = (1, 2, ..., n)$. The sample mean

$$\bar{X} = \sum_{1}^{n} X_i/n = (X_1 + X_2 + ... + X_n)/n \tag{5.1}$$

is an estimator of $\mu$. For repeated samples, the expected value of this estimator becomes

$$E(\bar{X}) = (1/n)\sum_{1}^{n} E(X_i) = (1/n)(n\mu) = \mu. \tag{5.2}$$

Thus, $\bar{X}$ is an *unbiased estimator* of $\mu$. An estimator for a population parameter is unbiased if its expectation over repeated samples becomes equal to the parameter. Further, its variance becomes

$$V(\bar{X}) = E(\bar{X} - \mu)^2 = (1/n^2)\sum_{1}^{n} E(X_i - \mu)^2$$

$$= (1/n)^2 (n\sigma^2) = \sigma^2/n. \tag{5.3}$$

Note that the expectation of $(X_i - \mu_i)(X_j - \mu_j), (i \neq j)$, vanishes since the sample is selected independently.

The *Standard Error* of $\bar{X}$ is given by

$$S.E.(\bar{X}) = \sqrt{V(\bar{X})} = \sigma/\sqrt{n}. \tag{5.4}$$

The standard error of an estimator is the same as the standard deviation of its distribution.

Both the variance and S.E. of the sample mean decrease as the sample size increases. The probability of the sample mean approaching the population mean increases as its S.E. becomes small. This result can be formally seen from the *Tschebysheff's inequality* presented in Appendix A5.1

The *Coefficient of Variation* (C.V.) of $X$ is $(\sigma/\mu)$. The unit of measurement, for instance, dosage in milligrams, of $\mu$ and $\sigma$ is the same, but the C.V. of $X$ is devoid of it. The coefficient of variation of $\bar{X}$ is given by

$$C.V.(\bar{X}) = S.E.(\bar{X})/\mu = (\sigma/\sqrt{n})/\mu, \tag{5.5}$$

which is devoid of the unit of measurement of X. It expresses the $S.E.(\bar{X})$ as a percentage of the mean $\mu$.

## 5.3   Estimation of the variance and standard error

From the observations of a random sample, unbiased estimator of $\sigma^2$ and $V(\bar{X})$ are given by

$$S^2 = \sum_1^n (X_i - \bar{X})^2/(n-1) \tag{5.6}$$

and

$$V(\bar{X}) = S^2/n. \tag{5.7}$$

Estimates of $S.E.(\bar{X})$ and $C.V.(\bar{X})$ are obtained from $S/\sqrt{n}$ and $(S/\sqrt{n})/\bar{X}$. They are however, not unbiased.

From the observed sample, $(x_1, x_2, ..., x_n)$, the mean and variance in (5.1) and (5.6) are obtained from $\bar{x} = \sum_1^n x_i/n$ and $s^2 = \sum_1^n (x_i - \bar{x})^2/(n-1)$, and the variance in (5.7) is estimated from $v(\bar{X}) = s^2/n$. Now, $S.E.(\bar{X})$ and $C.V.(\bar{X})$ are obtained from $s/\sqrt{n}$ and $(s/\sqrt{n})/\bar{x}$.

*Example 5.1*   For a random sample of $n = 16$ adults, the mean variance and standard deviation of the SBPs were found to be $\bar{x} = 131.3$, $s^2 = 102$ and $s = 10.1$ respectively. If the population variance of the SBPs is known to be $\sigma^2 = 98$, from (5.3) and (5.4), $v(\bar{X}) = 98/16 = 6.125$   and   $S.E.(\bar{X}) = 2.47$. From the estimate 102 for $\sigma^2$, $v(\bar{X}) = (102/16) = 6.375$ and $S.E.(\bar{X}) = 2.52$. In this case, the estimate of the standard error does not differ much from the actual value of 2.47. The estimate of the $C.V.(\bar{X})$ becomes $2.52/131.3 = 0.019$ or 1.9 percent.

The expectation of the alternative estimator $\hat{\sigma}^2 = \sum_1^n (X_i - \bar{X})^2/n = (n-1)S^2/n$ becomes equal to $(n-1)\sigma^2/n$ and hence it is not unbiased for $\sigma^2$. The bias of this estimator for $\sigma^2$ is $B(\hat{\sigma}^2) - \sigma^2 = -\sigma^2/n$, and it underestimates $\sigma^2$. This bias however becomes small as the sample size increases. Secondly, the biases of $S$ and $S/\sqrt{n}$ as estimators of $\sigma$ and $S.E.(\bar{X})$ become small with increasing sample size. As shown in Appendix A5.2, the *Mean Square Error (MSE)* of an estimator is the sum of its variance and the square of the bias. For an unbiased estimator, it becomes the same as the variance.

## 5.4    Confidence limits for the mean

When a random variable $X$ follows the normal distribution with mean $\mu$ and standard deviation $\sigma$, the standardized variable $Z = (X - \mu)/\sigma$ follows the *normal distribution* with zero mean and unit standard deviation. Similarly, $Z = (\bar{X} - \mu)/(\sigma/\sqrt{n})$ follows the standard normal distribution. As presented in Figure 4.1, the $(1 - \alpha)$ percent probability of this distribution falls between $-z_{\alpha/2}$ and $z_{\alpha/2}$. For instance, 90 percent of the area of this distribution falls between $-1.645$ and $1.645$ when $\alpha = 0.10$, and 95 percent between $-1.96$ and $1.96$ when $\alpha = 0.05$. This result can be expressed as

$$P\left[ -z_{\alpha/2} < \frac{\bar{X} - \mu}{\sigma/\sqrt{n}} < z_{\alpha/2} \right] = 1 - \alpha. \tag{5.8}$$

Following this coverage probability for the sample mean when $\sigma$ is known, $(1 - \alpha)$ percent confidence limits for $\mu$ are obtained from

$$\bar{X} \pm z_{\alpha/2}\left( \sigma/\sqrt{n} \right). \tag{5.9}$$

The upper and lower confidence limits are given by

$$C_u = \bar{X} + z_{\alpha/2}\left( \sigma/\sqrt{n} \right)$$

and

$$C_l = \bar{X} - z_{\alpha/2}\left( \sigma/\sqrt{n} \right). \tag{5.10}$$

With the observed sample mean $\bar{x}$, the upper and lower limits for $\mu$ are obtained from $C_u = \bar{x} + z_{\alpha/2}(\sigma/\sqrt{n})$ and $C_l = \bar{x} - z_{\alpha/2}(\sigma/\sqrt{n})$. Among the intervals in (5.9) obtained from the means of a large number of samples of size $n$, on the average $(1 - \alpha)$ percent enclose the unknown mean $\mu$. The confidence width

$$(C_u - C_l) = 2z_{\alpha/2}\left( \sigma/\sqrt{n} \right) \tag{5.11}$$

becomes small as $(\sigma/\sqrt{n})$ becomes small, that is, as the sample size increases. However, it becomes large as the confidence probability $(1 - \alpha)$ is increased. It is $2(1.645)$ $(\sigma/\sqrt{n}) = 3.29\,(\sigma/\sqrt{n})$ and $2(1.96)\,(\sigma/\sqrt{n}) = 3.92\,(\sigma/\sqrt{n})$ when $(1-\alpha) = 0.90$ and $0.95$ respectively.

To obtain the one-sided confidence limits, note that $P(Z < z_\alpha) = P(Z > z_\alpha) = (1-\alpha)$. From this result, the $(1 - \alpha)$ percent lower and upper confidence limits for $\mu$ are obtained from $\bar{x} - z_\alpha(\sigma/\sqrt{n})$ and $\bar{x} + z_\alpha(\sigma/\sqrt{n})$

When $X$ follows the normal distribution and $\sigma^2$ is estimated by $S^2$,

$$t_{n-1} = \frac{\bar{X} - \mu}{S/\sqrt{n}} \tag{5.12}$$

follows the *Student's t-distribution* with $(n-1)$ degrees of freedom (d.f.). The percentiles of this distribution for the coverage probability of $(1-\alpha)$ are given by – $t_{n-1,\alpha/2}$ and $t_{n-1,\alpha/2}$. For instance, for the $t$-distribution with $(n-1)=15$ d.f., $t_{\alpha/2}=1.753$ and 2.131 when $\alpha=0.10$ and 0.05 respectively. From the observed sample mean and standard deviation, $(1-\alpha)$ percent upper and lower confidence limits for $\mu$ are obtained from

$$C_u = \bar{x} + t_{n-1,\alpha/2}\left(s/\sqrt{n}\right)$$

and

$$C_l = \bar{x} - t_{n-1,\alpha/2}\left(s/\sqrt{n}\right). \tag{5.13}$$

and the confidence width becomes $2t_{n-1,\alpha/2}(s/\sqrt{n})$.

When $X$ follows a distribution other than the normal, from the *Central Limit Theorem*, the standardized variables $(\bar{X}-\mu)/(\sigma/\sqrt{n})$ as well as $(\bar{X}-\mu)/(S/\sqrt{n})$, approximately follow the standard normal distribution, provided $n$ is large. In such cases, confidence limits for $\mu$ can be obtained from $\bar{x} \pm z_{\alpha/2}(\sigma/\sqrt{n})$ if $\sigma$ is known and replacing it by $s$ when it is estimated.

*Example 5.2*   For the mean $\mu$ of the SBPs in Example 5.1 when $\sigma^2$ is known, 90 percent confidence limits are $C_l=[131.3-1.645(2.47)]=127.24$ and $C_u=[131.3+1.645(2.47)]=135.36$, resulting in the confidence width of $(135.36-127.24)=8.12$. Ninety-five percent limits are $C_l=[131.3-1.96(2.47)]=126.46$ and $C_u=[131.3+1.96(2.47)]=136.14$ with the confidence width of $(136.14-126.46)=9.68$. The 95 percent limits are wider than the 90 percent limits.

With the estimated variance of 102 and $t_{15,0.05}=1.753$, from (5.13), 90 percent confidence limits for the mean are $C_l=[131.3-1.753(2.52)]=126.88$ and $C_u=[131.3+1.753(2.52)]=135.72$. The confidence width now is $(135.72-126.88)=8.84$. With $t_{15,0.025}=2.131$, the 95 percent limits are $C_l=[131.3-2.131(2.52)]=125.93$ and $C_u=[131.3+2.131(2.52)]=136.67$. The confidence width $(136.67-125.93)=10.74$ is larger than the width for the 90 percent limits.

When $\sigma^2$ is known, one-sided 95 percent lower and upper confidence limits for $\mu$ are $[131.3-1.645(2.47)]=127.24$ and $[131.3+1.645(2.47)]=135.36$. When $\sigma^2$ is estimated, one-sided 95 percent limits are $[131.3-1.753(2.52)]=126.88$ and $[131.3+1.753(2.52)]=135.72$.

## 5.5   Estimator and confidence limits for the difference of two means

Consider the means $(\mu_1,\mu_2)$ and variances $(\sigma_1^2,\sigma_2^2)$ of the SBPs of adult male and female groups or populations. The means $(\bar{X}_1,\bar{X}_2)$ of random samples of sizes $(n_1,n_2)$ selected from these two groups are unbiased for $(\mu_1,\mu_2)$. The difference of the sample means $D = (\bar{X}_1 - \bar{X}_2)$ is unbiased for $\mu_d = (\mu_1 - \mu_2)$. If the two samples are selected independently, the variance of $D$ becomes

$$V(D) = V(\bar{X}_1) + V(\bar{X}_2) = \sigma_1^2/n_1 + \sigma_2^2/n_2, \tag{5.14}$$

and the standard error of $D$, S.E. $(D)$ is given by $\sqrt{V(D)}$.

If the above type of diagnostic measurements in both the groups can be considered to follow the normal distributions, $Z = (D - \mu_d)/S.E.(D)$ follows the standardized normal distribution. For non-normal distributions, $Z$ follows this distribution approximately, provided the sample sizes in the two groups are not too small. If $(\sigma_1^2, \sigma_2^2)$ are known, with the difference $d = (\bar{x}_1 - \bar{x}_2)$ of the observed sample means, $(1-\alpha)$ percent confidence limits for $\mu_d$ are obtained from

$$d \pm z_{\alpha/2} S.E.(D). \tag{5.15}$$

*Example 5.3*    For samples of sizes 15 and 10 from two groups of adult males and females, the means of the DBPs were found to be (95, 85). If it is known that the variances of the DBPs for these groups are $\sigma_1^2 = 36$ and $\sigma_2^2 = 16$, $V(D) = (36/15 + 16/10) = 4$ and $S.E.(D) = 2$. From (5.15), 95 percent confidence limits for $\mu_d$ are $10 - 1.96(2) = 6.08$ and $10 + 1.96(2) = 13.92$.

In several experimental situations, the variances $\sigma_1^2$ and $\sigma_2^2$ for the groups are not known, but they may be assumed to be equal. A statistical test of hypothesis to examine this assumption will be presented later. If the two variances are the same, from the sample variances of the two groups, an unbiased estimator for the common variance $\sigma^2$ is given by the pooled estimator

$$S_p^2 = \frac{(n_1 - 1) S_1^2 + (n_2 - 1) S_2^2}{(n_1 + n_2 - 2)}. \tag{5.16}$$

Now, the estimator for $V(D)$ becomes

$$v(D) = S_p^2(1/n_1 + 1/n_2), \tag{5.17}$$

and S.E. $(D)$ is obtained from $\sqrt{v(D)}$.

With the sample variances $(s_1^2, s_2^2)$, the pooled variance in (5.16) is estimated from $s_p^2 = [(n_1 - 1)s_1^2 + (n_2 - 1)s_2^2]/(n_1 + n_2 - 2)$. An estimate of the variance in (5.17) is obtained from $v(d) = s_p^2(1/n_1 + 1/n_2)$ and the standard error $S.E.(d)$ from $\sqrt{v(d)}$. The $(1 - \alpha)$ percent confidence limits for the difference $\mu_d$ of the two means are obtained from

$$d \pm t_{n_1 + n_2 - 2, \alpha/2} S.E.(d). \tag{5.18}$$

*Example 5.4*    Consider the comparisons of the means $\mu_1$ and $\mu_2$ of the DBPs of the two groups in Example 5.3 with samples of sizes $(n_1, n_2) = (15, 10)$, means $(\bar{x}_1, \bar{x}_2) = (100, 90)$, their difference $d = (100 - 90) = 10$ and variances $(s_1^2, s_2^2) = (25, 36)$. If it can be assumed that the variances $\sigma_1^2$ and $\sigma_2^2$ are the same, the estimate of the common variance is $s_p^2 = [14(25) + 9(36)]/23 = 29.30$. Now, $v(d) = 29.3(1/15 + 1/10) = 4.88$ and $S.E.(d) = 2.21$. For the $t$-distribution with 23 d.f., $t_{23, 0.025} = 2.069$. The 95 percent confidence limits for $\mu_d$ are $[10 - 2.069(2.21)] = 5.43$ and $[10 + 2.069(2.21)] = 14.57$, with the confidence width of $(14.57 - 5.43) = 9.14$.

# 5.6    Approximate confidence limits for the difference of two means

If $(\sigma_1^2, \sigma_2^2)$ are not equal and estimated by $(s_1^2, s_2^2)$, approximate confidence limits for $\mu_d$ can be obtained through the following procedures.

## 5.6.1    Large samples

When $(\sigma_1^2, \sigma_2^2)$ are not known, an unbiased estimate for $V(d)$ is given by $v(d) = s_1^2/n_1 + s_2^2/n_2$ and $S.E.$ $(d)$ is obtained from $\sqrt{v(d)}$. The approximate $(1 - \alpha)$ percent confidence limits for $\mu_d$ are obtained from $d \pm z_{\alpha/2}\sqrt{v(d)}$. For the DBPs in Example 5.4, $v(d) = [(25/15) + (36/10)] = 5.27$ and $S.E.(d) = 2.3$. Now, 95 percent confidence limits for $\mu_d$ are $[10 - 1.96(2.3)] = 5.49$ and $[10 + 1.96(2.3)] = 14.51$.

## 5.6.2    Welch-Aspin approximation (1949, 1956)

With the above estimator for the $S.E.$ $(d)$, from this approximation, $t = (d - \mu_d)/S.E.(d)$ follows the $t$-distribution with degrees of freedom

$$f = \frac{(w_1 + w_2)^2}{w_1^2/(n_1 - 1) + w_2^2/(n_2 - 1)}. \tag{5.19}$$

In this expression, $w_1 = (s_1^2/n_1)$ and $w_2 = 1/(s_2^2/n_2)$.

For the two groups in Example 5.4, we find that $f$ is close to 17. With this d.f., $t_{17, 0.025} = 2.11$. Ninety-five percent confidence limits for the difference of the two means are $[10 - 2.11(2.3)] = 5.147$ and $[10 + 2.11(2.3)] = 14.853$. These limits are close to the above limits obtained through the normal approximation.

## 5.6.3    Cochran's approximation (1964)

For this approximation, the percentile $t_w$ is found from

$$t_w = \frac{w_1 t_1 + w_2 t_2}{w_1 + w_2}, \tag{5.20}$$

where $t_1$ and $t_2$ are the percentiles of the $t$-distribution with $(n_1 - 1)$ and $(n_2 - 1)$ d.f. respectively. The confidence limits for $\mu_d$ are obtained from $d \pm t_w$ S.E.$(d)$. For the above example, when $\alpha = 0.05$, $t_1 = 2.145$, $t_2 = 2.262$, and $t_w = 2.225$. Now the 95 percent confidence limits for $\mu_d$ are $[10 - 2.225(2.3)] = 4.88$ and $[10 + 2.225(2.3)] = 15.12$. These limits are also close to the limits found above in Sections (5.6.1) and (5.6.2).

An important observation of this approximation is that when $n_1$ and $n_2$ are the same and equal to $m$, $t_1$ and $t_2$ are the same and $t_w$ becomes the percentile of the $t$-distribution with m d.f.

## 5.7   Matched samples and paired comparisons

The efficacy of a treatment can be examined from the measurements obtained before and after administering it to a sample of $n$ units. With $X$ and $Y$ denoting the measurements on the two occasions, the expected value and variance of the difference $d = (Y - X)$ are given by

$$\mu_d = E(Y - X) = E(Y) - E(X) = \mu_y - \mu_x \tag{5.21}$$

and

$$\sigma_d^2 = E(d - \mu_d)^2 = \sigma_y^2 + \sigma_x^2 - 2\rho\sigma_x\sigma_y. \tag{5.22}$$

The covariance and correlation of $X$ and $Y$ are $\sigma_{xy} = E(X - \mu_x)(Y - \mu_y)$ and $\rho = \sigma_{xy}/\sigma_x\sigma_y$.

From the sample observations $(X_i, Y_i), i = (1, 2, \ldots, n)$, and their differences $D_i = Y_i - X_i$, unbiased estimators of $\mu_d$ and $\sigma_d^2$ respectively are given by

$$D = \sum_1^n D_i/n = \sum_1^n (Y - X_i)/n = \bar{Y} - \bar{X} \tag{5.23}$$

and

$$S_d^2 = \sum_1^n (D_i - D)^2/(n - 1) = S_y^2 + S_x^2 - 2S_{xy}. \tag{5.24}$$

In (5.23), $\bar{X} = \sum_1^n X_i/n$ and $\bar{Y} = \sum_1^n Y_i/n$ are the sample means of $(X_i, Y_i)$. In (5.24), $S_x^2 = \sum_1^n (X_i - \bar{X})^2/(n - 1)$ and $S_y^2 = \sum_1^n (Y_i - \bar{Y})^2/(n - 1)$ are their sample variances, and $S_{xy} = \sum_1^n (X_i - \bar{X})(Y_i - \bar{Y})/(n - 1)$ is their sample covariance. Note that $S_{xy} = rS_xS_y$, where $r$ is the sample correlation coefficient.

The variance and standard error of $D$ are $V(D) = \sigma_d^2/n$ and $S.E.(D) = \sigma_d/\sqrt{n}$. Their estimators are given by $v(D) = S_d^2/n$ and $S_d/\sqrt{n}$. When $(X, Y)$ follow the *bivariate normal distribution*,

$$t_{n-1} = \frac{(D - \mu_d)}{S_d/\sqrt{n}} \qquad (5.25)$$

follows the $t$-distribution with $(n - 1)$ d.f. The mean and variance of the differences $d_i = (y_i - x_i)$, $i = (1,2,...,n)$, of the observed sample are $\bar{d} = (\bar{y} - \bar{x})$ and $s_d^2 = \sum_1^n (d_i - \bar{d})^2/(n-1)$. The $(1 - \alpha)$ percent confidence limits for $\mu_d$ are obtained from

$$\bar{d} \pm t_{n-1,\alpha/2}\left(s_d/\sqrt{n}\right). \qquad (5.26)$$

Note that $s_d^2 = s_x^2 + s_y^2 - 2s_{xy}$, where $s_x^2 = \sum_1^n (x_i - \bar{x})^2/(n-1)$ and $s_y^2 = \sum_1^n (y_i - \bar{y})^2/(n-1)$ are the sample variances of $x_i$ and $y_i$ respectively, and $s_{xy} = \sum_1^n (x_i - \bar{x})(y_i - \bar{y})/(n-1)$ is their sample covariance. The sample correlation is obtained from $r = s_{xy}/s_x s_y$.

*Example 5.5*   Consider the DBPs $(X_i, Y_i)$ of a sample of $n = 16$ adults before and after a medical treatment. If the observed sample means are $\bar{x} = 100$ and $\bar{y} = 85$, $d = (85 - 100) = -15$. If the sample variances of the DBPs before and after the treatment are $(225, 100)$ and the sample correlation is 0.5, $s_d^2 = [225 + 100 - 2(0.5)(10)(15)] = 175$ and $s_d = 13.23$. Since $t_{15,0.025} = 2.131$, for the $t$-distribution with $(n - 1) = 15$ d.f., 95 percent confidence limits for the average decrease in the DBP are $[15 - 2.131(13.23/4)] = 7.95$ and $[15 + 2.131(13.23/4)] = 22.05$.

## 5.8   Confidence limits for the variance

As seen in Section 5.3, the variance $S^2$ of a sample of size $n$ is unbiased for the population variance $\sigma^2$. If the population follows the normal distribution,

$$U = (n-1)S^2/\sigma^2 \qquad (5.27)$$

follows the chisquare $(\chi^2)$ distribution with $(n - 1)$ d.f. If $(\alpha/2)$ percent of this distribution falls below **a** and above **b** respectively, $(1 - \alpha)$ percent confidence limits for $\sigma^2$ are given by

$$C_l = (n-1)S^2/b \text{ and } C_u = (n-1)S^2/a \qquad (5.28)$$

and they are obtained with the observed sample variance $s^2$.

*Example 5.6*   For the SBPs of the 16 adults in Example 5.1, $s^2 = 102$. For the Chisquare distribution with 15 d.f., the lower and upper percentiles are $a = 6.262$ and $b = 27.49$ when $(1 - \alpha) = 0.95$. Ninety-five percent confidence limits for $\sigma^2$ are $15(102)/27.49 = 55.66$ and $15(102)/6.262 = 244.33$.

## 5.9    Confidence limits for the ratio of two variances

In Example 5.4, it was assumed that the variances $\sigma_1^2$ and $\sigma_2^2$ of the SBPs of the two groups are the same. In similar situations, the confidence intervals for their ratio can be first examined. Consider the measurements of two groups or populations following the normal distributions. The variances $S_1^2$ and $S_2^2$ of independent samples of sizes $n_1$ and $n_2$ from these populations are unbiased for their variances $\sigma_1^2$ and $\sigma_2^2$. The ratio

$$F = \frac{S_1^2/\sigma_1^2}{S_2^2/\sigma_2^2}$$  (5.29)

follows the $F$-distribution with $(n_1 - 1)$ and $(n_2 - 1)$ d.f. A percentage $(\alpha/2)$ of this distribution falls below $F_l$ and above $F_u$, and the latter is tabulated. The percentile $F_l$ is obtained from $1/F_u$ of the $F$-distribution with $(n_2 - 1)$ and $(n_1 - 1)$ d.f. as described in Section 4.4.8. Some software programs provide both $F_l$ and $F_u$. The lower and upper $(1 - \alpha)$ percent confidence limits for $(\sigma_1^2/\sigma_2^2)$ are given by

$$C_l = \frac{S_1^2}{S_2^2}\frac{1}{F_u}$$

and

$$C_u = \frac{S_1^2}{S_2^2}\frac{1}{F_l},$$  (5.30)

and they are obtained with the observed variances $(s_1^2, s_2^2)$.

*Example 5.7*   For the first sample in Example 5.4, $n_1 = 15$ and $s_1^2 = 25$. For the second sample, $n_2 = 10$ and $s_2^2 = 36$. For the $F$-distribution with 14 and 9 d.f., $F_{0.025} = 0.312$ and $F_{0.975} = 3.798$. From (5.30), 95 percent confidence limits for $(\sigma_1^2/\sigma_2^2)$ are $(25/36)/3.798 = 0.183$ and $(25/36)/0.312 = 2.226$.

## 5.10    Least squares and maximum likelihood methods of estimation

In the above sections, the population mean and variance $(\mu, \sigma^2)$ are estimated by the sample mean and variance $(\bar{X}, S^2)$. Consider a random sample $(X_1, X_2, \ldots, X_n)$ from the population, following the model

$$X_i = \mu + \varepsilon_i \tag{5.31}$$

with $E(\varepsilon_i) = 0$ and $V(\varepsilon_i) = \sigma^2$. For the *Least Squares (LS)* method of estimating $\mu$,

$$\phi = \sum_1^n \varepsilon_i^2 = \sum_1^n (X_i - \mu)^2 \tag{5.32}$$

is minimized with respect to $\mu$. Since $d\phi/d\mu = (-2)\sum_1^n (X_i - \mu) = 0$, the estimator for $\mu$ becomes $\hat{\mu} = \sum_1^n X_i/n = \bar{X}$. Further, since $d^2\phi/d\mu^2$ is non-negative, the minimum of (5.32) is obtained at $\hat{\mu}$. This sample mean is *unbiased* for $\mu$ since $E(\bar{X}) = \mu$. Several *linear* estimators of the form $(l_1 X_1 + l_2 X_2 + \ldots + l_n X_n)$, for specified constants $(l_1, l_2, \ldots, l_n)$ with $(l_1 + l_2 + \ldots + l_n) = 1$, are unbiased for $\mu$, but their variance will not be smaller than the variance $V(\bar{X}) = \sigma^2/n$ of this LS estimator. For instance, $(X_1 + X_2)/2$ is unbiased for $\mu$, but its variance $\sigma^2/2$ is clearly larger than $(\sigma^2/n)$ for $n > 2$. Thus, the sample mean $\bar{X}$ is the *Best Linear Unbiased Estimator* for $\mu$. The sample variance $S^2$ in (5.6) is formulated to be unbiased for the population variance $\sigma^2$, but the sample standard deviation $S$ is not unbiased for $\sigma$.

The *Maximum Likelihood* (ML) method offers a fundamental procedure for estimating the population parameters such as $\mu$, $\sigma^2$ and $\sigma$ for specified probability distribution of the random variable. For instance, if the random variable $X$ follows the normal distribution with mean $\mu$ and variance $\sigma^2$, the joint distribution of the sample observations $(X_1, X_2, \ldots, X_n)$ is given by

$$f(X_1, X_2, \ldots, X_n | \mu, \sigma^2) = \frac{e^{-\sum_1^n (X_i - \mu)^2/2\sigma^2}}{(2\Pi)^{n/2} (\sigma^2)^{n/2}}. \tag{5.33}$$

The *Likelihood function*

$$L = f(\mu, \sigma^2 | X_1, X_2, \ldots, X_n) \tag{5.34}$$

is the same as the right-hand side of (5.33). The ML estimators of $\mu$ and variance $\sigma^2$ are obtained by maximizing this expression with respect to these parameters. For this case of the normal distribution and similar exponential type distributions, the ML estimators can be obtained by maximizing $lnL$.

The ML estimators of $(\mu, \sigma^2)$ become $\hat{\mu} = \bar{X}$ and $\hat{\sigma}^2 = \sum_1^n (X_i - \bar{X})^2/n = (n-1)S^2/n$.

Notice that $\hat{\mu}$ is unbiased for $\mu$, but the expected value of $\hat{\sigma}^2$ becomes $(n-1)\sigma^2/n$, and it underestimates $\sigma^2$. The bias can be removed by considering $(n-1)\hat{\sigma}^2/n = S^2$ as the estimator.

Some properties of the ML estimators are as follows:

1. The ML estimator of a function of a parameter is the same function of the estimator. For instance, the ML estimators of $\sigma$ and $\mu^2$ are $\left[\sum_{1}^{n}(X_i-\bar{X})^2/n\right]^{1/2}$ and $\bar{X}^2$ respectively. The bias in the later case can be removed by considering $(\bar{X}^2 - S^2/n)$ as the estimator for $\mu^2$.

2. The probability of the ML estimator approaching the parameter increases as the sample size increases, that is, it becomes *consistent*.

3. The ML estimator is *asymptotically normal*; that is, it approaches the normal distribution as the sample size increases.

4. For some distributions of the random variable $X$, iterations are needed to obtain the ML estimator. For the gamma distribution $f(x|\alpha) = [1/(\alpha-1)!]e^{-x}x^{\alpha-1}$, iterations would be needed to obtain the estimator for $\alpha$.

# Exercises

**5.1.** Find 95 percent confidence limits for the population means of the heights, weights and BMIs of the ten-year-old boys and girls from the 20 sample observations in T1.1 and T1.2 and the summary figures in the solution to Exercise 1.1. Assume normality for the three characteristics.

**5.2.** As in Exercise 5.1, find the 95 percent confidence limits for the differences of the means of the *10-year*-old boys and girls for the three characteristics.

**5.3.** With the sample standard deviations in column (c) of Table T5, find 95 percent confidence limits for the ratios of the variances of the percentages of *private* expenditures of (1) Asia and Africa, and (2) South East Asia and Europe.

**5.4.** With the sample standard deviation in column (d) of Table T5, find 95 percent confidence limits for the ratio of the variances of the *total* expenditures of (1) Asia and Africa, and (2) South East Asia and Europe.

**5.5.** From the sample means and standard deviations in column (c) of Table T5, find 95 percent confidence limits for the difference of the average percentages of the *private* expenditures of Asia and Africa.

**5.6.** From the sample means and standard deviations in column (d) of Table T5, find 95 percent confidence limits for the difference of the average percentages of the *total* expenditures of Asia and Africa.

**5.7.** Poduri et al. (1996) examined the Functional Independence Measure (FIM) score at admission and discharge, Length of Stay (LOS) and Efficiency Ratio (ER) of stroke patients admitted to an inpatient medical rehabilitation unit. ER is the change in FIM from admission to discharge as a ratio of the LOS in days. For the $n_1 = 60$ "appropriate" patients, Group 1, the mean and standard deviation of the ERs were (0.81, 0.50). For the $n_2 = 10$ "inappropriate patients," Group 2, they were (0.36, 0.33). Find 95 percent confidence limits for (a) difference of the population means of the ERs of the two groups and (b) ratio of their population variances.

**5.8.** Cushman et al. (1995) presented the following means and standard deviations for the change in FIM from admission to discharge, LOS and ER (see Exercise 57) for the stroke patients in an inpatient medical rehabilitation unit for the pre-functional measure score (PFM) of less than or equal to 30 and greater than 30, Groups 1 and 2.

|  | Group 1 ($n = 15$) | | Group 2 ($n = 23$) | |
| --- | --- | --- | --- | --- |
|  | Mean | S.D. | Mean | S.D. |
| FIM change | 22.55 | 9.6 | 19.7 | 12.4 |
| LOS | 44.70 | 16.2 | 24.7 | 10.9 |
| ER | 0.56 | 0.31 | 0.93 | 0.53 |

Find 95 percent confidence limits for the ratios of the variances of the second and first groups for each of the three measures.

**5.9.** For the *Celiac* disease, Masselli (2010) et al. presented the results of the "evaluation with Dynamic Contrast - enhanced MR imaging." The mean and standard deviation of the "maximum enhancement of the duodenal wall" for (1) 60 patients with untreated celiac disease and (2) 45 patients treated for one year with a gluten-free diet respectively were (229.1, 46.4) and (109.8, 27.8). They were (94.7, 17.9) for the control group. "Mean duodenal wall thickness was not significantly different." Find 95 percent confidence limits for (a) the mean of the treated group and (b) difference of the population means of the untreated and treated groups.

# Appendix A5

## A5.1  Tschebycheff's inequality

For a random variable $X$, this inequality is given by

$$P\left[|X - E(X)| \le k\sqrt{V(X)}\right] \ge 1 - \left(1/k^2\right),$$

where $k$ is a positive constant. With $\varepsilon = k\sqrt{V(X)}$, this probability becomes the same as

$$P[|X - E(X)| \le \varepsilon] \ge 1 - V(X)/\varepsilon^2.$$

Thus, for a specified value of $k$, the probability of an unbiased estimator $X$ becoming closer to the mean $E(X)$ increases as its variance $V(X)$ decreases.

To apply the above inequality to the sample mean, replace $X$ by $\bar{X}$ and $\sigma^2$ by $V(\bar{X}) = \sigma^2/n$. For the standard normal distribution, $P[|Z| < 1.96] = 0.95$. From the above inequality, we find this probability to be $[1 - 1/(1.96^2)]$, which is approximately equal to 0.74.

## A5.2   Mean square error

As an illustration,

$$MSE\left(\hat{\sigma}^2\right) = E\left(\hat{\sigma}^2 - \sigma^2\right) = E\left\{\left[\hat{\sigma}^2 - E\left(\hat{\sigma}^2\right)\right] + \left[E\left(\hat{\sigma}^2\right) - \sigma^2\right]\right\}^2$$
$$= E\left[\hat{\sigma}^2 - E\left(\hat{\sigma}^2\right)\right]^2 + \left[E\left(\hat{\sigma}^2\right) - \sigma^2\right]^2.$$

The first term on the right-hand side is the variance of $\hat{\sigma}^2$, and the second term is the square of its bias. The bias of an estimator can be positive or negative. For an unbiased estimator, its MSE is the same as the variance.

# 6

# Proportions, odds ratios and relative risks: Estimation and confidence limits

## 6.1 Introduction

National and international organizations of health, clinical centers and laboratories present percentages related to the growth, vaccination and other aspects of children. Percentages related to cholesterol levels, hypertension, obesity, smoking habits and similar characteristics of the adult populations are frequently assessed. These types of proportions or percentages are estimated from the samples available or collected for specific purposes. The properties of the estimators for the proportions and their differences along with their confidence limits are presented in the following sections. The odds ratios and relative risks presented in Chapter 3 are of particular importance for various types of medical diagnosis and evaluations. Estimation and confidence limits of these measures are also presented and illustrated.

## 6.2 A single proportion

If a total number $X$ of individuals in a random sample from a population are hypertensive, an unbiased estimator of the proportion $p$ of the individuals to be hypertensive is $\hat{p} = X/n$. The variance and S.E. of this estimator are

$$V(\hat{p}) = pq/n \qquad (6.1)$$

*Statistical Methodologies with Medical Applications*, First Edition. Poduri S.R.S. Rao.
© 2017 John Wiley & Sons, Ltd. Published 2017 by John Wiley & Sons, Ltd.

and

$$S.E.(\hat{p}) = \sqrt{pq/n}, \tag{6.2}$$

where $q = (1-p)$ is the proportion of the normotensives in the population. An unbiased estimator of this proportion is given by $\hat{q} = (n-X)/n = (1-\hat{p})$; $V(\hat{q})$ and $S.E.(\hat{q})$ remain the same as (6.1) and (6.2). These results for $\hat{p}$ and $\hat{q}$ are obtained by first noting that $E(X) = np$ and $V(X) = npq$. The estimates of the variances and S.Es of $\hat{p}$ and $\hat{q}$ are obtained by replacing $p$ and $q$ with $\hat{p}$ and $\hat{q}$. With the observed value $x$ of the random variable $X$, the estimates $\hat{p}$ and $\hat{q}$ and their standard errors are obtained from $(x/n)$ and $(n - x)/n$.

## 6.3   Confidence limits for the proportion

The above results in Section 6.2 correspond to the binomial distribution presented in Section 4.3.2. Confidence limits for $p$ or $q$ can be obtained from the cumulative probabilities of this distribution, and they are also available in the software programs. If the sample size is not too small, from the *Central Limit Theorem*,

$$Z = (X - npq)/\sqrt{npq} = (\hat{p}-p)/\sqrt{pq/n} \tag{6.3}$$

follows the standardized normal distribution with zero mean and unit standard deviation. With the sample estimate $\sqrt{\hat{p}\hat{q}/n}$ for $S.E.(\hat{p})$, approximate $(1-\alpha)$ percent confidence limits for $p$ are obtained from

$$\hat{p} \pm z_{\alpha/2}\sqrt{\hat{p}\hat{q}/n}. \tag{6.4}$$

Similarly, the confidence limits for q are obtained from $\hat{q} \pm z_{\alpha/2}\sqrt{\hat{p}\hat{q}/n}$. These limits are also obtained by subtracting the upper and lower limits in (6.4) from one.

*Example 6.1*   If the number of hypertensives in a sample of $n = 500$ adults in the (40–60) years-of-age group was found to be $x = 200$, an estimate of the proportion $p$ of the hypertensives in this age group is $\hat{p} = (200/500) = 0.40$ or 40 percent. From this sample, $v(\hat{p}) = 0.40(0.60)/500 = 0.00048$ and $S.E.(\hat{p}) = 0.022$. From (6.4), approximate 95 percent confidence limits for $p$ are $[0.40 - 1.96(0.022)] = 0.357$ and $[0.40 + 1.96(0.022)] = 0.443$, that is, 35.7 and 44.3 percent.

The confidence width becomes $(44.3 - 35.7) = 8.6$ percent. Since $\hat{q} = 0.60$ and $S.E.(\hat{q}) = 0.022$, 95 percent confidence limits for q are $[0.60 - 1.96(0.022)] = 0.557$ and $[0.60 + 1.96(0.022)] = 0.643$, which are the same as $(1 - 0.443)$ and $(1 - 0.357)$.

## 6.4    Difference of two proportions or percentages

Consider the proportions of the hypertensives in the adult male and female populations to be $p_1$ and $p_2$. If $x_1$ males and $x_2$ females respectively were found to be hypertensive in samples of sizes $n_1$ and $n_2$ selected from these populations, unbiased
estimators of the two proportions are given by $\hat{p}_1 = x_1/n_1$ and $\hat{p}_2 = x_2/n_2$. An unbiased
estimator of the difference $D = (p_1 - p_2)$ of the proportions is $d = (\hat{p}_1 - \hat{p}_2)$. Its variance
and estimator of variance are

$$V(d) = V(\hat{p}_1 - \hat{p}_2) = V(\hat{p}_1) + V(\hat{p}_2)$$

$$= p_1(1-p_1)/n_1 + p_2(1-p_2)/n_2 \tag{6.5}$$

and

$$v(d) = \hat{p}_1(1-\hat{p}_1)/n_1 + \hat{p}_2(1-\hat{p}_2)/n_2 \tag{6.6}$$

The sample $S.E.(d)$ is obtained from the positive square root of this expression, and
the $(1-\alpha)$ percent confidence limits for $D$ are found from

$$d \pm z_{\alpha/2} S.E.(d). \tag{6.7}$$

*Example 6.2*    Consider random samples of sizes $n_1 = 300$ and $n_2 = 200$ selected
independently from large male and female adult populations in a community.
If the number of hypertensives in these samples were found to be $x_1 = 120$ and
$x_2 = 60$, an estimate of the difference $D = (p_1 - p_2)$ of the proportions of
hypertensives in these two groups is $d = [(120/300) - (60/200)] = (0.40 - 0.30) =$
$0.10$ or 10 percent. The sample estimate of the variance $V(d)$ is $v(d) =$
$[(0.4)(0.6)/300 + (0.3)(0.7)/200] = 0.00185$    and    $S.E.(d) = 0.043$.    Ninety-five
percent confidence limits for $D$ are $[0.10 - 1.96(0.043)] = 0.0157$ and $[0.10 + 1.96$
$(0.043)] = 0.1843$; that is, approximately 1.6 and 18.4 percent. The confidence
width of 16.8 in this case is rather large.

## 6.5    Combining proportions from independent samples

To assess the proportion $p$ of the adults with hypertension in a large population, $k$
independent samples of sizes $n_i$, $i = (1, 2, ..., k)$, may be selected. If $x_i$ of the adults
in these samples were observed to be hypertensive, the sample proportion $\hat{p}_i = (x_i/n_i)$
is an unbiased estimator of the population proportion $p$ with variance
$V(\hat{p}_i) = p(1-p)/n_i$. From the total sample of size $n = \sum_1^k n_i$, the overall estimator

for $p$ becomes $\hat{p} = \sum_1^k x_i/n = \sum_1^n n_i \hat{p}_i/n$. It is unbiased for $p$ with variance $V(\hat{p}) = p(1-p)/n$. For the estimate of this variance, $\hat{p}$ is substituted for $p$ in this expression.

## 6.6 More than two classes or categories

A population may consist of the adults with low, medium and high levels of systolic blood pressure. Similarly, other physical or medical characteristics such as weight, obesity, lipid levels may be classified into a suitable number of categories. In general, the population may be classified into $k$ categories in the proportions $(p_1, p_2, ..., p_k)$, $(p_1 + p_2 + ... + p_k) = 1$. If the numbers of adults $(X_1, X_2, ..., X_k)$ in these classes are observed in a random sample of size n from the population, an unbiased estimator of the proportion $p_i$, $i = (1, 2...k)$, is given by $\hat{p}_i = X_i/n$. The variance of this estimator becomes

$$V(\hat{p}_i) = p_i(1-p_i)/n. \tag{6.8}$$

An estimate of this variance is obtained by replacing $p_i$ with $\hat{p}_i$, and the S.E. of $\hat{p}_i$ is found from the square root of the estimated variance.

The observed numbers $(X_i, X_j)$ and the estimators $(\hat{p}_i, \hat{p}_j)$, $(i \pm j)$, are negatively correlated. The covariances of $(X_i, X_j)$, and of the estimators $(\hat{p}_i, \hat{p}_j)$ are given by

$$Cov(X_i, X_j) = -np_i p_j$$

and

$$Cov(\hat{p}_i, \hat{p}_j) = -p_i p_j/n. \tag{6.9}$$

The estimators of these covariances are obtained by replacing $(p_i, p_j)$ with $(\hat{p}_i, \hat{p}_j)$. The estimates of the proportions, their variances, S.E.s and the covariances are obtained from the observed values $(x_1, x_2, ..., x_k)$, $\sum_1^n x_i = n$.

The difference of the estimators $d = (\hat{p}_i - \hat{p}_j)$ is unbiased for $D = (p_i - p_j)$, $(i \pm j)$. Its variance and estimator of variance are

$$V(d) = [p_i(1-p_i) + p_j(1-p_j) + 2p_i p_j]/n \tag{6.10}$$

and

$$v(d) = [\hat{p}_i(1-\hat{p}_i) + \hat{p}_j(1-\hat{p}_j) + 2\hat{p}_i \hat{p}_j]/n. \tag{6.11}$$

The S.E.(d) is given by the square root of this estimated variance, and the $(1-\alpha)$ percent confidence limits for $D$ are obtained from

$$d \pm z_{\alpha/2}S.E.(d).$$    (6.12)

*Example 6.3*    Consider the observed numbers $x_1 = 250$, $x_2 = 150$ and $x_3 = 100$ found with Systolic Blood Pressure (SBP) in the ranges 130–140, 140–150 and >150 in a random sample of $n = 500$ from a large adult population. The estimates of the proportions of the adults in these ranges of the SBP are $\hat{p}_1 = (250/500) = 0.5$, $\hat{p}_2 = (150/500) = 0.3$ and $\hat{p}_3 = (100/500) = 0.2$. The estimate of the difference of the proportions $D = (p_1 - p_2)$ for the first two groups is $d = (0.5 - 0.3) = 0.2$ or 20 percent. From (6.11), $v(d) = [(0.5)(0.5) + (0.3)(0.7) + 2(0.5)(0.3)]/500 = 0.00152$ and hence $S.E.(d) = 0.039$. Ninety-five percent confidence limits for $D$ are $0.2 - 1.96(0.039) = 0.124$ and $0.2 + 1.96(0.039) = 0.276$; that is, 12.4 and 27.6 percent.

## 6.7    Odds ratio

Examination of the odds ratios and relative risks related to hypertension, lipid levels and other diagnostic characteristics, described in Chapter 3, is of importance to the medical profession as well as to the general public. The HDL levels of a sample of $n_1 = 400$ obese and an independent sample of $n_2 = 200$ non-obese male adults are presented in Table 6.1.

With the population proportions $p_1$ and $p_2$ of the adults with the HDL lower than 45 among the obese and non-obese adults respectively, the odds ratio is

$$OR = \frac{p_1/q_1}{p_2/q_2} = \frac{p_1 q_2}{p_2 q_1},$$    (6.13)

where $q_1 = (1 - p_1)$ and $q_2 = (1 - p_2)$. This ratio is obtained with the estimators $\hat{p}_1 = a/(a + b) = a/n_1$ and $\hat{p}_2 = c/(c + d) = c/n_2$.

For the case-control, retrospective and similar studies, $ln(OR)$ is related to the covariates such as age and length of a medical treatment. The estimators $\widehat{OR}$ and

Table 6.1    HDL of 400 obese and 200 nonobese adults.

| | HDL | | |
| --- | --- | --- | --- |
| | <45 | >45 | |
| Obese | $a = 280$ | $b = 120$ | $n_1 = 400$ |
| Nonobese | $c = 40$ | $d = 160$ | $n_2 = 200$ |

$ln(\widehat{OR})$ are obtained from (6.13) with $\hat{p}_1$ and $\hat{p}_2$. As shown in Appendix A6.1, $ln(\widehat{OR})$ is approximately unbiased for $ln(OR)$ with variance

$$V\left[ln\left(\widehat{OR}\right)\right] = (1/n_1 p_1 q_1 + 1/n_2 p_2 q_2). \tag{6.14}$$

The estimate of this variance is obtained from

$$v\left[ln\left(\widehat{OR}\right)\right] = (a+b)/ab + (c+d)/cd = (1/a + 1/b + 1/c + 1/d), \tag{6.15}$$

and S.E.($ln\widehat{OR}$) is obtained from the square root of this estimate.

From the figures in Table 6.1 for the HDL illustration, $\hat{p}_1 = (280/400) = 0.70$, $\hat{p}_2 = (40/200) = 0.20$, $\widehat{OR} = (280/120)/(40/160) = (28/3) = 9.33$ and $ln(\widehat{OR}) = 2.2332$. From (6.15), $v(ln\widehat{OR}) = [400/(280 \times 120) + 200/(40 \times 160)] = 0.0432$ and S.E.($ln\widehat{OR}$) = 0.2078. Ninety-five percent confidence limits for $ln(\widehat{OR})$ are $[2.2332 - 1.96(0.2078)] = 1.83$ and $[2.2332 + 1.96(0.2078)] = 2.64$. From these figures, confidence limits for the OR are (6.23, 14.01).

## 6.8  Relative risk

As described in Section 3.3, the relative risk RR for the obese and non-obese adults of the illustration in Section 6.7 is $RR = p_1/p_2$. Its estimator is given by

$$\widehat{RR} = (\hat{p}_1/\hat{p}_2) = \frac{a/(a+b)}{c/(c+d)}, \tag{6.16}$$

which is approximately unbiased for RR. As can be seen from Appendix A6.2, $ln(\widehat{RR})$ is approximately unbiased for $ln(RR)$ with variance

$$V\left(ln\widehat{RR}\right) = q_1/n_1 p_1 + q_2/n_2 p_2. \tag{6.17}$$

The estimate of this variance $v(ln\,\widehat{RR})$ is obtained from this expression by substituting $(\hat{p}_1, \hat{p}_2)$ for $(p_1, p_2)$.

From Table 6.1, the estimate of the relative risk for the obese and non-obese adults is $\widehat{RR} = (0.7/0.2) = 3.5$ and $ln(\widehat{RR}) = 1.2528$. With $(\hat{p}_1, \hat{p}_2) = (0.7, 0.2)$, $v(ln\,\widehat{RR}) = [0.3/(400)(0.7) + 0.8/(200)((0.2)] = 0.0211$, and S.E.($ln\widehat{RR}$) = 0.1453. Ninety-five percent confidence limits for $ln(RR)$ are $[1.2528 - 1.96(0.1453)] = 0.9686$ and $[1.2528 + 1.96(0.1453)] = 1.537$. From these figures, confidence limits for the RR are (2.63, 4.65).

## Exercises

**6.1.** Poduri et al. (1996) compared the "functional gains" of stroke patients admitted to an inpatient medical rehabilitation unit. Ninety-six percent of the ninety-six patients screened for admission by a nurse practitioner and 80 percent of the 100 screened by a physiatrist successfully met the functional goals. Find the 95 percent confidence limits for the (a) percentage gains of each group and (b) difference of the percentages.

**6.2.** For independent samples of sizes (100, 150, 250) of families in a large community, (25, 30, 45) respectively do not have adequate health insurance. Find the (a) combined estimate of the percentage, (b) its S.E., and (c) 95 percent confidence limits for the percentage.

**6.3.** In a random sample of 200 physicians of a university hospital, (20, 100, 70) respectively are (<30, 30–60, >60) years old. Estimate the difference and find the 95 percent confidence limits for (a) the percentages of the second and third groups and (b) the second group and the first and third groups together.

**6.4.** In a random sample of 200 adults of the U.S. population, (15, 25, 50) percent of the adults in the age groups (18–39, 40–59 and $\geq 60$) respectively were found to have low LDL. The population consists of approximately (35, 35, 15) percent of the adults in these age groups. Estimate the following percentages having low LDL and find the 95 percent confidence limits: (a) overall, (b) difference between the first two groups, and (c) difference between the third group and the first two groups together.

**6.5.** From the sample observations in Table 3.1, find the 95 percent confidence limits for the (a) odds ratio and (b) relative risk of hypertension for smokers versus nonsmokers.

# Appendix A6

## A6.1    Approximation to the variance of $ln\hat{p}_1$

From Taylor's series,

$$
\begin{aligned}
ln(\hat{p}_1) &= ln(p_1) + (\hat{p}_1 - p_1)(dln\hat{p}_1/dp_1) \text{ at } p_1 \\
&= ln(p_1) + (\hat{p}_1 - p_1)/p_1 + \ldots
\end{aligned}
\tag{A6.1}
$$

The expectation of the second term on the right hand side vanishes. The expectations of the remaining terms are of the form $(a_1/n_1 + a_2/n_1^2 + \ldots)$, where $(a_1, a_2, \ldots)$ depend on the second and higher-order moments of $\hat{p}_1$. These expectations become small when $n_1$ is not too small. In such a case, $ln(\hat{p}_1)$ becomes approximately unbiased for $ln(p_1)$. As a result, from the above expression,

$$
V(ln\,\hat{p}_1) = V(\hat{p}_1)/p_1^2 = (p_1 q_1/n_1)/p_1^2 = (q_1/n_1 p_1).
\tag{A6.2}
$$

Similarly, $V(ln\hat{p}_2) = (q_2/n_2 p_2)$.
Approximation to the variance of $ln(\hat{p}_1/\hat{q}_1)$:

As above,

$$ln\left(\frac{\hat{p}_1}{\hat{q}_1}\right) = ln\frac{p_1}{q_1} + \left(\frac{\hat{p}_1}{\hat{q}_1} - \frac{p_1}{q_1}\right)\left(\frac{d}{d\hat{p}_1}ln\frac{\hat{p}_1}{\hat{q}_1}\right) \text{ at } p_1 \tag{A6.3}$$

Now,

$$\frac{d}{d\hat{p}_1}\ ln\left(\frac{\hat{p}_1}{\hat{q}_1}\right) = \frac{d}{d\hat{p}_1}(ln\hat{p}_1 - ln\hat{q}_1) = 1 + \hat{p}_1 + 1/\hat{q}_1 = 1/\hat{p}_1\hat{q}_1, \tag{A6.4}$$

which becomes $1/p_1q_1$ at $p_1$. As a result,

$$ln\left(\frac{\hat{p}_1}{\hat{q}_1}\right) = ln\left(\frac{p_1}{q_1}\right) + \left(\frac{\hat{p}_1}{\hat{q}_1} - \frac{p_1}{q_1}\right)\frac{1}{p_1q_1} \tag{A6.5}$$

Further, $V(\hat{p}_1/\hat{q}_1) = V[\hat{p}_1/(1-\hat{p}_1)]$, which is approximately equal to $V(\hat{p}_1) = p_1q_1/n_1$. From (A6.3) and (A6.5),

$$V[ln(\hat{p}_1/\hat{q}_1)] = (p_1q_1/n_1)/(p_1q_1)^2 = 1/n_1p_1q_1. \tag{A6.6}$$

# 7

# Tests of hypotheses: Means and variances

## 7.1 Introduction

Statistical tests of hypotheses have become essential for scientific experiments and clinical trials. Some illustrations of the hypotheses of medical interest are as follows: (1) Exercise and non-fatty diets can reduce hypertension, increase HDL and decrease LDL. (2) The benefits of exercise are the same for both men and women. (3) Aspirin in small doses can be helpful to stroke patients, but may cause intestinal bleeding in large doses. (4) Air pollution and smoking can result in serious cardiovascular and respiratory problems. (5) Certain childhood vaccinations may have adverse effects. Some of these hypotheses are generated from observational and epidemiological studies on human populations. Hypotheses of frequent interest are related to the problems such as the effects of medical compounds and treatments, differences among the effects of treatments or dosages of drugs, and the side effects of certain treatments. The above types of hypotheses may be related to the means, variances, proportions, percentages, correlations and similar quantities of interest. The following sections present the statistical tests of hypotheses related to the means and variances.

The celebrated *Neyman-Pearson Lemma* (1933) and the associated *Likelihood Ratio procedure* provide the foundations for statistical tests of hypotheses with optimum properties. The tests of hypotheses presented in this chapter and elsewhere are derived from this procedure.

*Statistical Methodologies with Medical Applications*, First Edition. Poduri S.R.S. Rao.
© 2017 John Wiley & Sons, Ltd. Published 2017 by John Wiley & Sons, Ltd.

## 7.2    Principle steps for the tests of a hypothesis

Formulation of the null and alternative hypotheses, decision rule for the null hypothesis, and the Type I and II errors of rejecting a hypothesis when it is true and not rejecting it when it is false are presented in the following subsections. The $p$-value, which is the probability of obtaining an extreme value for the test statistic, is described. The power of a test, which is the probability of rejecting a false hypothesis, is illustrated.

### 7.2.1    Null and alternate hypotheses

For the examination of the mean $\mu$ of cholesterol, blood pressure or a similar diagnostic variable of a population of adults, the *null* and *alternative* hypotheses are specified as

$$H_0 : \mu = \mu_0$$

and

$$H_1 : \mu = \mu_1. \tag{7.1}$$

The null hypothesis specifies the *status quo*. The alternative hypothesis is the claimed change from the null hypothesis. The null hypothesis is always *simple* with the mean taking only one value. The alternative hypothesis can be simple with the mean taking only one value or *composite* with the mean possibly taking more than one value. For the right-sided, left-sided and two-sided alternative hypothesis, $\mu_1 > \mu_0, \mu_1 < \mu_0$ and $\mu_1 \neq \mu_0$ respectively. For instance, if it is claimed that the mean of the LDLs of a group of adults has increased from 100 mg/dl, $\mu_0 = 100$ and $\mu_1 > 100$. On the other hand, if the claim is that the mean has changed from 100, $\mu_1 \neq 100$. Similarly, if the claim is that the HDL has decreased from 40 mg/dl, $\mu_0 = 40$ and $\mu_1 < 40$.

### 7.2.2    Decision rule, test statistic and the Type I & II errors

For the above hypothesis regarding the mean of the LDL with the right-sided alternative, for instance, the sample mean $\bar{X}$ of a random sample of the adults can be considered as the *test statistic*. As a decision rule, the null hypothesis $H_0 : \mu = 100$ may be rejected if $\bar{X}$ exceeds 100 by a specified amount. This decision rule can lead to the errors of *rejecting $H_0$* when it is true and *not rejecting* it when it is false. They are respectively known as the Type I and Type II errors. The probabilities of committing these errors are

$$P(\text{Type I error}) = \alpha$$

And

$$P(\text{Type II error}) = \beta. \tag{7.2}$$

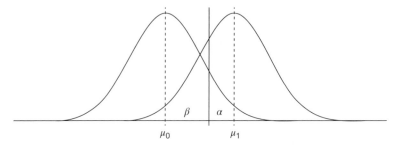

*Figure 7.1    Probabilities of Type I and II errors for the right-sided alternative.*

They can be formally expressed as follows:

Probabilities of the decision rule.

|  | $H_0$ is true | $H_0$ is false |
|---|---|---|
| Reject $H_0$ | $\alpha$ | $1-\beta$ |
| Do not reject $H_0$ | $1-\alpha$ | $\beta$ |

The probabilities $(\alpha, \beta)$ for the right-sided alternative are presented in Figure 7.1.

### 7.2.3    Significance level and critical region

The *Significance level* of the test is the same as $\alpha$. The test is considered highly significant if this probability is very small. In practice, it is set at a small value, for instance, 0.05 or 0.01. The *Critical Region (C.R.)* is the region of the test statistic for rejecting the null hypothesis when it is true. It is formed from the test statistic and the specified significance level.

### 7.2.4    The *p*-value

For the hypothesis on the LDL with the right-sided alternative mentioned in the above sections, the *p*-value is the probability of obtaining a value for $\bar{X}$ larger than the observed one. Similarly, with the sample mean as the test statistic for the hypothesis on the HDL with the left-sided alternative, it is the probability of obtaining a value for $\bar{X}$ smaller than the observed one. For the hypothesis on the LDLs with the two-sided alternative, it is the probability of obtaining a value for $\bar{X}$ larger or smaller than the observed one. The null hypothesis is less credible if the *p*-value is very small. Decisions regarding its rejection can be made from this probability without specifying the significance level.

### 7.2.5    Power of the test and the sample size

The power of a test $(1-\beta)$ is the probability of rejecting the null hypothesis when it is false. For the hypotheses in (7.1), it depends on the significance level for the test and the specified value of $\mu_1$. The Neyman-Pearson Lemma and the Likelihood Ratio provide the tests of hypotheses with the highest power for specified significance level.

For the hypotheses on the LDL and HDL in the above sections, the power of the test becomes an expression depending on the null and alternative values of the mean, significance level and sample size for obtaining $\bar{X}$. The sample size required for a specified power can be obtained from this expression.

## 7.3    Right-sided alternative, test statistic and critical region

Consider the claim that the mean $\mu$ of the LDLs of a large group of adults exceeds 100 mg/dl. In this case, the null and alternative hypotheses are specified as in (7.1) with $\mu_0 = 100$ and $\mu_1 > 100$. The null hypothesis is simple, and the alternative hypothesis is composite and right-sided. To examine the null hypothesis, the mean $\bar{X}$ of the LDLs of a random sample of size $n$ selected from the above adult population can be considered as the *test statistic*. If the LDLs follow the normal distribution with variance $\sigma^2$, the sample mean $\bar{X}$ follows the normal distribution with mean $\mu_0$ and standard error $S.E.(\bar{X}) = \sigma/\sqrt{n}$ when the null hypothesis is true: that is, $Z = (\bar{X} - \mu_0)/(\sigma/\sqrt{n})$ follows the standard normal distribution with zero mean and unit standard deviation.

For a specified significance level $\alpha$, the *Critical Region* for this null hypothesis is given by $\bar{X} \geq [\mu_0 + z_\alpha(\sigma/\sqrt{n})]$, where $z_\alpha$ is the $(1-\alpha)$th percentile of the standard normal distribution. With the observed value $\bar{x}$ of the sample mean, the critical region becomes

$$\bar{x} \geq \left[\mu_0 + z_\alpha\left(\sigma/\sqrt{n}\right)\right], \tag{7.3}$$

that is,

$$z = \frac{\bar{x} - \mu_0}{\sigma/\sqrt{n}} \geq z_\alpha. \tag{7.3a}$$

Equivalently, the null hypothesis is rejected if $\mu_0$ is smaller than the lower confidence limit

$$C_l = \left[\bar{x} - z_\alpha\left(\sigma/\sqrt{n}\right)\right] \text{ for } \mu.$$

## 7.3.1   The *p*-value

With the right-sided alternative, the *p-value* is the probability of finding the sample mean as large or larger than the observed mean $\bar{x}$ when $H_0$ is true. It is obtained from

$$P(\bar{X} \geq \bar{x} \mid \mu = \mu_0) = P\left(\frac{\bar{X} - \mu_0}{\sigma/\sqrt{n}} \geq \frac{\bar{x} - \mu_0}{\sigma/\sqrt{n}}\right)$$

$$= P\left[Z \geq \frac{\bar{x} - \mu_0}{\sigma/\sqrt{n}}\right] = P(Z \geq z). \qquad (7.4)$$

This probability is the same as the significance level corresponding to the observed sample mean $\bar{x}$.

*Example 7.1*    Consider the above hypotheses for the mean of the LDL with $\mu_0 = 100$ and $\mu_1 > 100$. For a random sample of $n = 16$ adults, the mean and standard deviation were found to be $\bar{x} = 116.99$ and $s = 25.04$. If the population standard deviation $\sigma$ is assumed to be 24, $S.E.(\bar{X}) = (24/4) = 6$ and $z = (116.99 - 100)/6 = 2.83$. If the significance level $\alpha$ is 0.05, $z_\alpha = 1.645$. Since $z$ exceeds 1.645, the null hypothesis is rejected at the 5 percent significance level.

The Critical Region and the lower 95 percent confidence limit for the mean are

$$CR : [100 + 1.645(6)] = 109.87$$

and

$$C_l : [116.99 - 1.645(6)] = 107.12.$$

The sample mean 116.99 exceeds 109.87, and $\mu_0$ is smaller than 107.12. Either of these results leads to the rejection of the null hypothesis at the 5 percent significance level. The *p*-value for the test becomes $P(Z \geq 2.83) = 0.0023$, which is very small and leads to the rejection of the null hypothesis.

## 7.3.2   Power of the test

For a specified significance level $\alpha$, the power of the above test at the mean $\mu_1$ is given by

$$P\left\{\bar{X} \geq \left[\mu_0 + z_\alpha\left(\sigma/\sqrt{n}\right)\right] \mid \mu = \mu_1\right\}$$

$$= P\left\{\frac{\bar{X} - \mu_1}{\sigma/\sqrt{n}} \geq \left[\frac{\mu_0 - \mu_1}{\sigma/\sqrt{n}} + z_\alpha\right]\right\}$$

$$= P\left\{Z \geq \left[\frac{\mu_0 - \mu_1}{\sigma/\sqrt{n}} + z_\alpha\right]\right\} \qquad (7.5)$$

Table 7.1    Power of the test for the mean of the LDL
with the right-sided alternative when $\alpha = 0.05$.

| $\mu_1$ | $(\mu_0 - \mu_1)/(\sigma/\sqrt{n}) + 1.645$ | Power |
|---|---|---|
| 100 | 1.645 | 0.050 |
| 105 | 0.812 | 0.208 |
| 110 | −0.022 | 0.509 |
| 115 | −0.855 | 0.804 |
| 120 | −1.688 | 0.954 |
| 125 | −2.522 | 0.994 |
| 130 | −3.355 | 0.999 |

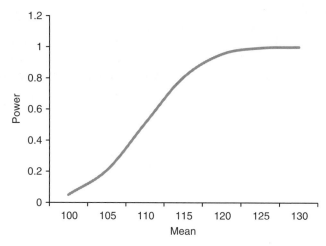

*Figure 7.2    Power of the test for the mean with the right-sided alternative when the
standard deviation is known.*

The power increases as the mean $\mu_1$ under $H_1$ increases from the mean $\mu_0$ of $H_0$. It
is presented in Table 7.1 and Figure 7.2 for the right-sided alterative in Example 7.1.

### 7.3.3    Sample size required for specified power

For the specified power $(1-\beta)$, from (7.5),

$$\left[(\mu_0 - \mu_1)/(\sigma/\sqrt{n})\right] + z_\alpha = z_{1-\beta}. \tag{7.6}$$

If the power of the test should be at least $(1-\beta)$, from this expression, the required
sample size is given by

$$n \geq \left(z_{1-\beta} - z_\alpha\right)^2/\delta^2 = \left(z_\beta + z_\alpha\right)^2/\delta^2, \tag{7.7}$$

where $\delta = (\mu_0 - \mu_1)/\sigma$. For a given $\delta$, as expected, the required sample size increases as the power increases. For the hypotheses in Example 7.1, if the significance level and power are considered to be 5 and 90 percent, $z_\alpha = 1.645$ and $z_{1-\beta} = -1.282$. At the alternative value of 115 for the mean, $\delta = (100 - 115)/24 = -(5/8)$. From (7.7), $n \geq (1.28 + 1.645)^2/(5/8)^2 = 21.90$ or close to 22. As can be seen from Table 7.1, with the sample of size 16, the power at the alternative value of 115 for the mean is only 80.4 percent.

## 7.3.4   Right-sided alternative and estimated variance

When $\sigma^2$ is estimated by the sample variance $S^2 = \sum_1^n (X_i - \bar{X})^2/(n-1)$, $t_{n-1} = (\bar{X} - \mu_0)/(S/\sqrt{n})$ follows the Student's $t$-distribution with $(n-1)$ d.f. Note that $S/\sqrt{n}$ is an estimate of the standard error $(\sigma/\sqrt{n})$ of the sample mean $\bar{X}$. The Critical Region for the null hypothesis in (7.1) with the right-sided alternative now is given by $\bar{X} \geq [\mu_0 + t_{n-1,\alpha}(S/\sqrt{n})]$, where $t_{n-1,\alpha}$ is the $(1-\alpha)$th percentile of the Student's $t$-distribution with $(n-1)$ d.f. With the estimated mean $\bar{x}$ and variance $s^2 = \sum_1^n (x_i - \bar{x})^2/(n-1)$, the critical region for rejecting the null hypothesis is given by

$$\bar{x} \geq \left[\mu_0 + t_{n-1,\alpha}\left(s/\sqrt{n}\right)\right], \qquad (7.8)$$

that is,

$$t = \frac{\bar{x} - \mu_0}{s/\sqrt{n}} \geq t_{n-1,\alpha}. \qquad (7.8a)$$

Equivalently, $H_0$ is rejected if $\mu_0$ is smaller than the lower $(1-\alpha)$ percent confidence limit $[\bar{x} - t_{n-1,\alpha}(s/\sqrt{n})]$ for $\mu$. The $p$-value is obtained from $P[t_{n-1} \geq (\bar{x} - \mu_0)/(s/\sqrt{n})] = P(t_{n-1} \geq t)$.

*Example 7.2*   When $\alpha = 0.05$, $t_{15, 0.05} = 1.753$. Since the standard deviation for the sample of the 16 adults in Example 7.1 is $s = 25.04$, the estimate of the standard error becomes $(s/\sqrt{n}) = (25.04/4) = 6.26$. Now, $t = (116.99 - 100)/6.26 = 2.71$ which exceeds 1.753, and hence the null hypothesis is rejected at the 5 percent significance level. The Critical Region for the sample mean and the lower confidence limit for the population mean are

$$CR: [100 + 1.753(6.26)] = 110.97$$

and

$$C_l: [116.99 - 1.753(6.26)] = 106.02.$$

Table 7.2    Power of the $t$-test for the mean of the LDL with estimated variance: Right-sided alternative.

| $\mu_1$ | Power | $\mu_1$ | Power |
|---|---|---|---|
| 100 | 0.050 | 120 | 0.937 |
| 105 | 0.198 | 125 | 0.990 |
| 110 | 0.419 | 130 | 0.999 |
| 115 | 0.770 | | |

The sample mean exceeds 110.97, and $\mu_0$ is smaller than 106.02. Both these results lead to the rejection of the null hypothesis at the 5 percent significance level. The $p$-value becomes $P(t_{15} \geq 2.71) = 0.0008$, which is very small and suggests the rejection of the null hypothesis.

### 7.3.5    Power of the test with estimated variance

When $\mu = \mu_1$ under $H_1$, $t'_{n-1} = (\bar{X} - \mu_1)/(S/\sqrt{n})$ follows the *noncentral* $t$-distribution with $(n-1)$ d.f. and *noncentrality parameter* $\phi = (\mu_0 - \mu_1)/(\sigma/\sqrt{n})$. The power of the above test for specified values of the sample size, significance level and this parameter are available through some of the computer software programs. The power of the above test for $\mu_0 = 100$ with $\sigma = 24$ and $n = 16$ and the 5 percent significance level obtained from MINITAB is presented in Table 7.2 for increasing values of $\mu_1$.

   In practice, LDLs and similar measurements may not follow the normal distribution. In such cases, following the *Central Limit Theorem*, $H_0$ is rejected if $\bar{x}$ exceeds $[\mu_0 + z_\alpha(\sigma/\sqrt{n})]$ when $\sigma$ is known or if it exceeds $[\mu_0 + z_\alpha(s/\sqrt{n})]$ when it is estimated by $s$. If $n$ is large, the power of the test for the case of the non-normal distributions can be obtained from (7.5).

## 7.4    Left-sided alternative and the critical region

For the claim that the mean of the HDL of an adult population does not exceed 40 mg/dl, the null and alternative hypotheses are specified as in (7.1) with $\mu_0 = 40$ and $\mu_1 < 40$. When $\sigma$ isknown, for specified significance level $\alpha$, the critical region for rejecting the null hypothesis becomes $\bar{X} \leq [\mu_0 - z_\alpha(\sigma)/\sqrt{n}]$. With the observed sample mean, the null hypothesis is rejected if

$$\bar{x} \leq [\mu_0 - z_\alpha(\sigma/\sqrt{n})], \tag{7.9}$$

that is,

$$z = \frac{\bar{x} - \mu_0}{\sigma/\sqrt{n}} \leq -z_\alpha. \tag{7.9a}$$

Equivalently, the null hypothesis is rejected if $\mu_0$ exceeds the upper confidence limit $C_u = \bar{x} + z_\alpha(\sigma/\sqrt{n})$ for $\mu$.

## 7.4.1    The $p$-value

This probability is obtained from

$$P(\bar{X} \leq \bar{x} | \mu = \mu_0) = P\left(\frac{\bar{X} - \mu_0}{\sigma/\sqrt{n}} \leq \frac{\bar{x} - \mu_0}{\sigma/\sqrt{n}}\right) \tag{7.10}$$

$$= P(Z \leq z).$$

*Example 7.3*   For a random sample of $n = 16$ adults, the sample mean and standard deviation of the HDLs were found to be $\bar{x} = 38.14$ and $s = 5.6$. If the population standard deviation $\sigma$ is known to be 5.2, $S.E.(\bar{X}) = (5.2/4) = 1.3$ and $z = (38.14 - 40)/1.3 = -1.43$. Since it is larger than $-1.645$, the null hypothesis $H_0:$ $\mu = 40$ is not rejected at the 5 percent significance level. The Critical Region in (7.9) and the 95 percent upper confidence limit for the mean become

$$CR: 40 - (1.645)(1.3) = 37.862$$

and

$$C_u: 38.14 + 1.645(1.3) = 40.279.$$

The null hypothesis value of 40 for the mean exceeds the critical value 37.862 and it is smaller than the upper confidence limit 40.279. Both these results suggest not rejecting the null hypothesis at the 5 percent significance level. The $p$-value of the test is $P(Z < -1.43) = 0.076$.

## 7.4.2    Power of the test

The power of the test for the values of the mean lower than the null hypothesis value is given by

$$P\{\bar{X} \leq [\mu_0 - z_\alpha(\sigma)/\sqrt{n}] | \mu = \mu_1\}$$

$$= P\left[\frac{\bar{X} - \mu_1}{\sigma/\sqrt{n}} \leq \left(\frac{\mu_0 - \mu_1}{\sigma/\sqrt{n}} - z_\alpha\right)\right] \tag{7.11}$$

$$= P\left[Z \leq \left(\frac{\mu_0 - \mu_1}{\sigma/\sqrt{n}} - z_\alpha\right)\right].$$

The power of the test for values of the mean lower than the null hypothesis value of 40 are presented in Table 7.3 and Figure 7.3. The power increases as the mean $\mu_1$ becomes smaller than the mean $\mu_0$ under $H_0$.

Table 7.3    Power of the test for the mean of the HDL with the left-sided alternative when $\alpha = 0.05$.

| $\mu_1$ | $(\mu_0 - \mu_1)/1.3 - 1.645$ | Power |
|---|---|---|
| 40 | −1.645 | 0.050 |
| 39 | −0.876 | 0.191 |
| 38 | −0.107 | 0.457 |
| 37 | 0.663 | 0.746 |
| 36 | 1.432 | 0.924 |
| 35 | 2.201 | 0.986 |
| 34 | 2.970 | 0.999 |

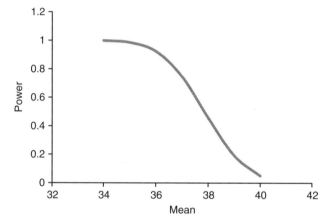

*Figure 7.3    Power of the test for the mean with the left-sided alternative when the standard deviation is known.*

### 7.4.3    Sample size for specified power

For the power of $(1-\beta)$, from (7.11), $[(\mu_0 - \mu_1)/(\sigma/\sqrt{n}) - z_\alpha] = z_\beta$. The required sample size becomes $n \geq (z_\beta + z_\alpha)^2/\delta^2$, which is the same as (7.7). From Example 7.3, for specified power of 90 percent at $\mu_1 = 37$ for the alternative value of the mean, $n \geq (1.282 + 1.645)^2/(3/5.2)^2 = 25.74$ or close to 26. From Table 7.3, the power at this alternative value for the mean is only 74.6 percent with the sample of size 16.

### 7.4.4    Left-sided alternative with estimated variance

With the estimates $(\bar{X}, S)$, the Critical Region for rejecting the above hypothesis becomes $\bar{X} \leq [\mu_0 - t_{n-1,\alpha}(S/\sqrt{n})]$. With the observed sample mean and standard deviation $(\bar{x}, s)$, it becomes

Table 7.4    Power for the t-test for the
mean of the HDL with the left-sided
alternative when $\alpha = 0.05$; estimated
variance.

| $\mu_1$ | Power |
|---|---|
| 40 | 0.050 |
| 39 | 0.181 |
| 38 | 0.430 |
| 37 | 0.711 |
| 36 | 0.901 |
| 35 | 0.978 |
| 35 | 0.978 |
| 34 | 0.997 |

$$\bar{x} \le \left[\mu_0 - t_{n-1,\alpha}\left(s/\sqrt{n}\right)\right], \tag{7.12}$$

that is,

$$t = \frac{\bar{x} - \mu_0}{s/\sqrt{n}} \le -t_{n-1,\alpha}. \tag{7.12a}$$

The null hypothesis is rejected if $\mu_0$ exceeds the $(1-\alpha)$ percent upper confidence limit $\left[\bar{x} + t_{n-1,\alpha}(s/\sqrt{n})\right]$ for $\mu$. The p-value for the test is obtained from $P(t_{n-1} \le t)$.

With the estimates of the mean and standard deviation in Example 7.3, $(s/\sqrt{n}) = 5.6/4 = 1.4$ and $t = (38.14 - 40)/1.4 = -1.329$, which is larger than $t_{15, 0.95} = -1.753$. As a result, the null hypothesis $H_0 : \mu = 40$ is not rejected at the 5 percent level of significance. The p-value for the test is $P(t_{15} \le -1.329) = 0.102$. At least a significance level of this amount is needed to reject the null hypothesis. The Power for the t-test with the estimated variance at different values of the mean obtained from the MINITAB are presented in Table 7.4.

## 7.5    Two-sided alternative, critical region and the p-value

To examine whether the mean of the LDLs has exceeded 100, the right-sided alternative was considered in Sections 7.3. Similarly, to examine whether the mean of the HDL has become lower than 40, the left-sided alternative was considered in Sections 7.4. To investigate whether the mean of the LDLs has changed from 100, the null and alternative hypotheses can be specified as (7.1) with $H_0 : \mu = 100$ and $H_1 : \mu \ne 100$. The significance level is now split into two equal halves ($\alpha/2$). If $\sigma$ is known, the critical region for rejecting $H_0$ becomes $|\bar{X} - \mu_0| > z_{\alpha/2}(\sigma/n)$. With the observed sample mean, the null hypothesis is rejected if

$$\bar{x} \geq \left[\mu_0 + z_{\alpha/2}\left(\sigma/\sqrt{n}\right)\right] \text{ or } \bar{x} \leq \left[\mu_0 - z_{\alpha/2}\left(\sigma/\sqrt{n}\right)\right], \tag{7.13}$$

that is,

$$|z| = \frac{|\bar{x} - \mu_0|}{\sigma/\sqrt{n}} \geq z_{\alpha/2}. \tag{7.13a}$$

The null hypothesis is rejected if $\mu_0$ falls outside the $(1-\alpha)$ percent confidence interval $\left[\bar{x} - z_{\alpha/2}(\sigma/\sqrt{n}), \bar{x} + z_{\alpha/2}(\sigma/\sqrt{n})\right]$ for $\mu$. The $p$-value for the test is obtained from $P(|Z| \geq z)$.

From Example 7.1, the null hypothesis $H_0 : \mu = 100$ *versus* $H_1 : \mu \neq 100$ is rejected at the 5 percent significance level since $z = 2.83$ exceeds $z_{0.025} = 1.96$. The $p$-value for the test is $P(Z \geq 2.83) + P(Z \leq -2.83) = 2(0.0023) = 0.0046$.

### 7.5.1   Power of the test

The power of the above test at the alternative value $\mu = \mu_1$ is given by $P = (P_1 + P_2)$, where

$$P_1 = P\left\{\bar{X} > \left[\mu_0 + z_{\alpha/2}\left(\sigma/\sqrt{n}\right)\right] | \mu = \mu_1\right\} = P\left(Z > \frac{\mu_0 - \mu_1}{\sigma/\sqrt{n}} + z_{\alpha/2}\right)$$

and

$$P_2 = P\left\{\bar{X} < \left[\mu_0 - z_{\alpha/2}\left(\sigma/\sqrt{n}\right)\right] | \mu = \mu_1\right\} = P\left(Z < \frac{\mu_0 - \mu_1}{\sigma/\sqrt{n}} - z_{\alpha/2}\right). \tag{7.14}$$

The power of the test for $\mu_1 \geq \mu_0$ at $\alpha = 0.05$ is presented in Table 7.5.

As can be seen from Table 7.5, $P_2$ is negligible. With the expressions in (7.14), the power for $\mu_1 < \mu_0$ becomes $P = (P_2 + P_1)$, and $P_1$ becomes negligible. For the values of

Table 7.5   Power of the test for the mean of the LDL with the two-sided alternative; $\mu_1 \geq \mu_0$.

| $\mu_1$ | $(\mu_0 - \mu_1)/(\sigma/\sqrt{n}) + 1.96$ | $P_1$ | $(\mu_0 - \mu_1)/(\sigma/\sqrt{n}) - 1.96$ | $P_2$ | Power $(P1 + P2)$ |
|---|---|---|---|---|---|
| 100 | 1.96 | 0.025 | −1.96 | 0.025 | 0.050 |
| 105 | 1.127 | 0.133 | −2.793 | 0.003 | 0.136 |
| 110 | 0.293 | 0.385 | −3.627 | 0 | 0.385 |
| 115 | −0.540 | 0.705 | −4.460 | 0 | 0.705 |
| 120 | −1.373 | 0.915 | −5.293 | 0 | 0.915 |
| 125 | −2.207 | 0.986 | −6.127 | 0 | 0.986 |
| 130 | −3.040 | 0.999 | −6.96 | 0 | 0.999 |

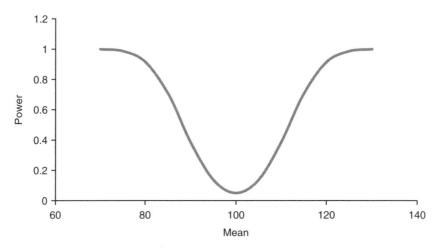

*Figure 7.4   Power for the test for the mean with the two-sided alternative.*

$\mu_1 = (100, 95, 90, 85, 80, 75, 70)$, the power for this case becomes the same as in the above table. For both the cases of $\mu_1 \geq \mu_0$ and $\mu_1 \geq \mu_0$, the power is presented in Figure 7.4.

## 7.5.2   Sample size for specified power

As seen above, $P_2$ in (7.14) is negligible for the power at the alternative value $\mu_1$ larger than $\mu_0$. With $P_1$ for the power, the required sample size becomes $n \geq \left(z_\beta + z_{\alpha/2}\right)^2 / \delta^2$. For the power of 90 percent at $\mu_1 = 115$, the required sample size becomes $n \geq (1.282 + 1.96)^2 / (15/24)^2 = 26.9$ or close to 27. The same sample size is required for the power of 90 percent at $\mu_1 = 85$. From Table 7.5, the power at $\mu_1 = 115$ or 85 is 70.5 percent with the sample of size 16.

## 7.5.3   Two-sided alternative and estimated variance

When the population variance is estimated, the Critical Region becomes $|\bar{X} - \mu_0| > t_{n-1,\alpha/2}(s/\sqrt{n})$.

With the estimated mean and standard deviation $(\bar{x}, s)$, the null hypothesis is rejected if

$$\bar{x} \geq \left[\mu_0 + t_{n-1,\alpha/2}\left(s/\sqrt{n}\right)\right] \quad \text{or} \quad \bar{x} \leq \left[\mu_0 - t_{n-1,\alpha/2}\left(s/\sqrt{n}\right)\right], \tag{7.15}$$

that is,

$$|t| = \frac{|\bar{x} - \mu_0|}{s/\sqrt{n}} \geq t_{n-1,\alpha/2}. \tag{7.15a}$$

Table 7.6   Power for the two-side
alternative for the mean of the LDL
with estimated variance.

| $\mu_1$ | Power |
|---|---|
| 100 | 0.050 |
| 105 | 0.122 |
| 110 | 0.345 |
| 115 | 0.647 |
| 120 | 0.876 |
| 125 | 0.973 |
| 130 | 0.997 |

The power for $\mu_1 = (95, 90, \dots, 70)$ are
the same as $(0.122, 0.345, \dots, 0.997)$.

Equivalently, the null hypothesis is rejected if $\mu_0$ falls outside the $(1 - \alpha)$ percent confidence limits $\left[\bar{x} - t_{n-1,\alpha/2}(s/\sqrt{n}), \bar{x} + t_{n-1,\alpha/2}(s/\sqrt{n})\right]$ for $\mu$.

From Example 7.2, $t = 2.71$, which exceeds $t_{15,\,0.025} = 2.49$. Hence the null hypothesis $H_0 : \mu = 100$ with the two-sided alternative is rejected at the 5 percent level of significance. The p-value for the test becomes $P(t_{15} > 2.71) + P(t_{15} < -2.71) = 2(0.008) = 0.016$, which is very small suggesting the rejection of the null hypothesis.

The power of the above test with the estimated standard deviation obtained from the MINITAB is presented in Table 7.6.

## 7.6   Difference between two means: Variances known

Several medical experiments are conducted to examine the differences of the effects of two or more treatments, for instance, on the adults of a selected group, or to compare the effect of a single treatment on two age groups. As in Section 5.5, consider the difference $\mu_d = (\mu_1 - \mu_2)$ of the means of two normal populations with variances $(\sigma_1^2, \sigma_2^2)$. To test the difference between the two means, the null and alternative hypotheses are specified as

$$H_0 = \mu_d = \mu_{d0}$$

and

$$H_1 : \mu_d = \mu_{d1}. \tag{7.16}$$

For the right-sided, left-sided and two-sided alternatives, $\mu_{d1} > \mu_{d0}, \mu_{d1} < \mu_{d0}$ and $\mu_{d1} \neq \mu_{d0}$ respectively.

As noted in Section 5.5, the difference $D = (\bar{X}_1 - \bar{X}_2)$ of the means of independent samples of sizes $(n_1, n_2)$ from the two groups is unbiased for $\mu_d$ with variance

$V(D) = \left(\sigma_1^2/n_1 + \sigma_2^2/n_2\right)$ and $S.E.(D) = \sqrt{V(D)}$. With the difference of the observed sample means $d = (\bar{x}_1 - \bar{x}_2)$, the test statistic for the above null hypothesis becomes

$$z = \frac{d - \mu_{d0}}{S.E.(D)}. \qquad (7.17)$$

For the specified significance level, the null hypothesis for the three cases of the alternative is rejected if $z > z_\alpha$, $z < -z_\alpha$ and $|z| \neq z_{\alpha/2}$ respectively. The $p$-values for these three cases are given by $P(Z \geq z)$, $P(Z \leq -z)$ and $[P(Z \geq z) + P(Z \leq -z)]$.

The power at $\mu_{d1}$ for the right-sided and left-sided alternatives is given by $P\{Z > [(\mu_{d0} - \mu_{d1})/S.E.(D) + z_\alpha]\}$ and $P\{Z < [(\mu_{d0} - \mu_{d1})/S.E.(D) - z_\alpha]\}$ respectively. For the two-sided alternative, it is given by

$$P\{Z > [(\mu_{d0} - \mu_{d1})/S.E.(D) + z_{\alpha/2}]\} + P\{Z < [(\mu_{d0} - \mu_{d1})/S.E.(D) - z_{\alpha/2}]\}.$$

To test the hypothesis that there is no difference between the means of the two groups, $\mu_{d0} = 0$ and $\mu_{d1}$ takes a specified value other than zero.

*Example 7.4*  Consider the sample in Examples 7.1 and 7.2 as that of the LDLs of an adult group with mean $\mu_1$ and standard deviation $\sigma_1 = 24$. The mean and standard deviation of the LDLs of a sample of size $n_1 = 16$ for this group were $\bar{x}_1 = 116.99$ and $s_1 = 25.04$. Consider a control group with mean $\mu_2$ and standard deviation of $\sigma_2 = 20$ for the LDLs, and the mean and standard deviation $(\bar{x}_2, s_2) = (104, 22)$ for a sample of size $n_2 = 20$. With the known standard deviations, $V(D) = [(484/16) + (400/20)] = 50.25$ and $S.E.(D) = 7.09$. The test statistic for the hypothesis of equality of the means of the two groups becomes $z = (116.99 - 104)/7.09 = 1.83$. Since $z_{0.05} = 1.645$, the null hypothesis $\mu_d = 0$ versus the alternative hypothesis $\mu_d > 0$ is rejected at the 5 percent level of significance. The $p$-value for the test is $P(Z \geq 1.83) = 0.0336$.

At the 5 percent significance level, the power of the above test at $(\mu_1 - \mu_2) = 5$ is $P\{Z \geq [(-5/7.09) + 1.645]\} = P(Z \geq 0.94) = 0.174$. The power at $(\mu_1 - \mu_2) = 10$ is

$$P[Z > (-10/7.09 + 1.645)] = P(Z > 0.2346) = 0.41.$$

## 7.6.1   Difference between two means: Variances estimated

When the variances of both the populations are the same, the common variance is estimated as in Section 5.5 from $s_p^2 = [(n_1 - 1)s_1^2 + (n_2 - 1)s_2^2]/(n_1 + n_2 - 2)$. The variance of the difference of the sample means is estimated from $v(d) = s_p^2(1/n_1 + 1/n_2)$ and S.E. $(d)$ is obtained from the square root of the estimated variance. The test statistic for the null hypothesis $H_0 : \mu_d = \mu_{d0}$ is given by

$$t = \frac{d - \mu_0}{S.E.(d)}. \qquad (7.18)$$

At the significance level $\alpha$, the null hypothesis is rejected if $t > t_{n1+n2-2, \alpha}$, $t < t_{n1+n2-2, \alpha}$ and $|t| > t_{n1+n2-2, \alpha/2}$ respectively for the three cases of the alternative hypothesis mentioned above. The $p$-value of the test for the right-sided and left-sided alternatives is obtained from $P(t_{n1+n2-2} > t)$ and $P(t_{n1+n2-2} < -t)$ respectively. For the two-sided alternative, it is obtained from $[P(t_{n1+n2-2} > t) + P(t_{n1+n2-2} < -t)]$. The power of the above test for alternative values of $\mu_d$ can be obtained from some of the software programs.

With the sample variances in Example 7.4, $s_p^2 = \left[15(25.04)^2 + 19(22)^2\right]/34 = 547.09$, $v(d) = 547.09(1/16 + 1/20) = 61.55$ and S.E.$(d) = 7.85$. The test statistic $t = [(116.99 - 104) - 0]/7.85 = 1.655$ does not exceed $t_{34, 0.05} = 2.3$. The null hypothesis that $\mu_d = 0$ versus the alternative $\mu_d > 0$ is not rejected at the 5 percent level of significance. The $p$-value of the test is $P(t_{34} > 1.655) = 0.0536$.

For the case of $\sigma_1^2 \neq \sigma_2^2$, $v(d) = [(25.04)^2/16 + (22)^2/20] = 63.38$ and S.E.$(d) = 7.96$. From Welch-Aspin approximation in Section 5.6.2, the statistic $t = d/$S.E.$(d)$ approximately follows the $t$-distribution with $f = 30.16$ or close to 30 d.f. The difference of the two means can be examined as above through the $t$-test with 30 d.f. For this illustration, $t = [(116.99 - 104) - 0]/7.96 = 1.63$ which does not differ much from the above value of $t = 1.655$ with 34 d.f. Cochran's (1964) approximation in Section 5.6.3 can also be employed to test the above null hypothesis of equality of the two means. The test for $H_0 : \mu_1 = \mu_2$ versus $H_1 : \mu_1 \neq \mu_2$ is known as the Beherens-Fisher test, Beherens (1964) and Fisher (1941). It can be examined through the above approximations.

## 7.7    Matched samples and paired comparison

As in Section 5.7, consider the measurements $(X, Y)$ before and after administering a treatment, with the means $(\mu_x, \mu_y)$ and their difference $\mu_d = (\mu_y - \mu_x)$. It is frequently of interest to test the hypothesis $H_0 : \mu_d = 0$. The alternative hypothesis can be one-sided or two-sided. From the paired sample observations $(x_i, y_i)$, $i = (1, 2, \ldots, n)$, the test statistic for this hypothesis is given by $t_{n-1} = (\bar{d} - \mu_d)/(s_d/\sqrt{n})$.

For the DBPs in Example 5.5, $H_0 : \mu_d = 0$ versus $H_1 : \mu_d < 0$ can be considered. From the sample means (100, 85) of the sixteen units, $\bar{d} = -15$ and $s_d = 13.23$. The test statistic becomes, $t_{15} = (-15 - 0)/(13.23/4) = -4.54$ with the p-value of 0.0004. The null hypothesis that the treatment does not decrease the DBP can be rejected.

## 7.8    Test for the variance

The null and alternative hypotheses for the variance of a normal distribution can be specified as

$$H_0 : \sigma^2 = \sigma_0^2$$

and

$$H_1 : \sigma^2 = \sigma_1^2 \tag{7.19}$$

For the right-sided, left-sided and two-sided alternatives, $\sigma_1^2 > \sigma_0^2, \sigma_1^2 < \sigma_0^2$ and $\sigma_1^2 \neq \sigma_0^2$ respectively.

With the variance $S^2$ of a sample of size $n$, the test statistic is

$$U = (n-1)S^2/\sigma_0^2$$

which follows $\chi_{n-1}^2$, the Chisquare distribution with $(n-1)$ d.f. When the alternative hypothesis is right-sided, with the observed value $S^2$ of the sample variance, the Critical Region for rejecting the null hypothesis at the significance level $\alpha$ becomes

$$u = \frac{(n-1)s^2}{\sigma_0^2} \geq \chi_{n-1,\alpha}^2. \tag{7.20}$$

This decision is the same as rejecting the null hypothesis if $\sigma_0^2$ is smaller than the lower $(1-\alpha)$ percent confidence limit for $\sigma^2$. Similarly, when the alternative is left-sided, the null hypothesis is rejected if $u \leq \chi_{n-1,\alpha/2}^2$. For the two-sided alternative, the Critical Region for rejecting the null hypothesis is given by $u \geq \chi_{n-1,\alpha/2}^2$ or $u \leq \chi_{n-1,1-(\alpha/2)}^2$.

The $p$-value of the test for the right-sided and left-sided alternative hypotheses are given by $P(\chi_{n-1}^2 \geq u)$ and $P(\chi_{n-1}^2 \leq u)$ respectively. For the two-sided alternative, it is obtained from $2P(\chi_{n-1}^2 \geq u)$.

As an illustration, in Example 7.1 the standard deviation of the LDLs was assumed to be 24, and the standard deviation of the 16 sample units was 25.04. For this case, consider $H_0 : \sigma^2 = (24)^2 = 576$ and $H_1 : \sigma^2 > 576$. The test statistic $u = 15(25.04)^2/576 = 16.33$ does not exceed $\chi_{15,0.05}^2 = 25.0$, and hence the null hypothesis is not rejected at the 5 percent significance level. The $p$-value of the test is $P(\chi_{15}^2 \geq 16.33) = 0.36$, which is large.

## 7.9    Test for the equality of two variances

For the variances of two normal populations, consider the null and alternative hypotheses

$$H_0 : \sigma_1^2 = \sigma_2^2 \tag{7.21}$$

and

$$H_1 : \sigma_1^2 > \sigma_2^2. \tag{7.22}$$

With the variances $(S_1^2, S_2^2)$ of independent samples of sizes $(n_1, n_2)$, the ratio $(S_1^2/\sigma_1^2)/(S_2^2/\sigma_2^2)$ follows $F n_1 - 1, n_2 - 1$, the $F$-distribution with $(n_1 - 1, n_2 - 1)$ d.

f. With the observed sample variances $\left(s_1^2, s_2^2\right)$, the Critical Region for rejecting the null hypothesis at the significance level of $\alpha$ is given by

$$F = \left(s_1^2/s_2^2\right) \geq F_{(n_1-1,\, n_2-1),\,\alpha}. \tag{7.23}$$

If the alternative hypothesis is $H_1 : \sigma_1^2 < \sigma_2^2$, the null hypothesis is rejected if $F < F_{(n_1-1,\, n_2-1),(1-\alpha)}$.

For the case of the two-sided alternative $H_1 : \sigma_1^2 \neq \sigma_2^2$, the null hypothesis is rejected if $F > F_{(n_1-1,\, n_2-1),\,\alpha/2}$ or $F < F_{(n_1-1,\, n_2-1),(1-\alpha/2)}$.

As an example consider the null hypothesis that the variances of the weights of the 16-year-old boys (1) and girls (2) are the same. From Tables T1.3 and T1.4, the variances of the weights of boys and girls for samples of size 20 each are $(9.34)^2 = 87.24$ and $(12.04)^2 = 144.96$. In this case, $F = \left(s_2^2/s_1^2\right) = (144.96/87.24) = 1.66$ which is smaller than $F_{(19,\, 19),\, 0.025} = 2.53$. The null hypothesis that the variances of the weights are the same is not rejected at the 5 percent significance level. The $p$-value is $2(0.139) = 0.278$.

## 7.10    Homogeneity of variances

For the equality of the variances of $k \geq 2$ groups, the null hypothesis is specified as

$$H_0 : \sigma_1^2 = \sigma_2^2 = \cdots = \sigma_k^2, \tag{7.24}$$

with the alternative hypothesis that at least two of the variances are not the same. Consider the variances $s_i^2$, $i = (1, 2, \ldots, k)$, obtained from independent samples of sizes $n_i$ from the $k$ groups, with the total sample size of $n = \sum_1^k n_i$. The test statistic for this hypothesis obtained by Bartlett (1937) from the Likelihood Ratio procedure is given by

$$u = \left(f \ln s_p^2 - \sum f_i \ln s_i^2\right) \bigg/ \left\{1 + \left[\sum(1/f_i) - (1/f)\right]/3(k-1)\right\}. \tag{7.25}$$

In this expression, $f_i = (n_i - 1)$ are the degrees of freedom of the variance from the $k$th group, $f = \Sigma f_i = (n - k)$ and $s_p^2 = \sum f_i s_i^2/f$ is the pooled variance with $(n - k)$ degrees of freedom; logarithm with base $\mathbf{e}$ is denoted by $\mathbf{ln}$. The null hypothesis is rejected at the significance level of $\alpha$ if this statistic exceeds $\chi_{k-1,\alpha}^2$.

As an illustration, for samples of 20 each, the standard deviations of the weights of the $(10, 16, 20)$ year-old boys from Tables (T1.1, T1.3) and Table 1.2 are $(3.00, 9.34, 13.71)$. From these figures, $s_p^2 = 94.733$, $\ln s_p^2 = 4.551$, $\sum f_i \ln s_i^2 = 19(11.902) = 226.138$.

From (7.25), $u = (33.26/1.0234) = 32.50$, which is much larger than $\chi^2_{2,0.05} = 5.99$. The null hypothesis of the equality of the variances of the weights of the three groups is rejected at the 5 percent significance level. The $p$-value for the test is very small.

# Exercises

**7.1.** The standard deviation of the LDLs of a group of adults is known to be 25 mg/dl, and it was of interest to examine whether the mean has exceeded 100 mg/dl. The mean and standard deviation of the LDLs for a sample of 25 adults were found to be 108 mg/dl and 30 mg/dl. (a) Formulate the null and alternative hypotheses, test the null hypothesis at the 5 percent level of significance, and find the $p$-value of the test. (b) Find the power of the test at the alternative value of 110 mg/dl for the mean. (c) Find the sample size required for the test at the 5 percent significance level and the power of 95 percent. (d) Test the null hypothesis with the estimated standard deviation and find the p-value of the test.

**7.2.** It is of interest to examine whether the average HDL of a group of adults has decreased from 45 mg/dl. For a sample of 25 adults, the mean and standard deviation of the HDL were 35 and 30. The actual standard deviation was assumed to be 25. Formulate the null and alternative hypotheses. (a) Test the null hypothesis at the 5 percent level of significance, and find the $p$-value for the test. (b) Find the power of the test at the alternative value of 35 for the HDL. (c) Find the sample size required for the power of 95 percent at the alternative value of 35. (d) Test the null hypothesis with the estimated standard deviation and find the $p$-value of the test.

**7.3.** It is of interest to examine whether the LDL of a group of adults has changed from 100 mg/dl. For a sample of $n = 25$ adults, the mean and standard deviation of the LDL was found to be 110 and 40. The actual standard deviation was known to be 35. Formulate the null and alternative hypotheses. (a) Test the null hypothesis at the 5 percent level of significance and find the $p$-value of the test. (b) Find the power at the alternative value of 105 for the mean. (c) Find the sample size required for the power of 20 percent at that alternative value. (d) Test the null hypothesis with the estimated standard deviation and find the $p$-value of the test.

**7.4.** Sachs et al. (2009) randomly assigned 811 overweight adults to one of four diets consisting of high and low combinations of fat and protein. For 80 percent of the completing participants, the average weight loss was 4 kg; 14 to 15 percent lost at least 10 percent of their initial weight. For the 204 and 201 participants receiving the low-fat-average protein and high fat–high protein diets respectively, the means and standard deviations (in parentheses) for the cholesterol and blood pressure levels were as follows. Total cholesterol: 192 (37) and 202 (13). SBP: 117 (12) and 120 (14). DBP: 74 (9) and 76 (9). Test the difference of the means of the two diets for the cholesterol and blood pressure levels.

**7.5.** Test for the differences of the population means of the heights, weights and BMIs of the 16-*year*-old boys and girls from the sample observations. The sample observations along with the means and standard deviations are presented in Tables T1.3 and T1.4.

**7.6.** In Example 7.3, the standard deviation $\sigma$ of the HDLs was assumed to be 5.2, and for the sample of $n = 16$ units $s = 5.6$. Test the hypothesis $H_0 : \sigma^2 = (5.2)^2 = 27.04$ *versus* $H_1 : \sigma^2 > 27.04$.

**7.7.** From Tables (T1.1, T1.3) and Table 1.2, the standard deviations of the heights of the (10, 16, 20) year-old boys from samples of size 20 are (5.12, 7.67, 7.16). The standard deviations for the BMIs are (1.76, 2.09, 2.56). Test the equality of the population variances for both the (a) heights and (b) BMIs.

**7.8.** As presented in Exercise 5.9 for the *celiac* disease, the mean and standard deviation of maximum enhancement of the duodenal wall for the 45 patients treated with *gluten-free* diet were (109.8, 27.8). Test the null hypothesis that the population mean for these patients is same as the mean of 94.7 for the control group *versus* it exceeds this value.

# 8

# Tests of hypotheses: Proportions and percentages

## 8.1 A single proportion

Proportions, percentages and probabilities of changes for men and women resulting from medical treatments or diet and exercise programs are of importance in clinical studies. Similarly, the percentages of children benefiting from or adversely affected by vaccination programs are of major interest. The formulation of the null and alternative hypothesis and the significance tests for proportions and percentages are similar to the procedures described in Chapter 7 for the means and variances. The null hypothesis is always *simple*. The alternative, the research hypothesis, can be simple or *composite*; right-sided or left-sided; it can also be simple.

## 8.2 Right-sided alternative

Consider the suggestion that the HDLs will be in the (40–60) range for at least 30 percent of a large group of adults participating in a treatment program. The null and alternative hypotheses for this percentage or proportion $p$ can be formulated as

$$H_0 : p = p_0$$

and

$$H_0 : p > p_0, \tag{8.1}$$

where $p_0 = 0.3$.

*Statistical Methodologies with Medical Applications*, First Edition. Poduri S.R.S. Rao.
© 2017 John Wiley & Sons, Ltd. Published 2017 by John Wiley & Sons, Ltd.

As a decision rule, $H_0$ may be rejected if the HDLs fall in that range for 10 or more adults in a random sample of size $n = 20$ receiving the treatment. If $H_0$ is true, the number of adults with the HDLs falling in that range can be considered to be the number of successes $X$ of the binomial distribution with probability $p_0 = 0.3$ and $n = 20$ trials. From this distribution $P(X \geq 10|n = 20, p_0 = 0.3) = 0.048$.

For large n, under the null hypothesis, $X$ follows the normal distribution approximately with mean $\mu = np_0$ and standard deviation $\sigma = \sqrt{np_0q_0}$, where $q_0 = (1 - p_0)$. In this case, the sample proportion $(X/n)$ approximately follows the normal distribution with mean $p_0$ and standard deviation $\sqrt{p_0q_0/n}$. The standardized variable

$$Z = (X - np_0)/\sqrt{np_0q_0} = [(X/n) - p_0]/\sqrt{(p_0q_0/n)} \tag{8.2}$$

follows the normal distribution with zero mean and unit standard deviation. For the above illustration, under the null hypothesis, the mean and standard deviation of $X$ are $np_0 = 20(0.3) = 6$ and $\sqrt{np_0q_0} = [20(0.3)(0.7)]^{1/2} = 2.0494$. For the sample proportion $(X/n)$, they are $p_0 = 0.3$ and $\sqrt{p_0q_0/n} = 0.1025$ respectively. From the above approximation, with the continuity correction for the discrete random variable $X$, $P(X \geq 10)$ becomes

$$P[X \geq (10 - 0.5) = P[Z \geq (9.5 - 6)/2.0494] = P(Z \geq 1.71) = 0.0436.$$

The above decision rule has resulted in a chance of almost 5 percent of rejecting the null hypothesis when it is true. This probability will decrease if $X$ is increased to 11 or more.

## 8.2.1   Critical region

In general, inference regarding the above type of hypothesis is made from the number of outcomes or successes $X$ in a random sample of size $n$. For the above illustration, $X$ is the number of adults with their HDLs falling in the $(40–60)$ range. For a specified significance level $\alpha$, for instance 0.05 or 0.01, the critical value of $X$ for rejecting the null hypothesis is obtained from the binomial distribution. From the normal approximation, $H_0$ is rejected if $Z$ in (8.2) exceeds $z_\alpha$. With the observed value $x$ of the random variable $X$, the Critical Region for rejecting $H_0$ is given by

$$x \geq \left(np_0 + z_\alpha \sqrt{np_0q_0}\right), \tag{8.3}$$

that is,

$$z = \frac{x - np_0}{\sqrt{np_0q_0}} = \frac{\hat{p} - p_0}{\sqrt{p_0q_0/n}} \geq z_\alpha, \tag{8.3a}$$

where $\hat{p} = (x/n)$ is the estimate of the proportion of the successes or outcomes. Equivalently, $H_0$ is rejected if $p_0$ is smaller than the $(1 - \alpha)$ percent lower confidence limit $C_l = \left(\hat{p} - z_\alpha \sqrt{p_0q_0/n}\right)$ for p.

With the continuity correction, $x$ and $\hat{p}$ in the above expressions and for the confidence limit are replaced by $(x - 1/2)$ and $(\hat{p} - 1/2n)$. Since the discrete binomial variable is approximated by the normal variable, as described by Snedecor and Cochran (1967, Sec. 8.6), the *continuity correction* is applied for finding the critical region and the confidence limits. Similar corrections are applied in the following sections for the left-sided and two-sided hypotheses.

## 8.2.2    The $p$-value

When $H_0$ is true, the $p$-value, which is the probability of observing a value $x$ or a larger value for the number of successes $X$ in a sample of size $n$, is given by

$$P = P(X \geq x | n, p_0). \tag{8.4}$$

With the normal approximation, this probability is obtained from $P(Z \geq z)$, where $z = (\hat{p} - p_0) / \sqrt{p_0 q_0 / n}$ as above. With the continuity correction, $\hat{p}$ is replaced by $(\hat{p} - 1/2n)$.

## 8.2.3    Power of the test

For a specified significance level $\alpha$, the probability of rejecting $H_0$ at $p = p_1 > p_0$ is given by the probability of $X$ exceeding the critical value, which is obtained from the binomial distribution with $n$ trials and probability of success $p_1$. With the normal approximation, this probability becomes

$$P\left[X \geq \left(np_0 + z_\alpha \sqrt{np_0 q_0} | n, p_1\right)\right]$$

$$= P\left\{\frac{X - np_1}{\sqrt{np_1 q_1}} \geq \left[\frac{n(p_0 - p_1)}{\sqrt{np_1 q_1}} + z_\alpha \frac{\sqrt{np_0 q_0}}{\sqrt{np_1 q_1}}\right]\right\}$$

$$= P\left[Z \geq \left(\frac{p_0 - p_1}{\sqrt{p_1 q_1 / n}} + z_\alpha \frac{\sqrt{p_0 q_0}}{\sqrt{p_1 q_1}}\right)\right], \tag{8.5}$$

where $q_1 = (1 - p_1)$.

## 8.2.4    Sample size for specified power

For the significance level $\alpha$, if the power of the test at the alternate value $p_1$ for the proportion is specified to be $(1 - \beta)$, from (8.5),

$$z_{1-\beta} = \frac{p_0 - p_1}{\sqrt{p_1 q_1 / n}} + z_\alpha \frac{\sqrt{p_0 q_0}}{\sqrt{p_1 q_1}}. \tag{8.6}$$

From this expression, the required sample size becomes

$$n \geq \left(z_{1-\beta} \sqrt{p_1 q_1} - z_\alpha \sqrt{p_0 q_0}\right)^2 / (p_0 - p_1)^2. \tag{8.7}$$

*Example 8.1*    Consider the above null hypothesis $H_0 : p = 0.3$ *versus* $H_1 : p > 0.3$ for the HDLs, and the significance level of 5 percent. If the HDLs of $x = 8$ adults in a sample of 20 were found to be in the above (40–60) range, from (8.3a), with the continuity correction for $x$, $z = (7.5 - 6)/(2.0494) = (0.375 - 0.30)/(0.1025) = 0.73$. Since this value for the test statistic is smaller than $z_{0.05} = 1.645$, the null hypothesis that $p_0 = 0.3$ is not rejected at the 5 percent significance level.

With the continuity correction, the lower 95 percent confidence limit for $p$ is $[0.375 - 1.645(0.1025)] = 0.21$. The null hypothesis value of 0.3 is not smaller than this limit and it results in the same conclusion as above.

From (8.4), the *p*-value for the test statistic is $P[Z \geq (7.5 - 6)/2.0494] = 0.23$, which is not very small and supports the above conclusion.

From (8.5), the power of the test at the alternative value of $p = 0.5$, for instance, becomes $P\{Z \geq [(- 0.2/0.1118) + 1.645(0.9165)]\} = P(Z \geq - 0.28) = 0.61$.

If it is required that with $\alpha = 0.05$ the power at $p = 0.5$ should be at least 0.80, $z_\alpha = 0.05$ and $z_{1-\beta} = -0.85$, and from (8.7) $n \geq [-0.85(0.5) - 1.645(0.4583)]^2 / 0.04 = 34.75$. At least, a sample of size 35 is needed.

## 8.3    Left-sided alternative

If the HDLs of at most 60 percent of the adults are considered to be in the (40–60) range, the null and alternative hypotheses are formulated as

$$H_0 : p = p_0$$

and

$$H_1 : p < p_0, \tag{8.8}$$

where $P_0 = 0.6$.

### 8.3.1    Critical region

For specified significance level $\alpha$, the critical value of the number of adults $X$ for rejecting the above null hypothesis is found from the binomial distribution. With the normality assumption for $X$ and its observed value $x$, the critical region becomes

$$x \leq \left( np_0 - z_\alpha \sqrt{np_0 q_0} \right), \tag{8.9}$$

that is,

$$z = \frac{x - np_0}{\sqrt{np_0 q_0}} = \frac{\hat{p} - p_0}{\sqrt{p_0 q_0/n}} \le -z_\alpha. \tag{8.9a}$$

This decision for rejecting the null hypothesis is the same as rejecting it if $p_0$ exceeds the upper $(1-\alpha)$ percent confidence limit $C_u = \hat{p} + z_\alpha \sqrt{p_0 q_0/n}$ for $p$. With the continuity correction, $x$ and $\hat{p}$ in these expressions are replaced by $(x + 1/2)$ and $(\hat{p} + 1/2n)$.

## 8.3.2   The $p$-value

When $H_0$ is true, the probability of observing a value $x$ or a smaller value for the outcomes $X$ in a sample of size $n$ is

$$P = P(X \le x | n, p_0). \tag{8.10}$$

With the normal approximation, this probability is given by $P(Z \le z)$, where $z(\hat{p} - p_0)/\sqrt{p_0 q_0/n}$ as before. With the continuity correction, $\hat{p}$ is replaced by $\hat{p} + 1/2n$.

## 8.3.3   Power of the test

The probability of rejecting $H_0$ at $p = p_1 < p_0$ is given by the probability of $X$ becoming smaller than the critical value for the specified significance level, which is obtained from the binomial distribution with n trials and probability of success $p_1$. With the normal approximation, this probability becomes

$$P\left[X \le \left(np_0 - z_\alpha \sqrt{np_0 q_0}\right) | n, p_1\right]$$
$$= P\left[Z \le \left(\frac{p_0 - p_1}{\sqrt{p_1 q_1/n}} - z_\alpha \frac{\sqrt{p_0 q_0}}{\sqrt{p_1 q_1}}\right)\right]. \tag{8.11}$$

## 8.3.4   Sample size for specified power

For the significance level $\alpha$, if the power of the test at the alternate value $p_1$ for the proportion is specified to be $(1-\beta)$, from (8.11),

$$z_{1-\beta} = \frac{p_0 - p_1}{\sqrt{p_1 q_1/n}} - z_\alpha \frac{\sqrt{p_0 q_0}}{\sqrt{p_1 q_1}}. \tag{8.12}$$

From this expression, the required sample size becomes

$$n \ge \left(z_{1-\beta} \sqrt{p_1 q_1} - z_\alpha \sqrt{p_0 q_0}\right)^2 / (p_0 - p_1)^2. \tag{8.13}$$

*Example 8.2*    Consider the left-sided hypothesis in (8.8) with $p_0 = 0.6$, with the 5 percent significance level. If the HDLs of $x = 7$ adults were found to be in the (40–60) range in a sample of $n = 20$ adults, with the normal approximation, $z = (7.5 - 12)/\sqrt{20(0.24)} = -2.05$. This value for the test statistic is smaller than $-z_{0.05} = -1.645$ and leads to the rejection of the null hypothesis at the 5 percent significance level.

With $\hat{p} = (7/20) = 0.35$ and the continuity correction, the upper 95 percent confidence level for p becomes $C_u = [(0.35 + 0.025) + 1.645(0.1095)] = 0.555$. The null hypothesis value of 0.6 for the proportion is clearly larger than this upper limit.

With the normal approximation and the continuity correction, from (8.10), the p-value is $P\{Z \leq (7.5 - 12)/[20(0.24)]^{1/2}\} = P(Z \leq -2.05) = 0.0202$.

With the significance level of $\alpha = 0.05$, from (8.11), the power of the test at the alternative value of $p_1 = 0.4$, for instance, becomes $P(Z \leq 0.18) = 0.571$.

For the power of 80 percent, $z_{1-\beta} = -0.85$. For the 5 percent significance level, and this value for the power at $p_1 = 0.4$, from (8.13), the required sample size becomes $n \geq \left[-0.85\sqrt{(0.4)(0.6)} - 1.645\sqrt{(0.6)(0.4)}\right]^2/(0.04) = 37.35$. A sample of at least 38 adults is required.

## 8.4    Two-sided alternative

If the HDLs for 50 percent of the adults are suspected to have changed from the (40–60) range, the null and alternative hypothesis can be formulated as

$$H_0 : p = p_0$$

and

$$H_1 : p \neq p_0, \tag{8.14}$$

where $p_0 = 0.50$.

The nature of the problem under investigation suggests whether the alternative hypothesis should be one-sided or two-sided. For instance, from the responses of a small sample of medical students, Colton et al. (1968) examined whether caffeine intake prevents noncaffeine drinkers from falling asleep. The null hypothesis in this case was that there is a 50 percent chance that it prevents sleep, that is, $H_0 : p = 0.5$. The alternative hypothesis may be specified as $H_1 : p > 0.5$ or as $H_1 : p \neq 0.5$.

### 8.4.1    Critical region

The specified significance level $\alpha$ is divided into two equal parts, $\alpha/2$ each for $p > p_0$ and $p < p_0$, and the critical values of $X$ for rejecting the null hypothesis can be found from the binomial distribution. With the normality assumption for X and its observed value $x$, the critical region becomes

$$x \geq \left( np_0 + z_{\alpha/2} \sqrt{np_0 q_0} \right) \tag{8.15a}$$

or

$$x \leq \left( np_0 - z_{\alpha/2} \sqrt{np_0 q_0} \right). \tag{8.15b}$$

With the continuity correction, $x$ in (8.15a) and (8.15b) are replaced by $(x - 1/2)$ and $(x + 1/2)$ respectively. With this correction, the null hypothesis is rejected if

$$z = \frac{(\hat{p} - 1/2n) - p_0}{\sqrt{p_0 q_0 / n}} \geq z_{\alpha/2} \tag{8.16a}$$

or

$$z = \frac{(\hat{p} + 1/2n) - p_0}{\sqrt{p_0 q_0 / n}} \leq -z_{\alpha/2}. \tag{8.16b}$$

This decision for rejecting the null hypothesis is the same as rejecting it (a) if $p_0$ becomes smaller than the lower $(1 - \alpha)$ percent confidence limit $C_l = (\hat{p} - 1/2n) - z_{\alpha/2} \sqrt{p_0 q_0 / n}$ or (b) if it exceeds the upper $(1 - \alpha)$ percent confidence limit $C_u = (\hat{p} + 1/2n) + z_{\alpha/2} \sqrt{p_0 q_0 / n}$.

### 8.4.2    The $p$-value

When $H_0$ is true, the probability of observing a value $x$ larger or smaller for the outcome $X$ in a sample of size $n$ is

$$P = P(X \geq x | n, p_0) + P(X \leq x | n, p_0) \tag{8.17}$$

With the normality approximation, this probability is given by

$$P(Z \geq z) + P(Z \leq -z), \tag{8.18}$$

where $z = (\hat{p} - p_0) / \sqrt{p_0 q_0 / n}$ as before. With the continuity correction, $\hat{p}$ is replaced by $(\hat{p} - 1/2n)$ and $(\hat{p} + 1/2n)$ in the first and second expressions respectively. Snedecor and Cochran (1967, pp. 209–213) describe and illustrate the application of the continuity correction for the normal approximation to the discrete binomial variable.

### 8.4.3    Power of the test

The probability of rejecting $H_0$ at $p = p_1 \neq p_0$ is given by the probability of $X$ becoming larger or smaller than the critical values for the specified significance level, which can be obtained from the binomial distribution with $n$ trials and probability of success $p_1$. With the normal approximation, this probability becomes

$$P\{X \geq [np_0 + z_{\alpha/2}\sqrt{np_0q_0}] \mid n, p_1\} + P\{X \leq [np_0 - z_{\alpha/2}\sqrt{np_0q_0}] \mid n, p_1\}$$

$$= P\left[\hat{p} \geq \left(p_0 + z_{\alpha/2}\sqrt{p_0q_0/n}\right) \mid n, p_1\right] + P\left[\hat{p} \leq \left(p_0 - z_{\alpha/2}\sqrt{p_0q_0/n}\right) \mid n, p_1\right]$$

$$= P\left[Z \geq \left(\frac{p_0 - p_1}{\sqrt{p_1q_1/n}} + z_{\alpha/2}\sqrt{\frac{p_0q_0}{p_1q_1}}\right)\right] + P\left[Z \leq \left(\frac{p_0 - p_1}{\sqrt{p_1q_1/n}} - z_{\alpha/2}\sqrt{\frac{p_0q_0}{p_1q_1}}\right)\right].$$
$$(8.19)$$

### 8.4.4   Sample size for specified power

The probability in the second expression on the right-hand side of (8.19) becomes small when $p_1$ is larger than $p_0$, and large when it is smaller than $p_0$. In the first case, the sample size for specified significance level $\alpha$ and the power of $(1-\beta)$ at the alternate value $p_1$ for the proportion is obtained from

$$\left(\frac{p_0 - p_1}{\sqrt{p_1q_1/n}} + z_{\alpha/2}\sqrt{\frac{p_0q_0}{p_1q_1}}\right) = z_{1-\beta}.$$
$$(8.20)$$

As a result, the solution to the required sample size is obtained from

$$n \geq \left(z_{1-\beta}\sqrt{p_1q_1} - z_{\alpha/2}\sqrt{p_0q_0}\right)^2 / (p_0 - p_1)^2.$$
$$(8.21)$$

In the second case,

$$\left(\frac{p_0 - p_1}{\sqrt{p_1q_1/n}} - z_{\alpha/2}\sqrt{\frac{p_0q_0}{p_1q_1}}\right) = z_\beta.$$
$$(8.22)$$

The required sample size is obtained from the same expression in (8.21).

*Example 8.3*   For the above two-sided hypothesis of the HDLs, consider the null hypothesis value $p_0 = 0.5$ with the 5 percent significance level and sample size $n = 20$. From the normal approximation, the critical values become (1) $x \geq [9.5 + 1.96\sqrt{20(0.5)(0.5)}] = 13.883$   or   (2)   $x \leq [10.5 - 1.96\sqrt{20(0.5)(0.5)}] = 6.117$, that is, $\hat{p} \geq 0.694$ or $\hat{p} \leq 0.306$.

If the observed value is $x = 13$, $\hat{p} = 0.65$ and the null hypothesis is not rejected. In this case, from (8.16a), $z = 1.118$ which is smaller than $z_{0.025} = 1.96$ and the same conclusion is drawn.

When $x = 13$, the upper and lower 95 percent confidence limits for p are $C_u = (0.65 + 0.025) + 1.96\sqrt{(0.5)(0.5)/20} = 0.6753$   and   $C_l = (0.65 - 0.025) - 1.96\sqrt{(0.5)(0.5)/20} = 0.4059$. The null hypothesis value of $p_0 = 0.50$ is smaller than the upper limit, and hence it is not rejected.

From (8.18), $P(Z \geq 1.118) = 0.13$ and hence the $p$-value for the test becomes $2(0.13) = 0.26$. From (8.19), the power at $p_1 = 0.80$ becomes $P(Z \geq -0.90) + P(Z \leq -5.8) = 0.8159$.

For the 5 percent significance level and the power of 90 percent at $p_1 = 0.80$, from (8.21), the required sample size becomes $n \geq [-1.29(0.4) - 1.96(0.5)]^2 / (0.09) = 24.9$, or close to 25.

## 8.5   Difference of two proportions

Consider the following statements : (1) The proportion of the adults with increased HDLs resulting from a medical treatment is higher for the (40–60) age group than for the older adults, (2) Exercise reduces the hypertension to a smaller proportion of the older adults than the younger ones, and (3) The proportions of the adults with weight reduction is not the same for men and women in certain age groups.

Denoting the above type of proportions for the two groups by $p_1$ and $p_2$, the null hypothesis for each of these situations is $H_0 : p_1 = p_2$. The alternative right - sided, left-sided and two-sided research hypotheses $H_1$ are formulated as $p_1 > p_2, p_1 < p_2$ and $p_1 \neq p_2$ respectively. The significance tests for these three cases are described in the following sections.

### 8.5.1   Right-sided alternative: Critical region and $p$-value

For this case, as described above, the null and alternative hypothesis are

$$H_0 : p_1 = p_2$$

and

$$H_1 : p_1 > p_2. \tag{8.23}$$

Consider a medical treatment for increasing the HDL administered to independent random samples of sizes $(n_1, n_2)$ from two groups of adults. Denote by $(X_1, X_2)$ the numbers of adults in the two samples with increased HDLs. The estimators $(X_1/n_1)$, $(X_2/n_2)$ and $[(X_1/n_1) - (X_2/n_2)]$ are respectively unbiased for the proportions $(p_1, p_2)$ with increased HDLs and the difference $(p_1 - p_2)$ of the proportions. Their variances are $p_1 q_1/n_1$, $p_2 q_2/n_2$ and $(p_1 q_1/n_1 + p_2 q_2/n_2)$ respectively, where $q_1 = (1-p_1)$ and $q_2 = (1-p_2)$.

When the null hypothesis in (8.21) is valid, $p_1$ and $p_2$ take the common value p, and the variance of $(X_1/n_1)-(X_2/n_2)$ becomes $pq(1/n_1 + 1/n_2)$, where $q = (1-p)$. From this result,

$$Z = \frac{(X_1/n_1 - X_2/n_2) - 0}{[pq(1/n_1 + 1/n_2)]^{1/2}} \tag{8.24}$$

follows the standard normal distribution for large $(n_1, n_2)$. At the specified significance level $\alpha$, the null hypothesis is rejected if $Z \geq z_\alpha$. With the observed values $(x_1, x_2)$ of the outcomes, estimates of the two proportions and their common value are obtained from $\hat{p}_1 = x_1/n_1$, $\hat{p}_2 = x_2/n_2$ and $\hat{p} = (x_1 + x_2)/(n_1 + n_2) = [(n_1/n)\hat{p}_1 + (n_2/n)\hat{p}_2]$, where $n = (n_1 + n_2)$ is the total sample size. The Critical Region for rejecting the null hypothesis becomes

$$z = \frac{(\hat{p}_1 - \hat{p}_2) - 0}{[\hat{p}\hat{q}(1/n_1 + 1/n_2)]^{1/2}} \geq z_\alpha. \tag{8.25}$$

The $p$-value of the test is the probability of observing $[(X_1/n_1)-(X_2/n_2)]$ as large or larger than $(\hat{p}_1 - \hat{p}_2)$ when $p_1 = p_2$ and it is given by

$$P = P\left[\frac{X_1/n_1 - X_2/n_2}{\{V[(X_1/n_1) - (X_2/n_2)]\}^{1/2}} \geq \frac{\hat{p}_1 - \hat{p}_2}{\{V[(X_1/n_1) - (X_2/n_2)]\}^{1/2}}\Big|p_1 = p_2\right]$$

$$= P\left[Z \geq \frac{\hat{p}_1 - \hat{p}_2}{\{V[(X_1/n_1) - (X_2/n_2)]\}^{1/2}}\right]. \tag{8.26}$$

Estimating $V[(X_1/n_1)-(X_2/n_2)]$ in this expression by $\hat{p}\hat{q}(1/n_1 + 1/n_2)$, the $p$-value is obtained from $P = P(Z \geq z)$.

*Example 8.4*    Consider the above hypothesis that the increase of the HDL is higher for the younger than older adults. If it has increased for 15 in a random sample of $n_1 = 20$ younger adults, and for 12 in an independent random sample of $n_2 = 30$ older adults, estimates of the proportions are $\hat{p}_1 = (15/20) = 0.75$ and $\hat{p}_2 = (12/30) = 0.40$. Under the null hypothesis, the estimate of the common proportion is $\hat{p} = (15 + 12)/50 = 0.54$, and $\hat{q} = (1-\hat{p}) = 0.46$. The estimate of the variance and S.E. of the difference of the two proportions are $(0.54)(0.46)/(1/20 + 1/30) = 0.0207$ and $(0.0207)^{1/2} = 0.1439$ respectively. The test statistic in (8.23) for the null hypothesis of equality of the two proportions becomes $z = [(0.75-0.40)-0]/(0.1439) = 2.43$, which is larger than $z_{0.05} = 1.645$. The null hypothesis is rejected at the 5 percent significance level.

The $p$-value for the test is $P(Z > 2.43) = 0.0075$, which is notably small suggesting the rejection of the null hypothesis.

### 8.5.2    Right-sided alternative: Power and sample size

The power of the above test for specified $(p_1, p_2)$ is given by

$$P = P[(X_1/n_1 - X_2/n_2) \geq z_\alpha\sqrt{v_0}|p_1, p_2]$$

$$= P\{[(X_1/n_1 - X_2/n_2) - (p_1 - p_2)]\} \geq [z_\alpha\sqrt{v_0} - (p_1 - p_2)]\}$$

$$= P\{Z \geq [z_\alpha\sqrt{v_0} - (p_1 - p_2)]/\sqrt{v_1}\}. \tag{8.27}$$

In this expression, $n = (n_1 + n_2)$, $p = (n_1 p_1 + n_2 p_2)/n$, $q = (1-p)$, $v_0 = pq(1/n_1 + 1/n_2)$, $q_1 = (1-p_1)$, $q_2 = (1-p_2)$ and $v_1 = (p_1 q_1/n_1 + p_2 q_2/n_2)$. When both the sample sizes are equal to $m$, (8.27) becomes

$$P = P\left\{Z \geq \frac{z_\alpha(2pq/m)^{1/2} - (p_1 - p_2)}{[(p_1 q_1 + p_2 q_2)/m]^{1/2}}\right\}, \tag{8.28}$$

where $p = (p_1 + p_2)/2$ and $q = (1-p)$.

The sample sizes required for specified significance level $\alpha$ and power of $(1-\beta)$ at $(p_1, p_2)$ can be obtained from (8.27). When both the sample sizes are equal, from (8.28),

$$\frac{z_\alpha(2pq/m)^{1/2} - (p_1 - p_2)}{[(p_1 q_1 + p_2 q_2)/m]^{1/2}} = z_{1-\beta}. \tag{8.29}$$

From this expression,

$$m \geq \left[z_\alpha(2pq)^{1/2} - z_{1-\beta}(p_1 q_1 + p_2 q_2)^{1/2}\right]^2 / (p_1 - p_2)^2. \tag{8.30}$$

As an illustration, consider the above right-sided alternative with the significance level $\alpha = 0.05$ when $n_1 = n_2 = 20$, and $(p_1, p_2) = (0.6, 0.4)$. In this case $p = (0.6 + 0.4)/2 = 0.5$, $pq(1/n_1 + 1/n_2) = 2(0.25)/20 = 0.025$, and $(p_1 q_1/n_1 + p_2 q_2/n_2) = 0.024$. From (8.28), the power at the specified proportions becomes $P\left\{Z \geq \left[1.645(.025)^{1/2} - (0.2)\right]/(.024)^{1/2}\right\} = P(Z \geq 0.39) = 0.35$ or 35 percent.

For the power of $(1-\beta) = 0.80$, $z_{1-\beta} = -0.85$. With $\alpha = .05$ and this value for the power at $(p_1, p_2) = (0.6, 0.4)$, from (8.30), the sample size required for each group is $m \geq \left[1.645(0.5)^{1/2} + (0.85)(0.48)^{1/2}\right]^2 / (.04) = 76.75$ or approximately 77.

## 8.5.3    Left-sided alternative: Critical region and $p$-value

The null and alternative hypotheses in this case are

$$H_0 : p_1 = p_2$$

and

$$H_1 : p_1 < p_2. \tag{8.31}$$

With the significance level of $\alpha$, the Critical Region for rejecting the null hypothesis is given by

$$z = \frac{\hat{p}_1 - \hat{p}_2}{[\hat{p}\hat{q}(1/n_1 + 1/n_2)]^{1/2}} \leq -z_\alpha. \tag{8.32}$$

The $p$-value is obtained from $P(Z \leq z)$.

*Example 8.5*   For the increase in the HDL for the two groups, consider the null and alternative hypotheses in (8.31) with the 5 percent significance level. If it increases for 10 and 20 younger and older adults in independent random samples of 20 and 30 respectively, $p_1 = (10/20) = 0.5$ and $\hat{p}_2 = (20/30) = 0.67$. Under the null hypothesis, the estimate of the common proportion is $\hat{p} = (10 + 20)/50 = 0.6$, and the sample variance and S.E. of $(\hat{p}_1 - \hat{p}_2)$ are $(0.6)(0.4)(1/20 + 1/30) = 0.02$ and $0.1414$. From (8.32), $z = (0.5 - 0.67)/(0.1414) = -1.20$, which is not smaller than $-z_{0.05} = -1.645$, and hence the null hypothesis is not rejected at the 5 percent significance level. The $p$-value for this test is $P(Z < -1.20) = 0.1151$, which is too large to reject the null hypothesis.

### 8.5.4   Left-sided alternative: Power and sample size

The power of the test at $(p_1, p_2)$ with the significance level $\alpha$ is obtained from (8.27) by replacing $z_\alpha$ with $-z_\alpha$. When the sample sizes are equal to $m$, it becomes

$$P = P\left\{ Z \le \frac{-z_\alpha (2pq/m)^{1/2} - (p_1 - p_2)}{[(p_1 q_1 + p_2 q_2)/m]^{1/2}} \right\}. \tag{8.33}$$

From this expression, the sample size $m$ for specified $\alpha$, power $(1 - \beta)$ and $(p_1, p_2)$ is obtained by equating the right side expression to $z_\beta = -z_{1-\beta}$, and becomes the same as (8.30).

As an illustration, consider the above left-sided alternative with the significance level $\alpha = 0.05$ when $n_1 = n_2 = 20$ and $(p_1, p_2) = (0.4, 0.6)$. In this case, $p = (0.4 + 0.6)/2 = 0.5$, $pq(1/n_1 + 1/n_2) = 2(0.25)/20 = 0.025$, and $(p_1 q_1/n_1 + p_2 q_2/n_2) = 0.024$. From (8.33), the power at the specified proportions becomes $P\left\{ Z \le \left[ -1.645(.025)^{1/2} + (0.2) \right]/(.024)^{1/2} \right\} = P(Z \le -0.39) = 0.35$.

For the power $(1 - \beta) = 0.80$, $z_{1-\beta} = -0.85$. With $\alpha = 0.05$ and this value for the power at $(p_1, p_2) = (0.4, 0.6)$, from (8.30), the sample size required for each group becomes $m \ge \left[ 1.645(0.5)^{1/2} + 0.85(0.48)^{1/2} \right]^2/(0.04) = 76.75$ or approximately 77.

### 8.5.5   Two-sided alternative: Critical region and $p$-value

The null and alternative hypotheses in this case are

$$H_0 : p_1 = p_2$$

and

$$H_1 : p_1 \ne p_2. \tag{8.34}$$

With the significance level of $\alpha$, the Critical Region is given by

$$|z| \geq z_{\alpha/2}, \qquad (8.35)$$

that is, $z \geq z_{\alpha/2}$ or $z \leq -z_{\alpha/2}$, where $z$ is the same as in (8.25) or (8.32). The $p$-value of this test is obtained from $2P(Z \geq z)$.

*Example 8.6*    As in Example 8.4, consider the increase of HDL for 15 in a random sample of 20 younger adults and for 12 in an independent random sample of 30 older adults. In this case, $\hat{p}_1 = (15/20) = 0.75$, $\hat{p}_2 = (12/30) = 0.40$, and under the null hypothesis $\hat{p} = (15 + 12)/50 = 0.54$. With these estimates, $z = 2.43$, as found in the above example, which is larger than $z_{0.025} = 1.96$. The null hypothesis is rejected at the significance level of 5 percent. Since $P(Z \geq 2.43) = 0.0075$, the $p$-value becomes $2(.0075) = 0.015$, which is too small and suggests the rejection of the null hypothesis.

For the continuity correction, the numerator of the larger of $\hat{p}_1$ and $\hat{p}_2$ is decreased and the smaller increased by $(1/2)$. The estimate $\hat{p}\hat{q}(1/n_1 + 1/n_2)$ of the variance remains the same.

For this Example, with the corrected proportions $(14.5/20) = 0.725$ and $(12.5/30) = 0.4167$, $z = (0.725 - 0.4167)/0.1439 = 2.14$. The null hypothesis is rejected at the 5 percent level of significance since $z > 1.96$. Since $P(Z > 2.14) = 0.016$, the $p$-value becomes $2(0.016) = 0.032$.

## 8.5.6    Power and sample size

Following the Critical Region in (8.35), the power for specified $(p_1, p_2)$ at the significance level $\alpha$ is given by

$$P\{Z \geq [z_{\alpha/2}\sqrt{v_0} - (p_1 - p_2)]/\sqrt{v_1}\} + P\{Z \leq [-z_{\alpha/2}\sqrt{v_0} - (p_1 - p_2)]/\sqrt{v_1}\}. \quad (8.36)$$

When the sample size for each group is equal to $m$, this probability becomes

$$P = P\left[Z \geq \frac{z_{\alpha/2}(2pq/m)^{1/2} - (p_1 - p_2)}{(p_1q_1/m + p_2q_2/m)^{1/2}}\right] + P\left[Z \leq \frac{-z_{\alpha/2}(2pq/m)^{1/2} - (p_1 - p_2)}{(p_1q_1/m + p_2q_2/m)^{1/2}}\right],$$
$$(8.37)$$

where $p = (p_1 + p_2)/2$.

The probabilities in the first and second expressions become small if $p_1 < p_2$ and $p_1 > p_2$ respectively. Ignoring the smaller probability, the required sample size for specified significance level $\alpha$, power of $(1 - \beta)$ at $(p_1, p_2)$ is given by

$$m \geq \left[z_{\alpha/2}(2pq)^{1/2} - z_{1-\beta}(p_1q_1 + p_2q_2)^{1/2}\right]^2 / (p_1 - p_2)^2. \quad (8.38)$$

For the illustration, consider the power for the above two-sided alternative at $(p_1, p_2) = (0.6, 0.4)$ when $n_1 = n_2 = 20$ and $\alpha = 0.05$. In this case, $p = 0.5$, and from (8.37), the power becomes $[P(Z \geq 0.71) + P(Z \leq -3.29)] = (0.2389 + 0.0005) = 0.24$.

At the 5 percent significance level, for the power of 80 percent at $(p_1, p_2) = (0.6, 0.4)$, from (8.38), the required sample size is given by

$$m \geq \left[ 1.96(0.5)^{1/2} + (0.85)(0.48)^{1/2} \right]^2 / (0.04) = 97.5 \text{ or close to } 98.$$

## 8.6    Specified difference of two proportions

In Section 8.5, the equality of two proportions was examined. In some applications, with a specified difference $\delta$, the null hypothesis takes the form

$$H_0 : (p_1 - p_2) = \delta. \tag{8.39}$$

For the alternative hypothesis, $(p_1 - p_2)$ can be larger, smaller or not equal to $\delta$. With the estimates $(\hat{p}_1, \hat{p}_2)$ from independent samples of sizes $(n_1, n_2)$, the test statistic is given by

$$z = \frac{(\hat{p}_1 - \hat{p}_2) - \delta}{(\hat{p}_1 \hat{q}_1 / n_1 + \hat{p}_2 \hat{q}_2 / n_2)^{1/2}}. \tag{8.40}$$

For the significance level of $\alpha$, the Critical Region becomes $z \geq z_\alpha$, $z \leq -z_\alpha$ and $|z| \geq z_{\alpha/2}$ for the right-sided, left-sided and two-sided alternative hypothesis respectively. The $p$-values for these three cases are given by $P(Z \geq z)$, $P(Z \leq z)$ and $2P(Z \geq z)$.

*Example 8.7*    Consider the increase of the HDLs in Example 8.4 for the younger and older adults with the hypotheses $H_0 : (p_1 - p_2) = 0.10$ and $H_1 : (p_1 - p_2) > 0.10$. With estimates 0.75 and 0.40 from samples of sizes (20, 30) for the two groups, the sample variance and S.E. of $(\hat{p}_1 - \hat{p}_2)$ are $[(0.75)(0.25)/20 + (0.40)(0.60)/30] = 0.0174$ and 0.1319. The test statistic in (8.40) becomes $z = (0.25/0.1319) = 1.90$, which exceeds $z_{0.05} = 1.645$. As a result, the null hypothesis that the difference of the percentages for the younger and older adults is 10 percent *versus* it exceeds this value is rejected at the 5 percent significance level. The $p$-value for the test is, $P(Z \geq 1.90) = 0.029$ which is small and suggests the rejection of the null hypothesis.

## 8.7    Equality of two or more proportions

Clinical experiments are conducted to examine whether k treatments, for instance, for the relief of sinus problems, are equally effective. With $p_i$, $i = (1, 2, ..., k)$, denoting the probability effectiveness for the $k$th treatment, the null hypothesis becomes $H_0 : p_1 = p_2 = ... = p_k$ with the alternative hypothesis $H_1$ that at least one of the $k$ probabilities is different from the rest.

As described in Section (8.5.5) for the case of $k = 2$ treatments, the test statistic for the null hypothesis is given by the standardized normal variate in (8.25) or (8.32). The estimators $(\hat{p}_1, \hat{p}_2)$ for $(p_1, p_2)$ are obtained from independent samples of sizes $(n_1, n_2)$ for the two treatments and $\hat{p} = (n_1\hat{p}_1 + n_2\hat{p}_2)/n$ for the common proportion p from the combined sample of size $n = (n_1 + n_2)$. From (8.25) or (8.32), $z^2$ is the same as $\left[n_1(\hat{p}_1 - \hat{p})^2 + n_2(p_2 - \hat{p})^2\right]/\hat{p}\hat{q}$, where $\hat{q} = (1 - \hat{p})$, and it follows the chisquare distribution with a single degree of freedom.

Similarly, for the above hypothesis for $k \geq 2$ proportions,

$$U = \frac{n_1(\hat{p}_1 - \hat{p})^2 + n_2(\hat{p}_2 - \hat{p})^2 + \ldots + n_k(\hat{p}_k - \hat{p})^2}{\hat{p}\hat{q}} = \frac{\sum_1^n n_i(\hat{p}_i - \hat{p})^2}{\hat{p}\hat{q}} \qquad (8.41)$$

follows the chisquare distribution with $(k-1)$ d.f. In this expression $\hat{p}_i$, $i = (1, 2, \ldots, k)$, are the estimators for $p_i$ obtained from independent samples of sizes $n_i$. The estimator for $p$ from the total sample of size $n = \sum_1^k n_i$ is $\hat{p} = \sum_1^n n_i p_i / n$ and $\hat{q} = (1 - \hat{p})$.

*Example 8.8*    Consider the hypothesis that four pain relief medications are equally effective. If they are effective for (70, 90, 80, 50) percent of the patients respectively in samples of sizes (10, 10, 20, 20), with the total sample of size $n = 60$, the estimate of the overall proportion becomes $\hat{p} = (7 + 9 + 16 + 10)/60 = 0.7$. From (8.41), $U = [10(0) + 10(0.04) + 20(0.01) + 20(0.04)]/(0.21) = 6.67$ with 3 d.f. and does not exceed $\chi^2_{3, 0.05} = 7.81$. The hypothesis that the four medications are equally effective is not rejected at the 5 percent level of significance.

## 8.8    A common proportion

If the null hypothesis is that the $k \geq 2$ proportions in the above section are all equal to a specified proportion $p_0$, the test statistic

$$Z = \frac{|\hat{p} - p_0| - (1/2n)}{\sqrt{p_0 q_0 / n}}, \qquad (8.42)$$

where $q_0 = (1 - p_0)$, approximately follows the standard normal distribution. Equivalently, $U = Z^2$ follows the chisquare distribution with a single degree of freedom.

If the null hypothesis is that each of the medications in Example 8.8 is effective for 80 percent of the patients, from (8.42), $Z = [-0.1 - (1/120)]/(0.16/60)^{1/2} = -2.098$ and $U = 4.40$ with the $p$-value of $2(0.018) = 0.036$. The null hypothesis that the four medications are effective for 80 percent of the patients is rejected at the 5 percent level of significance.

The test statistics in (8.41) and (8.42) are presented in Snedecor and Cochran (1967, p. 248) with illustrations of the Mendelian hypothesis of inheritance.

# Exercises

**8.1.** In Example 8.1, for the HDLs, $H_0 : p = 0.3$ and $H_1 : p > 0.3$ was considered. (a) Test this null hypothesis at the 5 percent significance level exactly and through the normal approximation if the HDL was found to be in the (40–60) mg/dl for 15 adults in a sample of 30. With the normality assumption for the HDLs, find (a) the $p$-value of the test, (b) power of the test at $p = 0.5$, and (c) the sample size required for the 5 percent significance level and the power of 0.80 at $p = 0.5$.

**8.2.** For the hypothesis of the HDLs in Example 8.2 with the left-sided alternative, find (a) the $p$-value of the test for $x = 7$ and (b) the power of the test at $p = 0.4$ from the binomial distribution, and compare them with the results obtained from the normal approximation.

**8.3.** For the hypothesis in Example 8.3 for the HDL with $H_0 : p = 0.5$ and the two-sided alternative, find the (a) critical values from the binomial distribution if the significance level should not exceed 5 percent, (b) $p$-value for the test at $x = 14$ and (c) power at $p_1 = 0.8$. Compare the results in (b) and (c) with those obtained from the normal approximation.

**8.4.** From Example 6.2, independent samples of sizes $n_1 = 300$ males and $n_2 = 200$ females, $x_1 = 120$ and $x_2 = 60$ respectively were found to be hypertensive. For the corresponding population proportions $p_1$ and $p_2$, test the hypothesis $H_0 : p_1 = p_2$ *versus* $H_1 : p_1 > p_2$ at the 5 percent significance level, and find the $p$-value.

**8.5.** In Example 6.3, for a random sample of 500, the number of adults were $x_1 = 250$, $x_2 = 150$ and $x_3 = 100$ in the ranges 130–140, 140–150 and >150 of the SBPs. Test the hypothesis at the 5 percent significance level that the population percentages for the first two ranges are the same, and find the $p$-value of the test statistic.

**8.6.** Chrysant et al. (2009) presented the results of the treatment of isolated systolic hypertension (SBP $\geq 140$ mmHg and DBP $\leq 90$ mmHg) with hydrochlorothiazide and irbersartan. The treatment is considered to have controlled the hypertension if SBP is reduced to less than 140 mmHg ; less than 130 mmHg for the Type 2 diabetic patients. The results for male and female groups, older and younger than 65 years, and for the diabetic patients are as follows:

Test for the equality of the proportions controlled for (a) males and females and (b) for persons older and younger than 65 years of age, and (c) the proportions of the controlled and uncontrolled Type 2 diabetic patients.

|  | Males | Females | Total | $\leq 65$ years | 65 years | Total |
|---|---|---|---|---|---|---|
| Controlled | 156 | 174 | 330 | 104 | 226 | 330 |
| Not controlled | 68 | 45 | 113 | 47 | 66 | 113 |
| Total | 224 | 219 | 443 | 151 | 292 | 443 |

Type 2 diabetic patients:

|                | Yes | No  | Total |
|----------------|-----|-----|-------|
| Controlled     | 65  | 265 | 330   |
| Not controlled | 73  | 40  | 113   |
| Total          | 138 | 305 | 443   |

**8.7.** A treatment for hypertension was found to be effective for (40, 70, 70) percent respectively of the (30, 30, 40) persons of three age groups. Test the hypothesis that the percentage of effectiveness is the same for the three groups.

**8.8.** With the information in Exercise 8.7, test the hypothesis that the treatment is effective for 50 percent of each of the age groups.

# 9

# The Chisquare statistic

## 9.1 Introduction

The chisquare distribution plays a prominent role in several applications of statistics. It is widely used for statistical analyses in biological, genetic, medical and various other types of experiments and investigations. As seen in Sections 5.8 and 7.8, confidence limits and test of hypothesis for the variance of a normal distribution are derived from this distribution. The chisquare tests for the equality of proportions and percentages in Sections 8.7 and 8.8 are obtained as approximations.

The Chisquare Statistic presented in Section 9.2 evaluates the discrepancies between the observed frequencies of an attribute or categorical variable from those expected from a hypothesis. Larger values of this statistic lead to the rejection of the hypothesis. The tests of *Goodness of Fit* and *Independence and Contingency* in the following sections are important applications of this statistic.

## 9.2 The test statistic

Consider a total of n units classified into k groups or classes with observed numbers $(O_1, O_2, ..., O_k)$, $\sum_1^k O_i = n$. For a specified null hypothesis, denote the expected number of units in these classes by $(E_1, E_2, ..., E_k)$, $\sum_1^k E_i = n$. The *Pearson Chisquare Statistic*

$$U = \sum_1^k \frac{(O_i - E_i)^2}{E_i} = \sum_1^k \frac{O_i^2}{E_i} - n \qquad (9.1)$$

*Statistical Methodologies with Medical Applications*, First Edition. Poduri S.R.S. Rao.
© 2017 John Wiley & Sons, Ltd. Published 2017 by John Wiley & Sons, Ltd.

approximately follows the chisquare distribution with $(k-1)$ d.f., $\chi^2_{k-1}$. Larger values of this statistic suggest the rejection of the null hypothesis. With the continuity correction, this statistic is obtained from

$$U = \sum_1^k \frac{[|O_i - E_i| - 0.5]^2}{E_i}. \tag{9.1a}$$

## 9.2.1    A single proportion

Consider the hypothesis that 40 percent of a large adult population is obese. The corresponding null and alternative hypotheses are

$$H_0 : p = p_0$$

and

$$H_1 : p \neq p_0, \tag{9.2}$$

where $p_0 = 0.40$.

If 12 adults are found to be obese in a random sample of $n = 20$ from the above population, the observed and expected numbers of the obese and non-obese individuals can be expressed into two classes as follows.

| Class | Observed number ($O_i$) | Expected number ($E_i$) | $[|O_i - E_i| - 0.5]^2 / E_i$ |
|---|---|---|---|
| 1 | $O_1 = 12$ | $E_1 = 20(0.4) = 8$ | $(3.5)^2/8 = 1.53$ |
| 2 | $O_2 = 8$ | $E_2 = 20(0.6) = 12$ | $(3.5)^2/12 = 1.02$ |

From the right-hand side column, from (9.1a), $U = (1.53 + 1.02) = 2.55$. Since it does not exceed $\chi^2_{1, 0.05} = 3.84$, the null hypothesis that 40 percent of the above adult population is obese is not rejected.

As seen in Section 8.4, the test statistic for the above null hypothesis is $Z = [|\hat{p} - p_0| - (1/2n)]/\sqrt{p_0 q_0/n}$, which approximately follows the standard normal distribution. The Chisquare Statistic $U$ in (9.1a) is the same as $Z^2$. With the observed estimate $\hat{p} = (12/20) = 0.6$, $z = 1.597$ and $U = 2.55$.

Without the correction for continuity, from (9.1), $U = \left[(12-8)^2/8 + (8-12)^2/12\right] = (10/3) = 3.33$. For the normal approximation, $z = (0.6 - 0.4)/\sqrt{(0.4)(0.6)/20} = 1.826$ and $z^2 = 3.33$.

## 9.2.2    Specified proportions

Consider the hypothesis that the hypertension of an adult population in the mild, moderate and high ranges is 20, 30 and 50 percent. The number observed in these classes in a random sample of 200 of these adults and the corresponding numbers expected from the hypothesis are as follows:

| $O_i$: | 30 | 50 | 120 |
|---|---|---|---|
| $E_i$: | $200(0.2) = 40$ | $200(0.3) = 60$ | $200(0.5) = 100$ |

From (9.1a), $U = \left(9.5^2/40 + 9.5^2/60 + 19.5^2/100\right) = 7.56$, which is larger than $\chi^2_{2,0.05} = 5.992$ with the $p$-value of 0.0228. The null hypothesis is rejected with the significance level of 2.28 percent or smaller.

## 9.3    Test of goodness of fit

For statistical analysis and inference in several applications, it is frequently of interest to examine whether the observations of a sample follow a specified distribution such as the normal. The data are classified into $k$ groups with the observed numbers $O_i$, $i = (1,2,...,k)$, in the $k$th group, and the expected numbers are obtained from the specified distribution. In this case, the statistic $U$ in (9.1a) approximately follows the chisquare distribution with $(k - r - 1)$ d.f., $\chi^2_{k-r-1}$, where $r$ is the number of estimated parameters of the distribution. For the computation of this statistic, the classes with expected numbers smaller than five are combined with the adjacent classes.

As an illustration, the weights (in pounds) of $n = 400$ adults were grouped into $k = 15$ classes (125–130), (130–135),..., (195–200) of equal widths of five. The mean, variance and standard deviation of this frequency distribution were $\bar{x} = 163.325$, $s^2 = 236.67$ and $s = 15.384$. The standardized scores $z = (x - 163.325)/15.384$ for the end-values (125, 130, ...,200) and the corresponding cumulative probabilities of the standard normal distribution were found. The probabilities $p_i$ in the classes were obtained from these cumulative probabilities. The observed numbers $O_i$ and expected numbers $E_i = np_i$ for the 15 groups are presented in Table 9.1. From (9.1a), $U = 5.31$. Since the mean and variance were estimated, $r = 2$. For the Chisquare distribution with $(15 - 2 - 1) = 12$ d.f., $\chi^2_{12,0.05} = 21.03$. The value of 5.31 for $U$ is much smaller than 21.03 suggesting that the normal distribution with the above mean and variance can be fitted to the weights.

## 9.4    Test of independence: ($r$ x $c$) classification

This test is also known as the *Test of Association and Contingency*. It is frequently of interest to examine whether two attributes or characteristics, for instance, age and hypertension or weight and lipid levels are related. A sample of $n$ observed number of adults can be classified into $i = (1,2,...,r)$ rows and $j = (1,2,...,c)$ columns corresponding to the two attributes. Denote by $O_{ij}$ the observed number in the $i$th row and

Table 9.1  Observed and expected frequencies of the normal distribution of the 400 weights in 15 classes.

| $O_i$ | $E_i$ |
|-------|-------|
| 6 | 7 |
| 10 | 7 |
| 14 | 13 |
| 18 | 21 |
| 29 | 31 |
| 35 | 41 |
| 51 | 48 |
| 56 | 52 |
| 50 | 50 |
| 45 | 43 |
| 30 | 34 |
| 20 | 24 |
| 16 | 15 |
| 12 | 9 |
| 8 | 5 |

$j$th column. The totals of the rows and columns become $R_i = \sum_{j=1}^{c} O_{ij}$ and $C_j = \sum_{i=1}^{r} O_{ij}$, and

$$n = \sum_{1}^{r} R_i = \sum_{1}^{c} C_j$$

The probabilities of the $i$th row and $j$th column are $(R_i/n)$ and $(C_j / n)$. When the hypothesis that the row and column classifications are independent is valid, the probability $(E_{ij} / n)$ of the $(ij)$th cell becomes the same as $(R_i / n)(C_j / n)$, and as a result $E_{ij} = R_i C_j / n$.

Following (9.1), the test statistic for the null hypothesis is given by

$$U = \sum_{1}^{r} \sum_{1}^{c} \frac{(O_{ij} - E_{ij})^2}{E_{ij}} = \sum_{1}^{r} \sum_{1}^{c} \frac{O_{ij}^2}{E_{ij}} - n, \qquad (9.3)$$

which approximately follows the chisquare distribution with $(r - 1)(c - 1)$ d.f. With the continuity correction, this statistic is obtained from

$$U = \sum_{1}^{r} \sum_{1}^{c} \frac{\left[|O_{ij} - E_{ij}| - 0.5\right]^2}{E_{ij}}. \qquad (9.3a)$$

The following two examples illustrate the application of this test statistic.

*Example 9.1*   The observed and expected numbers (in parentheses) of 500 adults classified according to age and hypertension are given below.

| | Hypertension | | | | |
|---|---|---|---|---|---|
| Age | Low | Medium | High | Very high | Total |
| 50–65 | 75 (60) | 65 (80) | 35 (40) | 25 (20) | 200 |
| $\geq$65 | 75 (90) | 135 (120) | 65 (60) | 25 (30) | 300 |
| Total | 150 | 200 | 100 | 50 | 500 |

From (9.3a), $U = 12.75$ with the $p$-value of 0.005 from the chisquare distribution with $(2 - 1)(4 - 1) = 3$ d.f. This small $p$-value suggests the rejection of the hypothesis that hypertension levels are independent of age.

The test statistic $U$ for the hypothesis of equality of $k$ binomial proportions is presented in (8.41). This hypothesis is the same as that the successes-failures classification with $r = 2$ rows is independent of the column classification with $c = k$ corresponding to the binomial proportions. For this case, the test statistic (8.41) coincides with (9.3).

As an illustration, consider three treatments to be effective for (10, 24, 26) of the adults in samples of sizes (20, 30, 50) respectively. The estimates of the proportions for the effectiveness are $\hat{p}_1 = (10/20) = 0.5$, $\hat{p}_2 = (24/30) = 0.8$ and $\hat{p}_3 = (26/50) = 0.52$. When the hypothesis $H_0 : p_1 = p_2 = p_3$ is valid, estimate of the common proportion $p$ becomes $\hat{p} = (10 + 24 + 26)/100 = 0.6$. From (8.41), the test statistic for this hypothesis is $U = (1.72/0.24) = 7.167$.

The observed number of effective cases and their expected values (in parentheses) for the hypothesis of independence of the (row $\times$ column) classification are as follows:

| | Treatments | | | |
|---|---|---|---|---|
| | 1 | 2 | 3 | Total |
| Effective | 10 (12) | 24 (18) | 26 (30) | 60 |
| Not effective | 10 (8) | 6 (12) | 24 (20) | 40 |
| Total | 20 | 30 | 50 | 100 |

From (9.3), $U = [(4/12) + (36/18) + (16/30) + (4/8) + (36/12) + (16/20)] = 7.167$, same as the above value for the test statistic. In either case, the $p$-value for $U$ is very close to 0.05. The effectiveness of the three treatments is different at the 5 percent level of significance.

## 9.5    Test of independence: (2x2) classification

In several biological, genetic, medical and similar applications, the two characteristics of interest are classified into high–low, success–failure, effective–not effective, and similar categories. The observed numbers for the effectiveness of two treatments administered for hypertension to $n$ adults, for instance, may be classified as follows:

|               | Treatment 1    | Treatment 2    | Total            |
| ------------- | -------------- | -------------- | ---------------- |
| Effective     | $a$            | $b$            | $R_1 = (a+b)$    |
| Not effective | $c$            | $d$            | $R_2 = (c+d)$    |
| Total         | $C_1 = (a+c)$  | $C_2 = (b+d)$  | $n$              |

The hypothesis that both the treatments are equally effective is the same as the hypothesis that the row and column classifications are independent; that is, there is no association between the treatments and their effectiveness. When this hypothesis is valid, the expected numbers are given by $E_{11} = R_1 \times C_1/n$, $E_{12} = R_1 \times C_2/n$, $E_{21} = R_2 \times C_1/n$ and $E_{22} = R_2 \times C_2/n$. Following (9.3), the test statistic for the hypothesis is given by

$$U = \sum_1^2 \sum_1^2 \frac{(O_{ij} - E_{ij})^2}{E_{ij}} = \sum_1^2 \sum_1^2 \frac{O_{ij}^2}{E_{ij}} - n \qquad (9.4)$$

$$= \frac{n(ad - bc)^2}{R_1 R_2 C_1 C_2}, \qquad (9.4a)$$

which follows the chisquare distribution with $(2-1)(2-1) = 1$ d.f. If the expected value in one of the four cells is found, the remaining three are automatically determined since the row and column totals are fixed. With the continuity correction, the test statistic becomes

$$U = \sum_1^2 \sum_1^2 \frac{[|O_{ij} - E_{ij}| - (1/2)]^2}{E_{ij}} \qquad (9.5)$$

$$= \frac{n[|ad - bc| - (n/2)]^2}{R_1 R_2 C_1 C_2}. \qquad (9.5a)$$

The derivations of (9.4a) and (9.5a) are presented in Appendix A9.1.

The hypothesis of independence of the rows and columns is the same as the hypothesis that the column proportions are equal, that is, $H_0 : p_1 = p_2$; both the treatments are equally effective. It is also the same as the hypothesis that the row proportions are equal, that is, the effective and noneffective proportions for the first or second treatment are equal. This result is analytically presented in Appendix A9.2.

*Example 9.2*    The number of hypertensive patients with decreased systolic blood pressure (SBP) as a result of receiving a low or high dose of a treatment are as follows:

|  |  | Low | High | Total |
|---|---|---|---|---|
|  | 80–90 | 15 | 32 | 47 |
| SBP | >90 | 10 | 8 | 18 |
|  | Total | 25 | 40 | 65 |

The expected numbers in the cells are $E_{11} = (25 \times 47)/65 = 18.08$, $E_{12} = (40 \times 47)/65 = 28.92$, $E_{21} = (18 \times 25)/65 = 6.92$ and $E_{22} = (18 \times 40)/65 = 11.08$. Since the row and column totals are known, one of the four expected numbers determines the rest. From (9.5) or (9.5a), $U = 2.16$, which is smaller than $\chi^2_{1,0.05} = 3.843$. The hypothesis that the SBPs are the same for both the low and high doses is not rejected at the 5 percent level of significance.

## 9.5.1    Fisher's exact test of independence

If the Chisquare statistic $U$ in (9.4) or (9.5) is small, the $p$-value will be large and the hypothesis of independence or lack of association between the row and column effects is not rejected; that is, $H_0 : p_1 = p_2$ is not rejected. However, the approximation that $U$ follows the Chisquare distribution with one degree of freedom is found to be not valid if any of the four expected frequencies becomes five or smaller. In this case, Fisher 1915, (1925) recommended finding the exact $p$-value for the observed $(a, b, c, d)$ and more extreme values for the given marginal totals $(R_1, R_2, C_1, C_2)$. This probability for a set of $(a, b, c, d)$ follows the hypergeometric distribution

$$P(a,b,c,d) = \binom{R_1}{a}\binom{R_2}{c} / \binom{n}{C_1} = \binom{C_1}{a}\binom{C_2}{b} / \binom{n}{R_1} = \frac{R_1! R_2! C_1! C_2!}{a! b! c! d! n!}.$$

(9.6)

As an illustration, consider the following observed values for two treatments:

|  | Treatment 1 | Treatment 2 | Total |
|---|---|---|---|
| Effective | $a = 1$ | $b = 4$ | $R_1 = 5$ |
| Not effective | $c = 4$ | $d = 6$ | $R_2 = 10$ |
| Total | $C_1 = 5$ | $C_2 = 10$ | $n = 15$ |

The observations $(a, b, c)$ are considered small. For the same marginal totals, the different arrangements of the observations in the four cells are arranged in the following six tables.

| Tables of the arrangements | | | | | | | | | | | |
|---|---|---|---|---|---|---|---|---|---|---|---|
| (1) | | (2) | | (3) | | (4) | | (5) | | (6) | |
| 0 | 5 | 1 | 4 | 2 | 3 | 3 | 2 | 4 | 1 | 5 | 0 |
| 5 | 5 | 4 | 6 | 3 | 7 | 2 | 8 | 1 | 9 | 0 | 10 |

From (9.6), the probabilities for these six arrangements respectively are 0.0839, 0.3497, 0.3996, 0.1499, 0.0166 and 0.0003, with their total adding up to unity.

The p-value is the probability of the observed and more extreme frequencies. The arrangement in the first table is *more extreme in the same direction* as the observed table; its probability 0.0839 is smaller than 0.3497 for the observed table. The *p*-value in this case is $P_A = (0.0839 + 0.3497) = 0.4336$. The arrangements in Tables (3) – (6) are *more extreme in the opposite direction*. The p-value in this case is $P_B = (0.3497 + 0.3996 + \ldots + 0.0003) = 0.9161$. Finally, the p-value for the hypothesis of independence, that is, $H_0 : p_1 = p_2$ *versus* $H_1 : p_1 \neq p_2$, is given by the minimum of $(P_A, P_B)$ for the above arrangements. In this case, the p-value becomes 0.4336. Since it is large, the null hypothesis of the independence of the row and column factors is not rejected. Both the treatments can be considered to be equally effective.

For the above null hypothesis with the alternative $H_1 : p_1 < p_2$, the p-value becomes $P_A = 0.4336$. For the alternative $H_1 : p_1 > p_2$, it becomes $P_B = 0.9161$. *GraphPad*, for instance, can be used to find these p-values.

### 9.5.2    Mantel-Hanszeltest statistic

In some practical situations, the observations for the $2 \times 2$ classification become available for $k$ repetitions of an experiment or from stratification formed, for instance, from age groups. The observed numbers in the $k$th stratum are given as shown below.

| | Columns | | Total |
|---|---|---|---|
| | $a_i$ | $b_i$ | $R_{1i}$ |
| Rows | | | |
| | $c_i$ | $d_i$ | $R_{2i}$ |
| Total | $C_{1i}$ | $C_{2i}$ | $n_i$ |

For this situation, the statistic for the independence of the (Row × Column) classification obtained by Cochran (1954b), followed by Mantel and Haenszel (1959), is given by

$$\chi^2_{MH} = \frac{[|A - E| - 0.5]^2}{V}. \tag{9.7}$$

This statistic follows the chisquare distribution with a single degree of freedom. In this expression, $A = \sum_{1}^{k} a_i$, $E_i = R_{1i}C_{1i}/n_i$, $E = \sum_{1}^{k} E_i$, $V_i = R_{1i}R_{2i}C_{1i}C_{2i}/n_i^2(n_i-1)$ and $V = \sum_{1}^{k} V_i$.

*Example 9.3*    Consider the following decreases of the SBPs of three groups for the low and high levels of the dosages of a treatment

|  | Low | High |  | Low | High |  | Low | High |  |
|---|---|---|---|---|---|---|---|---|---|
|  | 1 | 2 | Total | 1 | 2 | Total | 1 | 2 | Total |
| 80–90 | 10 | 18 | 28 | 15 | 20 | 35 | 20 | 30 | 50 |
| SBP >90 | 12 | 40 | 52 | 20 | 45 | 65 | 20 | 50 | 70 |
| Total | 22 | 58 | 80 | 35 | 65 | 100 | 40 | 80 | 120 |

For these observations, $A = 45$, $E = (7.7 + 12.25 + 16.67) = 36.67$, $V = (3.67 + 5.23 + 6.54) = 15.44$. From (9.7), $\chi_{MH}^2 = (8.33 - 0.5)^2/15.44 = 3.97$, which exceeds $\chi_{1,0.05}^2 = 3.843$. The null hypothesis that the decrease for the two levels of the SBP is independent of the two dosage levels is rejected at the 5 percent level of significance.

# Exercises

**9.1.** A population is classified into eight groups with age (<10, 10–20, ..., 60–70, >70) years. The percentages of these groups expected to be affected by air pollution are (20, 15, 10, 5, 5, 10, 15, 20) respectively. In a random sample of 200 of this population, the number actually affected were (45, 25, 18, 15, 12, 25, 28, 32) respectively. Examine whether these observed numbers support the hypothesized expected numbers.

**9.2.** Average annual percentages of patients' emergency department visits in the United States during 2009–2010 for cold symptoms, injury, and other reasons were 27, 21 and 52 percent respectively. (*Source*: Health, United States, 2012, Figure 23, Chart book: Special Feature on Emergency Care, p. 25.). For a sample of 200 visits in one of the Northeastern cities, the number of visits for the three reasons were (60, 50, 90). Test the following hypotheses: (a) the percentages for this city do not differ from the national averages, and (b) the percentage for the cold symptoms does not significantly exceed that for injuries.

**9.3.** Among the 400 members of an educational institution (60, 70, 140) under 22, 22–60 and over 60 years of age received the flu vaccination, and (60, 30, 40) in these groups did not receive the vaccination. Examine whether age and receiving vaccination are associated.

**9.4.** The hypertension of 300 adults of three age groups is classified as follows. The expected numbers are presented in the parentheses. Test the hypothesis that age and hypertension are not related.

|       | Low     | Medium  | High    | Total |
|-------|---------|---------|---------|-------|
| 50–60 | 7(10)   | 12(15)  | 31(25)  | 50    |
| 60–70 | 13(20)  | 23(30)  | 64(50)  | 100   |
| >70   | 40(30)  | 55(45)  | 55(75)  | 150   |
| Total | 60      | 90      | 150     | 300   |

**9.5.** From the results presented in Exercise 8.6 for the systolic blood pressure treatment, examine through the chisquare test the difference of the proportions controlled for (a) males and females, and (b) younger and older than 65 years, and (c) the proportions of the controlled and uncontrolled Type 2 diabetic patients.

**9.6.** Olson et al. (2005) presented the following figures for the medical care of insured and uninsured children in the United States:

|                    | Delayed | Unmet |
|--------------------|---------|-------|
| Full- year insured | 744     | 590   |
| Part-year          | 1100    | 730   |
| ................   |         |       |
| Full-year coverage |         |       |
| Public             | 282     | 201   |
| Private            | 662     | 331   |

Test the following hypotheses: (a) Whether medical care is delayed or unmet does not differ for the full or part-year insured children. (b) Delayed or unmet medical care does not differ for the full-year public and private coverage.

**9.7.** The SBPs of three groups for two treatments are as follows. Test the hypothesis that the two treatments are equally effective.

|     |       | Treatment | | | Treatment | | | Treatment | | |
|-----|-------|---|----|-------|----|----|-------|----|----|-------|
|     |       | 1 | 2  | Total | 1  | 2  | Total | 1  | 2  | Total |
| SBP | 80–90 | 14 | 16 | 30   | 20 | 20 | 40    | 20 | 40 | 60    |
|     | >90   | 6  | 44 | 50    | 10 | 50 | 60    | 30 | 30 | 60    |
|     | Total | 20 | 60 | 80    | 30 | 70 | 100   | 50 | 70 | 120   |

# Appendix A9

## A9.1    Derivations of 9.4(a)

$(O_{11} - E_{11}) = (a - R_1C_1/n) = (ad - bc)/n$.    Similarly,    $(O_{12} - E_{12}) = -(ad - bc)/n$, $(O_{21} - E_{21}) = -(ad - bc)/n$ and $(O_{22} - E_{22})/n = (ad - bc)/n$. Further, $[(1/E_{11}) + (1/E_{12}) + (1/E_{21}) + (1/E_{22})] = n[(1/R_1C_1) + (1/R_2C_1) + (1/R_1C_2) + (1/R_2C_2)] = n[(1/C_1)((1/R_1 + 1/R_2) + (1/C_2((1/R_1 + 1/R_2)) = n^2(1/C_1R_1R_2 + 1/C_2R_1R_2) = n^2/R_1R_2C_1C_2$. From these expressions, (9.4) becomes the same as (9.4a).

For the correction factor, consider (a,d) to be larger than (b,c). The former pair are replaced by $(a - 1/2, d - 1/2)$ and the latter by $(b + 1/2, c + 1/2)$. Now, $(O_{11} - E_{11}) = (O_{22} - E_{22}) = [(ad - bc) - n/2]/n$ and $(O_{12} - E_{12}) = (O_{21} - E_{21}) = -[(ad - bc) - n/2]/n$. Sum of the expected frequencies remains the same as above. With these corrections, (9.4) becomes (9.5) and (9.5a).

## A9.2    Equality of the proportions

Consider the equality of the two column proportions. The estimates of the proportions are $\hat{p}_1 = a/C_1$, $\hat{p}_2 = b/C_2$ and $(\hat{p}_1 - \hat{p}_2) = (ad - bc)/C_1C_2$. When the null hypothesis of equality of the proportions is valid, the estimate of the common proportion is $\hat{p} = (a + b)/n$, $\hat{p}\hat{q}(1/C_1 + 1/C_2) = R_1R_2/nC_1C_2$, $Z = (\hat{p}_1 - \hat{p}_2)/[\hat{p}\hat{q}(1/C_1 + 1/C_2)]^{1/2} = (ad - bc)/(R_1R_2C_1C_2/n)^{1/2}$, and $U = Z^2 = n(ad - bc)^2/R_1R_2C_1C_2$.

If $\hat{p}_1$ is larger than $\hat{p}_2$, $(a, b)$ are replaced by $(a - 1/2, b + 1/2)$. Now, $(\hat{p}_1 - \hat{p}_2) = [(ad - bc) - (n/2)]/C_1C_2$. If $\hat{p}_2$ is larger than $\hat{p}_1$, $(a, b)$ are replaced by $(a + 1/2, b - 1/2)$. In this case, $(\hat{p}_1 - \hat{p}_2) = [-(ad - bc) - (n/2)/C_1C_2$. In either case, $Z = \{|(ad - bc)| - (n/2)\}/(R_1R_2C_1C_2/n)^{1/2}$ and $U = Z^2 = n[|ad - bc)| - (n/2)]^2/R_1R_2C_1C_2$.

# 10

# Regression and correlation

## 10.1 Introduction

Heights and weights of children increase with their age. Increase of weight may result in increased levels of hypertension of adults. The relationship of systolic blood pressure (SBP), for instance, on age, weight and other relevant factors can be examined through regression analysis. In this illustration, SBP is the *dependent* variable and age and weight are the *independent* or explanatory variables. The relationship between these variables may be linear or nonlinear. In some applications, one or both these variables may be categorical.

Linear and Multiple Regression, Least Squares Method of estimation, Analysis of Variance (ANOVA) tests for the significance of the regression, confidence limits for the regression coefficients, prediction intervals for the dependent variable and related topics are presented in the following sections. Logistic regression with dichotomous and continuous predictors and the estimation of the odds ratio are illustrated. The final sections present the simple, partial and multiple correlation coefficients, tests of hypotheses and confidence limits for the correlation between two random variables. The rank correlation coefficient is also described.

## 10.2 The regression model: One independent variable

To examine whether the SBPs of a population of adults significantly depend on their weights, they can be considered as the dependent and independent variables $Y$ and $X$ respectively, or as the criterion and predictor variables. For persons weighing 160 lbs,

*Statistical Methodologies with Medical Applications*, First Edition. Poduri S.R.S. Rao.
© 2017 John Wiley & Sons, Ltd. Published 2017 by John Wiley & Sons, Ltd.

for instance, the distribution of the SBPs may vary about the mean of 130 mm/Hg. Similarly, it may vary about the mean of 140 mm/Hg for persons weighing 170 lbs. Consider $k$ values $X_i$, $i = (1, 2, ..., k)$, of the weights with mean $E(Y|X_i)$ and variance $V(Y|X_i)$ at $X_i$. If the means fall on a straight line and the variances at each $X_i$ are the same, they can be expressed as

$$E(Y|X_i) = \beta_0 + \beta_1 X_i \tag{10.1a}$$

and

$$V(Y|X_i) = \sigma^2. \tag{10.1b}$$

The coefficient $\beta_1$ is the *slope* of the *regression line* in (10.1a), and it is the rate of change of $E(Y|X_i)$ with respect to $X$. If $X$ increases to $X_2$ from $X_1$, the rate of increase of $E(Y|X)$ becomes

$$\beta_1 = [E(Y|X_2) - E(Y|X_1)]/(X_2 - X_1), \tag{10.2}$$

which is the derivative of $E(Y|X_i)$ with respect to $X$. If $X$ decreases to $X_2$ from $X_1$, the rate of decrease of $E(Y|X)$ is obtained from replacing the denominator by $(X_1 - X_2)$. The *intercept* $\beta_0$ of this line is $E(Y|X_i)$ at $X_i = 0$. In some practical situations, the independent variable can be $X_i$ or one of its transformations, for instance, $X_i^2$ or $ln(X_i)$. For some applications, the variance $V(Y|X_i)$ need not be the same at each $X_i$, and the modification required for this case will be described later.

For a random sample $(Y_1, Y_2, ..., Y_n)$ of independent observations at $(X_1, X_2, ..., X_n)$ the *linear regression* equation becomes

$$Y_i = \beta_0 + \beta_1 X_i + \varepsilon_i. \qquad i = (1, 2, ..., n) \tag{10.3}$$

For an individual unit, the deviation from the mean

$$\varepsilon_i = Y_i - E(Y|X_i) = Y_i - (\beta_0 + \beta_1 X_i) \tag{10.3a}$$

is the *random error* at $X_i$ with the following assumptions:

1. $E(\varepsilon_i|X_i) = 0$,

2. $V(\varepsilon_i|X_i) = \sigma^2$, same at each $X_i$,

3. the random errors $\varepsilon_i$ at each $X_i$ are uncorrelated, and

4. these errors at different values of the independent variable are uncorrelated, that is, $Cov(\varepsilon_i, \varepsilon_j|X_i, X_j) = 0$ for $(i \neq j)$.

The first assumption follows from (10.3a) and the third and fourth follow from the independence of the sample observations $(Y_1, Y_2, ..., Y_n)$. Modifications to the model in (10.3) and these assumptions are made suitable to the applications.

Galton (1885) examined the linear relationship of the heights of 930 adult children on the heights of 250 of their respective mid-parent heights, averages of the heights of each parent. To correct for sex, heights of the female children were multiplied by 1.08. He found the offspring "to be smaller than the parents, if the parents were large; to be larger than the parents, if the parents were small." Children of taller parents tend to be taller, but shorter than their parents. Similarly, children of shorter parents tend to be shorter, but taller than their parents. Galton characterized this tendency as the *Regression to the Mean*. In his study, the average heights of both the parents ($X$) and sons ($Y$) were close to 68 inches, and their standard deviations were almost the same. The estimate of the slope coefficient was (2/3).With this slope, the estimate of the regression line for the sons becomes $(\hat{Y}-68) = (2/3)(X-68)$. If the height of a mid-parent's $X = 64$, for instance, smaller than the average of 68, their son's height is $\hat{Y} = 68 - (2/3)(4) = 65.33$ and the son is taller than the parent. On the other hand, if the height of the mid-parent is $X = 72$, larger than the average of 68, the son's height becomes $\hat{Y} = 68 + (2/3)4 = 70.67$ and the son is shorter than the parent. From these historical beginnings, *regression* analysis has become a commonplace in several types of statistical studies. From the above equation, estimates ($\hat{Y}$) of sons' heights at the heights of fathers ($X$) are as follows:

Galton's regression of son's height on father's height.

| Father's height ($X$): | 62 | 64 | 66 | 68 | 70 | 72 | 74 |
|---|---|---|---|---|---|---|---|
| Son's height ($\hat{Y}$) | 64 | 65.33 | 66.67 | 68 | 69.33 | 70.67 | 72 |

## 10.2.1   Least squares estimation of the regression

With the above assumptions for $\varepsilon_i$, the Least Squares (LS) Estimators of the intercept, slope and $E(Y|X_i)$ are obtained by minimizing

$$\phi = \sum_{1}^{n} (Y_i - \beta_0 - \beta_1 X_i)^2 \tag{10.4}$$

with respect to $\beta_0$ and $\beta_1$.

Setting the first derivatives of (10.4) with respect to these coefficients to zero results in the following equations for the estimators $\hat{\beta}_0$ and $\hat{\beta}_1$:

$$\sum_{1}^{n} (Y_i - \hat{\beta}_0 - \hat{\beta}_1 X_i) = 0 \tag{10.5a}$$

and

$$\sum_{1}^{n} (Y_i - \hat{\beta}_0 - \hat{\beta}_1 X_i) X_i = 0. \tag{10.5b}$$

These estimating equations are known as the *normal equations* although they are not in general related to the normal distribution.

As solutions of these two equations, the estimators become

$$\hat{\beta}_0 = \bar{Y} - \hat{\beta}_1 \bar{X} \tag{10.6a}$$

and

$$\hat{\beta}_1 = \frac{\sum_1^n (X_i - \bar{X})(Y_i - \bar{Y})}{\sum_1^n (X_i - \bar{X})^2} = \frac{\sum_1^n (X_i - \bar{X})(Y_i - \bar{Y})/(n-1)}{\sum_1^n (X_i - \bar{X})^2/(n-1)} = \frac{S_{xy}}{S_x^2}. \tag{10.6b}$$

The numerator and denominator of the right-hand side expression of (10.6b) are the sample covariance of $(X, Y)$ and variance of $X$. Notice that $\hat{\beta}_1 = S_{xy}/S_x^2 = r(S_x/S_y)$, where $r = S_{xy}/S_x S_y$ is the sample correlation of $X$ and $Y$. This estimator can also be expressed as $\sum_1^n x_i y_i / \sum_1^n x_i^2$ or $\left[\sum_i^n x_i y_i/(n-1)\right]/\left[\sum_1^n x_i^2/(n-1)\right]$, where $x_i = (X_i - \bar{X})$ and $y_i = (Y_i - \bar{Y})$. The estimator for the mean $E(Y|X_i)$ at $X_i$ is given by

$$\hat{Y}_i = \hat{\beta}_0 + \hat{\beta}_1 X_i = \bar{Y} + \hat{\beta}_1 (X_i - \bar{X}), \tag{10.7}$$

that is,

$$(\hat{Y}_i - \bar{Y}) = \hat{\beta}_1 (X_i - \bar{X}). \tag{10.7a}$$

These Least Squares Estimators for the intercept, slope and $E(Y|X_i)$ are linear functions of the observed values $Y_i$ of the dependent variable at the given or specified values $X_i$ of the independent variable. Note that $\sum_1^n (X_i - \bar{X})(Y_i - \bar{Y})$ is the same as $\sum_1^n (X_i - \bar{X}) Y_i$.

## 10.2.2    Properties of the estimators

From (10.3), the expectations of $\hat{\beta}_0$, $\hat{\beta}_1$ and $\hat{Y}_i$ are respectively equal to $\beta_0$, $\beta_1$ and $E(Y|X_i)$, that is, they are *unbiased* estimators. The variances of these estimators are

$$V(\hat{\beta}_0) = \sigma^2 \left[ \frac{1}{n} + \frac{\bar{X}^2}{\sum_1^n (X_i - \bar{X})^2} \right], \tag{10.8}$$

$$V(\hat{\beta}_1) = \frac{\sigma^2}{\sum_1^n (X_i - \bar{X})^2} \tag{10.9}$$

and

$$V(\hat{Y}_i) = (\sigma^2/n) + (X_i - \bar{X})^2 V(\hat{\beta}_1)$$

$$= \sigma^2 \left[ \frac{1}{n} + \frac{(X_i - \bar{X})^2}{\sum_1^n (X_i - \bar{X})^2} \right]. \tag{10.10}$$

These variances decrease as the dispersion $\sum_1^n (X_i - \bar{X})^2$ of the independent variable increases. The *precision* of an estimator increases as its variance decreases, and $X_i$ should be farther apart for these variances to become small. The Standard Errors (S.E.s) of $\hat{\beta}_0, \hat{\beta}_1$ and $\hat{Y}_i$ are given by $\sqrt{V(\hat{\beta}_0)}$, $\sqrt{V(\hat{\beta}_1)}$ and $\sqrt{V(\hat{Y}_i)}$. Additional related results are $Cov(\hat{\beta}_0, \hat{\beta}_1) = -\bar{X}V(\hat{\beta}_1)$, and $\hat{\beta}_1$ is uncorrelated with $\bar{Y}$.

The observed residuals are $e_i = Y_i - \hat{Y}_i$, $i = (1, 2, ..., n)$. The normal equations in (10.5a) and (10.5b) are the same as $\sum_1^n e_i = 0$ and $\sum_1^n e_i X_i = 0$. From these results, it can be seen that (a) the average of the residuals $\bar{e} = \sum_1^n e_i/n = 0$, that is, average of $\hat{Y}_i$ is the same as $\bar{Y}$, and (b) $e_i$ and $\hat{Y}_i$ are uncorrelated. The sample correlation of $(X, Y)$ is $r = (S_{xy}/S_x S_y)$. From (10.7), the square of the correlation of $Y_i$ and $\hat{Y}_i$ is the same as $r^2$, as shown in Appendix A10.1.

An unbiased estimator of $\sigma^2$ is given by

$$\hat{\sigma}^2 = \frac{\sum_1^n e_i^2}{n-2} = \frac{\sum_1^n (Y_i - \hat{Y}_i)^2}{n-2}, \tag{10.11}$$

with $(n-2)$ d.f. The estimates $v(\hat{\beta}_1), v(\hat{\beta}_0)$ and $v(\hat{Y}_i)$ of the variances in (10.8), (10.9) and (10.10) are obtained from replacing $\sigma^2$ by $\hat{\sigma}^2$ in these expressions. The sample S.E.s of $\hat{\beta}_0, \hat{\beta}_1$ and $\hat{Y}_i$ are obtained from the square roots of these sample variances.

## 10.2.3 ANOVA (Analysis of Variance) for the significance of the regression

With the observed $Y_i$ and the estimates $\hat{Y}_i$, the Total Sum of Squares (SST) can be expressed as

$$\sum_1^n (Y_i - \bar{Y})^2 = \sum_1^n \left[ (\hat{Y}_i - \bar{Y}) + (Y_i - \hat{Y}_i) \right]^2 = \sum_1^n (\hat{Y}_i - \bar{Y})^2 + \sum_1^n (Y_i - \hat{Y}_i)^2. \tag{10.12}$$

The sum of the cross products of the middle term vanishes. The right-hand side expressions are the Regression and Residual (Error) Sums of Squares, SSR and SSE respectively. The equations in (10.12) can be expressed as $SST = SSR + SSE$.

From (10.7), SSR is the same as $\hat{\beta}_1^2 \sum_1^n (X_i - \bar{X})^2 = \hat{\beta}_1 \sum_1^n (X_i - \bar{X})(Y_i - \bar{Y})$, and $r^2 = (SSR/SST)$. As shown in Appendix A10.1, $r^2$ is also the square of the correlation of $Y_i$ and $\hat{Y}_i$.

When $\varepsilon_i$ follows the normal distribution with zero mean and variance $\sigma^2$, the test for the *Significance of the Regression*, that is, $H_0 : \beta_1 = 0$ *versus* $H_1 : \beta_1 \neq 0$ is provided by the $F$-ratio with 1 and $(n-2)$ d.f. as presented in Table 10.1, the ANOVA (Analysis of Variance) table. The sums of squares are denoted by SS. The mean squares denoted by MS are obtained from dividing the SS by their respective d.f. Note that $F_{1,(n-2)} = t_{n-2}^2$.

As noted before, the Error Mean Square $\hat{\sigma}^2 = SSE/(n-2)$ in (10.11) is unbiased for $\sigma^2$. With one independent variable as in this case, the Regression Mean Square is the same as the Regression Sum of Squares. Its expected value, $\sigma^2 + \beta_1^2 \sum_1^n (X_i - \bar{X})^2$, becomes larger than $\sigma^2$ as the absolute value $|\beta_1|$ of the slope coefficient becomes larger than zero.

*Example 10.1*   Regression of LDL on weight : Age, weight, weekly time (minutes) for physical activity and exercise (FIT), LDL and HDL for a random sample of 20 adults along with their summary figures are presented in Tables T10.1(a)–T10.1 (d). For the regression of LDL (Y) on weight (X), from (10.6a), (10.6b) and (10.7),

$$\hat{\beta}_0 = -213.6, \; \hat{\beta}_1 = 2.23$$

and

$$\hat{Y}_i = -213.6 + 2.23 X_i.$$
$$(50.9) \; (0.3326)$$

The S.E.s of the estimates of the intercept and slope coefficients obtained from (10.8) and (10.9) are presented in the parentheses. The test statistics for the hypotheses that $\beta_0 = 0$ and $\beta_1 = 0$ are $t_{18} = -(213.6/50.9) = -4.2$ and $t_{18} = (2.23/0.3326) = 6.72$ respectively. The ANOVA and the $F$-test for the significance of the regression, that is $H_0 : \beta_1 = 0$ are presented in the following table.

ANOVA for the regression of LDL on weight.

| Source | d.f | SS | MS | F | p-value |
|---|---|---|---|---|---|
| Regression | 1 | 21266.93 | 21266.93 | 45.10 | $2.67 \times 10^{-6}$ |
| Residual | 18 | 8487.27 | 471.52 | | |
| Total | 19 | 29754.2 | | | |

The regression of LDL on weight is highly significant with the very small $p$-value. The discrepancy between $F = 45.10$ and $t^2 = (6.78)^2 = 45.16$ is due to the rounding-off of the decimals.

## 10.2.4    Tests of hypotheses, confidence limits and prediction intervals

It is of practical importance to examine whether the intercept and slope coefficients are significantly different from zero or they are equal to specified values. The null hypothesis $H_0 : \beta_0 = 0$ examines whether the regression line goes through the origin, and $H_0 : \beta_0 = \beta_0'$ is intended to test whether the intercept takes the specified value $\beta_0'$. Similarly, $H_0 : \beta_1 = 0$ and $H_0 : \beta_1 = \beta_1'$ respectively examine whether the regression of $Y$ on $X$ is significant and whether the slope coefficient takes the specified value $\beta_1'$. It is also of importance to investigate whether the mean $E(Y|X_i)$ takes a specified value $\mu_0$. The test statistics for the above hypotheses and confidence limits for $\beta_0$, $\beta_1$ and $E(Y|X_i)$ are presented in Table 10.2.

The alternative hypothesis in each case can be one-sided or two-sided. The test statistics follow the $t$-distribution with $(n-2)$ d.f, same degrees of freedom of the error mean square $\hat{\sigma}^2$. With one independent variable in the regression model, $t_{n-2}^2$ is the same as $F(1, n-2)$. The square of the Test Statistic for $H_0 : \beta_1 = 0$ is the same as the $F$-ratio in Table 10.1.

Table 10.1    ANOVA for the Significance of the Regression with one independent variable.

| Source | d.f | SS | MS | $F$ |
|---|---|---|---|---|
| Regression | 1 | SSR | SSR | $(SSR/1)/\hat{\sigma}^2$ |
| Residual | $n-2$ | SSE | $\hat{\sigma}^2 = SSE/(n-2)$ | |
| Total | $n-1$ | SST | | |

Table 10.2    Hypotheses, Test Statistics and Confidence Limits; regression on one independent variable.

| $H_0$ | Test statistic | $(1-\alpha)$ percent confidence limits |
|---|---|---|
| $\beta_0 = 0$ | $\hat{\beta}_0/\sqrt{v(\hat{\beta}_0)}$ | $\hat{\beta}_0 \pm t_{n-2,\alpha/2}\sqrt{v(\hat{\beta}_0)}$ |
| $\beta_0 = \beta_0'$ | $(\hat{\beta}_0 - \beta_0')/\sqrt{v(\hat{\beta}_0)}$ | |
| $\beta_1 = 0$ | $\hat{\beta}_1/\sqrt{v(\hat{\beta}_1)}$ | $\hat{\beta}_1 \pm t_{n-2,\alpha/2}\sqrt{v(\hat{\beta}_1)}$ |
| $\beta_1 = \beta_1'$ | $(\hat{\beta}_1 - \hat{\beta}_1')/\sqrt{v(\hat{\beta}_1)}$ | |
| $E(Y|X_i) = \mu_0$ | $(\hat{Y}_i - \mu_0)/\sqrt{v(\hat{Y}_i)}$ | $\hat{Y}_i \pm t_{n-2,\alpha/2}\sqrt{v(\hat{Y}_i)}$ |

As presented in Table 10.2, $(1-\alpha)$ percent confidence limits for $E(Y|X_i)$ are obtained from

$$\hat{Y}_i \pm t_{n-2,\alpha/2}\sqrt{v(\hat{Y}_i)}. \qquad (10.13)$$

At an individual or new value $X_{new}$ of the independent variable, the *predicted value* of the dependent variable $Y_i$ is

$$\hat{Y}_{new} = \hat{\beta}_0 + \hat{\beta}_1 X_{new}. \qquad (10.14)$$

The variance of the error of prediction becomes

$$V(\hat{Y}_{new} - Y_i) = V(\hat{Y}_{new}) + V(Y_i)$$

$$= \left[\frac{1}{n} + \frac{(X_{new}-\bar{X})^2}{\sum_1^n (X_i-\bar{X})^2}\right]\sigma^2 + \sigma^2. \qquad (10.15)$$

Replacing $\sigma^2$ in this expression by its estimator $\hat{\sigma}^2$ in (10.11), the $(1-\alpha)$ percent prediction limits for $Y_i$ at $X_{new}$ are obtained from

$$\hat{Y}_{new} \pm t_{n-2,\alpha/2}\hat{\sigma}\left[1 + \frac{1}{n} + \frac{(X_{new}-\bar{X})^2}{\sum_1^n (X_i-\bar{X})^2}\right]^{1/2}. \qquad (10.16)$$

As can be expected, the prediction interval in (10.16) for the individual value of the dependent variable is wider than the interval in (10.13) for the mean.

For the regression of LDL $(Y)$ on weight $(X)$, the estimate $\hat{Y}_i = \hat{\beta}_0 + \hat{\beta}_1 X_i$ for the regression equation (solid line), its 95 percent confidence and prediction limits for different values of the weight $(X)$ obtained from the *MINITAB* are presented in Figure 10.1. They are further examined in Example 10.2

*Example 10.2*   Inference for the regression of LDL on weight. For the regression of LDL $(Y)$ on weight $(X)$, the estimates of the intercept, slope, their S.E.s and related statistics are presented below:

| Coefficient | Estimate | S.E. | $t$ | $p$-value | Confidence limits $(\alpha = .05)$ |
|---|---|---|---|---|---|
| Intercept | −213.60 | 50.90 | −4.20 | 0.0005 | (−320.54, −106.66) |
| Slope | 2.23 | 0.3326 | 6.72 | $2.67 \times 10^{-6}$ | (1.53, 2.93) |

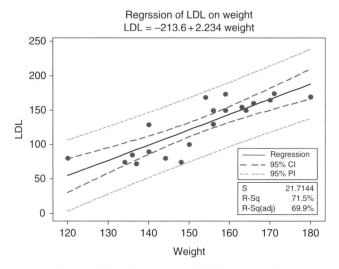

*Figure 10.1    Regression of LDL on weight.*

As can be seen from the t-statistic of 6.72 with 18 d.f. for the slope and the $F$-value of 45.10 with (1, 18) d.f. in the ANOVA table of Example 10.1, the regression of LDL on weight is highly significant.

From (10.7), the estimate of the mean $E(Y|X_i) = \beta_0 + \beta_1 X_i$ at the weight $X_i = 150$ is $\hat{Y}_i = -213.6 + 2.23(150) = 120.9$. With this value for the weight and $\hat{\sigma}^2 = 471.52$, from (10.10), $v(\hat{Y}_i) = 24.18$ and $S.E.(\hat{Y}_i) = 4.92$. With $t_{18,\,0.025} = 2.101$, from (10.13), 95 percent confidence limits for $E(Y|X = 150)$ are $120.9 - 2.101(4.92) = 110.56$ and $120.9 + 2.101(4.92) = 131.24$.

For a new value of $X_i = 160$, the predicted value is $\hat{Y}_{new} = -213.6 + 2.23(160) = 143.2$. With $\hat{\sigma}^2 = 471.52$, the estimate of the variance in (10.15) becomes $v(\hat{Y}_{new} - Y_{new}) = 471.52\left[1 + (1/20) + (160 - 152.35)^2/4262.65\right] = 501.57$. From (10.16), 95 percent prediction limits for the LDL at this value for the weight become $143.2 - 2.101(22.4) = 96.14$ and $143.2 + 2.101(22.4) = 190.26$.

## 10.3    Regression on two independent variables

In practice, a diagnostic or physical characteristic may depend on more than one independent variable, for instance, LDL ($Y$) on age ($X_1$) and weight ($X_2$). The means of $Y$ at given values ($X_{1i}, X_{2i}$) of these variables can be considered to lie on the plane with the equation

$$E(Y|X_{1i}, X_{2i}) = \beta_0 + \beta_1 X_{1i} + \beta_2 X_{2i}. \tag{10.17}$$

The slopes of this plane on the $X_1$ and $X_2$ axes are denoted by $(\beta_1, \beta_2)$ and its intercept with the $Y$ axis by $\beta_0$. The regression equation

$$Y_i = E(Y|X_{1i}, X_{2i}) + \varepsilon_i = \beta_0 + \beta_1 X_{1i} + \beta_2 X_{2i} + \varepsilon_i \tag{10.18}$$

represents the individual observations of the dependent variable at the fixed values $(X_{1i}, X_{2i})$ of the independent variables with $E(\varepsilon_i|X_{1i}, X_{2i}) = 0$. It is assumed that $V(\varepsilon_i|X_{1i}, X_{2i}) = \sigma^2$, same at each $(X_{1i}, X_{2i})$. From (10.18), note that $V(Y|X_{1i}, X_{2i}) = \sigma^2$.

The Least Squares Estimators $(\hat{\beta}_0, \hat{\beta}_1, \hat{\beta}_2)$ of the regression coefficients are obtained from minimizing

$$\phi = \sum_1^n \left(Y_i - \hat{\beta}_0 - \hat{\beta}_1 X_{1i} - \hat{\beta}_2 X_{2i}\right)^2 \tag{10.19}$$

with respect to these coefficients. The resulting *normal equations* obtained from the derivatives of (10.19) become

$$\sum_1^n \left(Y - \hat{\beta}_1 X_{1i} - \hat{\beta}_2 X_{2i}\right) = 0, \tag{10.20a}$$

$$\sum_1^n \left(Y - \hat{\beta}_0 - \hat{\beta}_1 X_{1i} - \hat{\beta}_2 X_{2i}\right) X_{1i} = 0 \tag{10.20b}$$

and

$$\sum_1^n \left(Y - \hat{\beta}_0 - \hat{\beta}_1 X_{1i} - \hat{\beta}_2 X_{2i}\right) X_{2i} = 0. \tag{10.20c}$$

Denoting $(Y, X_1, X_2)$ by the subscripts $(0, 1, 2)$, their sample variances can be expressed as $(S_{00}, S_{11}, S_{22})$ and the covariances as $(S_{01}, S_{02}, S_{12})$. From the above normal equations,

$$\hat{\beta}_0 = \bar{Y} - \hat{\beta}_1 \bar{X}_1 - \hat{\beta}_2 \bar{X}_2, \tag{10.21a}$$

$$\hat{\beta}_1 = (S_{10}S_{22} - S_{20}S_{21}) / (S_{11}S_{22} - S_{12}^2) \tag{10.21b}$$

and

$$\hat{\beta}_2 = (S_{20}S_{11} - S_{10}S_{12}) / (S_{11}S_{22} - S_{12}^2). \tag{10.21c}$$

The estimator for the mean $E(Y|X_{1i}, X_{2i})$ becomes

$$\hat{Y}_i = \hat{\beta} + \hat{\beta} X_{1i} + \hat{\beta}_2 X_{2i} = \bar{Y} + \hat{\beta}_1 x_{1i} + \hat{\beta}_2 x_{2i}, \tag{10.22}$$

where $x_{1i} = (X_{1i} - \bar{X}_1)$ and $x_{2i} = (X_{2i} - \bar{X}_2)$.

## 10.3.1    Properties of the estimators

The three estimators in (10.21a)–(10.21c) are *unbiased* for $(\beta_0, \beta_1, \beta_2)$ respectively. Further,

$$V(\hat{\beta}_1) = \sigma^2 / (1 - r_{12}^2) \sum_1^n x_{1i}^2, \tag{10.23a}$$

$$V(\hat{\beta}_2) = \sigma^2 / (1 - r_{12}^2) \sum_1^n x_{2i}^2 \tag{10.23b}$$

and

$$Cov(\hat{\beta}_1, \hat{\beta}_2) = -\sigma^2 \sum_1^n x_{1i} x_{2i} / (1 - r_{12}^2) \sum_1^n x_{1i}^2 \sum_1^n x_{2i}^2 \tag{10.23c}$$

where $r_{12} = S_{12} / (S_{11} S_{22})^{1/2}$ is the correlation of $(X_1, X_2)$. The covariances of $\hat{\beta}_1$ and $\hat{\beta}_2$ with $\bar{Y}$ are zero. From (10.21a),

$$V(\hat{\beta}_0) = \sigma^2 / n + \bar{X}_1^2 V(\hat{\beta}_1) + \bar{X}_2^2 V(\hat{\beta}_2) + 2\bar{X}_1 \bar{X}_2 Cov(\hat{\beta}_1, \hat{\beta}_2). \tag{10.24}$$

Further,

$$Cov(\hat{\beta}_0, \hat{\beta}_1) = -\bar{X}_1 V(\hat{\beta}_1) - \bar{X}_2 Cov(\hat{\beta}_1, \hat{\beta}_2) \tag{10.24a}$$

and

$$Cov(\hat{\beta}_0, \hat{\beta}_2) = -\bar{X}_2 V(\hat{\beta}_2) - \bar{X}_1 Cov(\hat{\beta}_1, \hat{\beta}_2). \tag{10.24b}$$

The S.E.s of $(\hat{\beta}_0, \hat{\beta}_1, \hat{\beta}_2)$ are obtained from the square roots of their variances given above. It is desirable that the S.E.s of $\hat{\beta}_1$ and $\hat{\beta}_2$ should be small. Notice from (10.23a) and (10.23b) that they decrease as the variances of $X_1$ and $X_2$ increase but their correlation decreases. The estimator $\hat{Y}_i$ in (10.22) is unbiased for $E(Y|X_{1i}, X_{2i})$ with variance

$$V(\hat{Y}_i | X_{1i}, X_{2i}) = (\sigma^2 / n) + x_{1i}^2 V(\hat{\beta}_1) + x_{2i}^2 V(\hat{\beta}_2) + 2x_{1i} x_{2i} Cov(\hat{\beta}_1, \hat{\beta}_2). \tag{10.25}$$

An unbiased estimator of $\sigma^2$ is given by

$$\hat{\sigma}^2 = \frac{\sum_1^n e_i^2}{n-3} = \frac{\sum_1^n (Y_i - \hat{Y}_i)^2}{n-3} \tag{10.26}$$

with $(n-3)$ d.f. The sample estimates $v(\hat{\beta}_0), v(\hat{\beta}_1)$ and $v(\hat{\beta}_2)$ of the variances of the coefficients and also of the covariance in (10.23c) are obtained by replacing $\sigma^2$

with $\hat{\sigma}^2$. The sample S.E.s of $(\hat{\beta}_0, \hat{\beta}_1, \hat{\beta}_2)$ are given by the square roots of these estimates. The sample estimate $v(\hat{Y}_i)$ of the variance in (10.25) and $S.E(\hat{Y}_i) = \sqrt{v(\hat{Y}_i)}$ are similarly obtained with $\hat{\sigma}^2$.

The observed residuals are $e_i = (Y_i - \hat{Y}_i)$. For the model in (10.18), from (10.20a),

$$\sum_1^n e_i = 0,$$ that is, their average $\bar{e} = \sum_1^n e_i/n = 0.$ Notice from (10.20b) and (10.20c) that the sample correlations of $e_i$ with $(X_{1i}, X_{2i})$ vanish. As in the case of the single independent variable, $e_i$ becomes uncorrelated with $\hat{Y}_i$.

## 10.3.2   ANOVA for the significance of the regression

The Total Sum of Squares SST can be expressed as

$$\sum_1^n (Y_i - \bar{Y})^2 = \sum_1^n (\hat{Y}_i - \bar{Y})^2 + \sum_1^n (Y_i - \hat{Y}_i)^2. \tag{10.27}$$

The first term on the right-hand side of this expression is the Regression Sum of Squares, which becomes

$$SSR = \hat{\beta}_1^2 \sum_1^n x_{1i}^2 + \hat{\beta}_2^2 \sum_1^n x_{2i}^2 + 2\hat{\beta}_1\hat{\beta}_2 \sum_1^n x_{1i}x_{2i} = \hat{\beta}_1 \sum_1^n x_{1i}y_i + \hat{\beta}_2 \sum_1^n x_{2i}y_i. \tag{10.28}$$

In this expression, $\sum_1^n x_{1i}y_i = \sum_1^n (X_{1i} - \bar{X})(Y_i - \bar{Y})$ and $\sum_1^n x_{2i}y_i = \sum_1^n (X_{2i} - \bar{X})(Y_i - \bar{Y})$. With the observed residuals $e_i = (Y_i - \hat{Y}_i)$, $i = (1, 2, \ldots, n)$, the second term of (10.27) is the Residual or Error Sum of Squares $SSE = \sum_1^n e_i^2$.

The null hypothesis to examine whether $Y$ significantly depends on $X_1$ and $X_2$ is $H_0: \beta_1 = 0$ and $\beta_2 = 0$, *versus* the alternative hypothesis $H_1$ that it does not depend on $X_1$ or $X_2$ or both, that is, either $\beta_1 \neq 0, \beta_2 \neq 0$ or $(\beta_1, \beta_2) \neq 0$. When $\varepsilon_i$ follows the normal distribution with zero mean and variance $\sigma^2$, the test statistic for this null hypothesis is provided by the $F$-ratio with 2 and $(n - 3)$ d.f. as shown in Table 10.3.

*Example 10.3*   ANOVA for the regression of LDL ($Y$) on age ($X_1$) and weight ($X_2$): From the sample observations in Table (T10.1). The means of the three variables are (126.7, 42.75, 152.35). From (10.21a)–(10.21c), $\hat{\beta}_0 = -176.44$, $\hat{\beta}_1 = 0.89$ and $\hat{\beta}_2 = 1.74$. The estimate for $E(Y|X_1, X_2)$ in (10.22) becomes $\hat{Y}_i = -176.44 + 0.89X_{1i} + 1.74X_{2i}$. The ANOVA for the significance of the regression is given below. The regression of LDL on age and weight is highly significant.

Table 10.3    ANOVA for the significance of the regression on two independent variables.

| Source | d.f | SS | MS | F |
|---|---|---|---|---|
| Regression | 2 | $\sum_{1}^{n}\left(\hat{Y}_i-\bar{Y}\right)^2$ | $\sum_{1}^{n}\left(\hat{Y}_i-\bar{Y}\right)^2/2$ | $\left[\sum_{1}^{n}\left(\hat{Y}_i-\bar{Y}\right)^2/2\right]/\hat{\sigma}^2$ |
| Residual | $(n-3)$ | $\sum_{1}^{n}\left(Y_i-\hat{Y}_i\right)^2$ | $\hat{\sigma}^2=\sum_{1}^{n}\left(Y_i-\hat{Y}_i\right)^2/(n-3)$ | |
| Total | $(n-1)$ | $\sum_{1}^{n}\left(Y_i-\bar{Y}\right)^2$ | | |

ANOVA for the regression of LDL ($Y$) on age ($X_1$) and weight ($X_2$).

| Source | d.f | SS | MS | F | $P$-value |
|---|---|---|---|---|---|
| Regression | 2 | 22132.96 | 11066 | 24.68 | $9.39\times10^{-6}$ |
| Residual | 17 | 7621.23 | 448.31 | | |
| Total | 19 | 29754.19 | | | |

### 10.3.3    Tests of hypotheses, confidence limits and prediction intervals

When the hypothesis that $Y$ does not depend on $X_1$ and $X_2$ is rejected through the $F$-test of the above ANOVA procedure, it can be further examined whether $Y$ depends significantly on either of these independent variables. The corresponding hypotheses for this purpose are $H_0:\beta_1=0$ versus $H_1:\beta_1\neq0$ and $H_0:\beta_2=0$ versus $H_1:\beta_2\neq0$.

An unbiased estimator of the difference $(\beta_1-\beta_2)$ of the slope coefficients is given by $(\hat{\beta}_1-\hat{\beta}_2)$ with variance

$$V\left(\hat{\beta}_1-\hat{\beta}_2\right)=V\left(\hat{\beta}_1\right)+V\left(\hat{\beta}_2\right)-2Cov\left(\hat{\beta}_1,\hat{\beta}_2\right). \qquad (10.29)$$

This variance can be obtained from (10.23a)–(10.23c). Its sample estimate $v\left(\hat{\beta}-\hat{\beta}_{21}\right)$ is obtained by replacing $\sigma^2$ with $\hat{\sigma}^2$. The sample $S.E.\left(\hat{\beta}_1-\hat{\beta}_2\right)$ is given by the square root of the resulting sample variance. The test statistic for $H_0:\beta_1=\beta_2$, that is, $(\beta_1-\beta_2)=0$ becomes $t_{n-3}=\left(\hat{\beta}_1-\hat{\beta}_2\right)/S.E.\left(\hat{\beta}_1-\hat{\beta}_2\right)$.

The test statistics for the above hypotheses and the confidence limits for the regression coefficients and the mean $E(Y|X_{1i},X_{2i})$. are presented in Table 10.4.

The *predicted value* $Y_{\text{new}}$ of the dependent variable at the individual or new values $\left(X_1',X_2'\right)$ of the independent variables is obtained from

Table 10.4   Hypotheses, Test Statistics and Confidence Limits for the regression on two independent variables.

| $H_0$ | Test Statistic | $(1-\alpha)$ percent Confidence Limits |
|---|---|---|
| $\beta_0 = 0$ | $\hat{\beta}_0 / \sqrt{v(\hat{\beta}_0)}$ | $\hat{\beta}_0 \pm t_{n-3,\alpha/2} \sqrt{v(\hat{\beta}_0)}$ |
| $\beta_0 = \beta_0'$ | $(\hat{\beta}_0 - \beta_0') / \sqrt{v(\hat{\beta}_0)}$ | |
| $\beta_1 = 0$ | $\hat{\beta}_1 / \sqrt{v(\hat{\beta}_1)}$ | $\hat{\beta}_1 \pm t_{n-3,\alpha/2} \sqrt{v(\hat{\beta}_1)}$ |
| $\beta_1 = \beta_1'$ | $(\hat{\beta}_1 - \beta_1') / \sqrt{v(\hat{\beta}_1)}$ | $\hat{\beta}_2 \pm t_{n-3,\alpha/2} \sqrt{v(\hat{\beta}_1 - \hat{\beta}_2)}$ |
| $\beta_2 = 0$ | $(\hat{\beta}_1 - \hat{\beta}_2) / \sqrt{v(\hat{\beta}_1 - \hat{\beta}_2)}$ | $(\hat{\beta}_1 - \hat{\beta}_2) \pm t_{n-3,\alpha/2} \sqrt{v(\hat{\beta}_1 - \hat{\beta}_2)}$ |
| $E(Y_i \mid X_{1i}, X_{2i}) = \mu_0$ | $(\hat{Y}_i - \mu_0) / \sqrt{v(\hat{Y}_i)}$ | $\hat{Y}_i \pm t_{n-3} \sqrt{v(\hat{Y}_i)}$ |

$$\hat{Y}_{new} = \hat{\beta}_0 + \hat{\beta}_1 X_1' + \hat{\beta}_2 X_2' = \bar{Y} + \hat{\beta}_1 (X_1' - \bar{X}_1) + \hat{\beta}_2 (X_2' - \bar{X}_2). \tag{10.30}$$

Further,

$$V(\hat{Y}_{new} - Y_{new}) = \sigma^2 + (\sigma^2/n) + (X_1' - \bar{X}_1)^2 V(\hat{\beta}_1) + (X_2' - \bar{X}_2)^2 V(\hat{\beta}_2)$$
$$+ 2(X_1' - \bar{X}_1)(X_2' - \bar{X}_2) Cov(\hat{\beta}_1, \hat{\beta}_2). \tag{10.31}$$

The sample estimate $v(\hat{Y}_{new} - Y_{new})$ of this variance is obtained by replacing $\sigma^2$ with $\hat{\sigma}^2$, and $(1-\alpha)$ percent prediction interval for $Y_i$ are obtained from $\hat{Y}_{new} \pm t_{n-3,\alpha/2} \sqrt{v(\hat{Y}_{new} - Y_{new})}$.

*Example 10.4*   Regression of LDL (Y) on age $(X_1)$ and weight $(X_2)$

| Coefficient | Estimate | S.E. | $t_{17}$ | $p$-value | Confidence limits $(\alpha = 0.05)$ |
|---|---|---|---|---|---|
| Intercept | −176.43 | 56.40 | −3.13 | 0.006 | (−295.44, −57.44) |
| Age | 0.89 | 0.64 | 1.39 | 0.183 | (−0.46, 2.24) |
| Weight | 1.74 | 0.48 | 3.61 | 0.002 | (0.73, 2.75) |

The coefficient $\beta_1$ of age is not significant at the 5 percent level. Its 95 percent confidence limits are $[0.89 - 2.11(0.64)] = -0.46$ and $[0.89 + 2.11(0.64)] = 2.24$. The coefficient $\beta_2$ of weight is significantly different from zero. With $t_{17, 0.025} = 2.11$, the 95 percent confidence limits for this coefficient are $[1.74 - 2.11(0.48)] = 0.73$ and $[1.74 + 2.11(0.48)] = 2.75$.

From the variances and covariances in Table T10.1(c), the correlation of age $(X_1)$ and weight $(X_2)$ is $r_{12} = 0.74$. From (10.23a)–(10.23c), the estimates of V$(\hat{\beta}_1)$, V$(\hat{\beta}_2)$

and $\text{Cov}(\hat{\beta}_1, \hat{\beta}_2)$ respectively are 0.41, 0.23 and $-0.23$. As a result, the estimate of $V(\hat{\beta}_1 - \hat{\beta}_2)$ becomes $v(\hat{\beta}_1 - \hat{\beta}_2) = [0.41 + 0.23 + 2(0.23)] = 1.1$ . Hence, the sample S.E. of $(\hat{\beta}_1 - \hat{\beta}_2)$ is 1.05 and the 95 percent confidence limits for $(\hat{\beta}_1 - \hat{\beta}_2)$ are given by $(0.89 - 1.74) \pm 2.11(1.05)$, that is, $(-3.07, 1.37)$. Since these limits enclose zero, $H_0 : \beta_1 = \beta_2$ is not rejected at the 5 percent significance level. From the above table, the statistic for this hypothesis is $t_{17} = [(0.89 - 1.74)/1.05] = -0.81$ with the $p$-value of 0.42. This high $p$-value also suggests that the hypothesis of equality of the two slope coefficients should not be rejected.

The estimate of the mean $E(Y|X_{1i} = 75, X_{2i} = 165)$ of the LDL at age 75 years and weight 165 lbs is $\hat{Y}_1 = [-176.43 + 0.89(75) + 1.74(165)] = 177.41$. From (10.25), its estimated variance becomes $v(\hat{Y}_i) = [(448.31/20) + (75 - 42.75)^2(0.41) + (165 - 152.35)^2(0.23) - 2(75 - 42.75)(165 - 152.35)(0.23)] = 297.98$, and hence the sample S.E.$(\hat{Y}_i) = 17.26$. The 95 percent confidence limits for the mean at age 75 years and weight 165 lbs become $177.41 \pm 2.11(17.26)$, that is, $(140.99, 213.83)$. At these values for age and weight, from (10.31), $v(\hat{Y}_{new} - Y_{new}) = (448.31 + 297.98) = 746.29$, and the 95 percent prediction limits for the LDL are $\left[ 177.41 - 2.11(746.21)^{1/2} \right] = 119.77$ and $\left[ 177.41 + 2.11(746.21)^{1/2} \right] = 235.05$. For this illustration, both the confidence and prediction intervals are wide.

From (10.30), the predicted value of the LDL for a 70-year-old individual with a weight of 170 lbs becomes $\hat{Y}_{new} = [-176.44 + 0.89(70) + 1.74(170)] = 181.66$. From (10.31), $v(\hat{Y}_{new} - Y_{new}) = [448.31(21/20) + (70 - 42.75)^2(0.41) + (170 - 152.35)^2 (0.23) - 2(70 - 42.75)(0.23)(170 - 152.35)] = 625.26$ and $\sqrt{v(\hat{Y}_{new} - Y_{new})} = 25.01$. The 95 percent prediction intervals for the LDL are $[181.66 \pm 2.11(25.01)]$, that is, $(128.89, 234.43)$. As above, the prediction interval is wide.

## 10.4  Multiple regression: The least squares estimation

For the health assessment and similar purposes, it is of interest to examine the effect of age, weight and similar predictors, the *independent variables*, on LDL, HDL, SBP, DBP and other diagnostic factors, the *dependent variables*. In clinical experiments, the responses on each dependent variable on a set of the predictors, independent variables, are examined. At the measurements $(X_{1i}, X_{2i}, \ldots X_{pi})$ of p of the predictors for the $i$th individual, the expected value and variance of the diagnostic variable Y can be considered to be of the form

$$E(Y|X_{1i}, X_{2i}, \ldots X_{pi}) = \beta_0 + \beta X_{1i} + \beta_2 X_{2i} + \ldots \beta_p X_{pi} \qquad (10.32)$$

and

$$V(Y|X_{1i}, X_{2i}, \ldots X_{pi}) = \sigma^2. \qquad (10.33)$$

The expected value in (10.32) is the equation to a hyperplane of p dimensions, with its slopes $(\beta_1, \beta_2, ..., \beta_p)$ and intercept $\beta_0$. The observations of a random sample of n units now can be expressed as the *Multiple Regression Equation*

$$Y_i = \beta_0 + \beta_1 X_{1i} + \beta_2 X_{2i} + ... + \beta_p X_{pi} + \varepsilon_i, \qquad (10.34)$$

$i = (1, 2, ..., n)$. For the random errors $\varepsilon_i$, $E(\varepsilon_i | X_{1i}, X_{2i}, ... X_{pi}) = 0$ and $V(\varepsilon_i | X_{1i}, X_{2i}, ..., X_{pi}) = \sigma^2$. They are assumed to be uncorrelated at $(X_{1i}, X_{2i}, ..., X_{pi})$ and at each of these independent variables.

The normal equations obtained by minimizing

$$\phi = \sum_1^n \left( Y_i - \beta_0 - \beta_1 X_{1i} - \beta_2 X_{2i} - ... \beta_p X_{pi} \right)^2 \qquad (10.35)$$

with respect to $(\beta_0, \beta_1, ..., \beta_p)$ and the resulting Least Squares Estimators $(\hat{\beta}_0, \hat{\beta}_1, \hat{\beta}_2, ..., \hat{\beta}_p)$ are presented in Appendix A10.2. With the sample means $(\bar{Y}; \bar{X}_1, \bar{X}_2, ..., \bar{X}_p)$, from the first normal equation, the estimator of the intercept becomes $\beta_0 = \bar{Y} - \hat{\beta}_1 \bar{X}_1 - \hat{\beta}_2 \bar{X}_2 - ... - \hat{\beta}_p \bar{X}_p$. The estimator for the mean in (10.32) becomes

$$\hat{Y}_i = \hat{\beta}_0 + \hat{\beta}_1 X_{1i} + \hat{\beta}_2 X_{2i} + ... + \hat{\beta}_p X_{pi}$$

$$= \bar{Y} + \hat{\beta}_1 (X_{1i} - \bar{X}_1) + \hat{\beta}_2 (X_{2i} - \bar{X}_2) + ... + \hat{\beta}_p (X_{pi} - \bar{X}_p) \qquad (10.36)$$

$$= \bar{Y} + \hat{\beta}_1 x_{1i} + \hat{\beta}_2 x_{2i} + ... + \hat{\beta}_p x_{pi},$$

where $x_{1i} = (X_{1i} - \bar{X}_1), ....., x_{pi} = (X_{pi} - \bar{X}_p)$. The observed residuals are $e_i = (Y_i - \hat{Y}_i)$, $i = (1, 2, ...., n)$. From the first normal equation in A10.2, the average $\bar{e} = \sum_1^n e_i / n$ of the residuals is zero. Further, as in the case of a single independent variable, the correlation of $e_i$ with $\hat{Y}_i$ becomes zero.

The expressions for the above estimators for the regression coefficients, and the variances and covariances of the estimators are presented in Appendix A10.2 in matrix notation. These Least Squares Estimators are linear functions of the observed values $Y_i$ of the dependent variable. The estimators $(\hat{\beta}_0, \hat{\beta}_1, \hat{\beta}_2, ..., \hat{\beta}_p)$ are unbiased for the intercept and the slope coefficients, and $\hat{Y}_i$ in (10.36) is unbiased for the mean in (10.32). It is shown through the *Gauss-Markov* theorem that their variances are smaller than any other linear unbiased estimators. Hence, they are known as the *Best Linear Unbiased Estimators, BLUEs*.

An unbiased estimator of $\sigma^2$ is given by

$$\hat{\sigma}^2 = \frac{\sum_1^n (Y_i - \hat{Y}_i)^2}{n - p - 1}. \qquad (10.37)$$

The variances and covariances of the above estimators are obtained by replacing $\sigma^2$ with this estimator.

## 10.4.1    ANOVA for the significance of the regression

The Total SS can be decomposed as the Regression SS and Residual SS, SSR and SSE as follows:

$$\sum_1^n (Y_i - \bar{Y})^2 = \sum_1^n (\hat{Y}_i - \bar{Y})^2 + \sum_1^n (Y_i - \hat{Y}_i)^2, \tag{10.38}$$

which can be expressed as $SST = SSR + SSE$. An expression relating SSR to the estimators of the regression coefficients is presented in Appendix A10.3. The null hypothesis to examine whether $Y$ significantly depends on $(X_1, X_2, \ldots, X_p)$ is $H_0 : \beta_1 = \beta_2 = \ldots = \beta_p = 0$. The alternative hypothesis $H_1$ is that it does not depend on at least one of these independent variables.

When $\varepsilon_i$ follows the normal distribution with zero mean and variance $\sigma^2$, the Test Statistic for this hypothesis is given by the $F$-ratio as shown in Table 10.5.

*Example 10.5*    Estimate and the ANOVA for the regression of LDL on Age ($X_1$), Weight ($X_2$) and Fitness ($X_3$):

From the sample of the 20 adults in Table T10.1(a), the estimate for $E(Y|X_1, X_2, X_3)$ is $\hat{Y} = -169.96 + 0.72X_1 + 1.79X_2 - 0.06X_3$. The different sums of squares and the $F$-test are as follows:

| Source | d.f. | SS | MS | F | p-value |
|---|---|---|---|---|---|
| Regression | 3 | 22146.50 | 7382.20 | 15.53 | $5.35 \times 10^{-5}$ |
| Residual | 16 | 7607.70 | 475.50 | | |
| Total | 19 | 29754.20 | | | |

Table 10.5    ANOVA for the significance of the regression on p independent variables.

| Source | d.f | SS | MS | F |
|---|---|---|---|---|
| Regression | $p$ | $\sum_1^n (\hat{Y}_i - \bar{Y})^2$ | $\sum_1^n (\hat{Y}_i - \bar{Y})^2 / p$ | $\left[ \sum_1^n (\hat{Y}_i - \bar{Y})^2 / p \right] / \hat{\sigma}^2$ |
| Residual | $n - p - 1$ | $\sum_1^n (Y_i - \hat{Y}_i)^2$ | $\sum_1^n (Y_i - \hat{Y}_i)^2 / (n-p-1)$ | |
| Total | $n - 1$ | $\sum_1^n (Y_i - \bar{Y})^2$ | | |

Note that $\hat{\sigma}^2 = \sum_1^n (Y_i - \hat{Y}_i)^2 / (n-p-1)$ as given in (10.37).

The very small p-value for the F-test indicates that the regression of LDL on the three diagnostic variables is highly significant. However, as will be seen from the t-statistics of Example 10.6 in the following section, only weight has a significant effect on the LDL but not age and fitness.

## 10.4.2    Tests of hypotheses, confidence limits and prediction intervals

To examine whether the regression goes through the origin, or any of the p slope coefficients are significantly different from zero, the null hypothesis takes the form of $H_0 : \beta_k = 0$, $k = (0, 1, 2, ..., p)$. The Test Statistic for this hypothesis is $t = \hat{\beta}_k / S.E.(\hat{\beta}_k)$, which follows the t-distribution with $(n - p - 1)$ d.f. Similarly, for $H_0 : \beta_k = \beta_k^*$, a specified value, $t = (\hat{\beta}_k - \beta_k^*) / S.E.(\hat{\beta}_k)$ also follows the t-distribution with $(n - p - 1)$ d.f. The $(1 - \alpha)$ percent confidence limits for $\beta_k$ are obtained from $\hat{\beta}_k \pm t_{n-p-1, \alpha/2} S.E.(\hat{\beta}_k)$. Confidence limits for the mean in (10.32) and prediction intervals for the dependent variable are found as in Sections (10.2.4) and (10.3.3).

An unbiased estimator of the difference of two of the regression coefficients or a linear combination, $L = l_1\beta_1 + l_2\beta_2 + ... l_r\beta_r$, $0 < r \leq p$, is given by $\hat{L} = l_1\hat{\beta}_1 + l_2\hat{\beta}_2 + ... + l_r\hat{\beta}_r$, with variance $V(\hat{L}) = \sigma^2 (l_1^2 C_{11} + l_2^2 C_{22} + ... + 2l_1 l_2 C_{12} + ...)$. The estimate $v(\hat{L})$ of this variance is obtained by replacing $\sigma^2$ with $\hat{\sigma}^2$ and the $S.E.(\hat{L})$ is given by $\sqrt{v(\hat{L})}$. The test statistic for the null hypothesis $H_0 : L = L^*$ for specified value of L is given by $t = (L - L*)/S.E.(\hat{L})$, which follows the t-distribution with $(n - p - 1)$ d.f. The $(1 - \alpha)$ percent confidence limits for L are obtained from $\hat{L} \pm t_{n-p-1, \alpha/2} S.E.(\hat{L})$.

*Example 10.6*    For the regression of LDL on Age, Weight and Fitness considered in Example 10.5, the estimates of the regression coefficients, their S.E.s and the t-statistics for testing their significance are presented below.

|           | Estimate | S.E.  | t      | p-value |
|-----------|----------|-------|--------|---------|
| Intercept | −169.96  | 68.53 | −2.48  | 0.025   |
| Age       | 0.717    | 1.18  | 0.61   | 0.552   |
| Weight    | 1.7869   | 0.56  | 3.17   | 0.006   |
| Fitness   | −0.0641  | 0.361 | − 0.18 | 0.861   |

Among the three independent variables, the effect of weight on LDL is highly significant.

At $X_1 = 50$, $X_2 = 166$ and $X_3 = 120$, $\hat{Y} = 154.85$ and $S.E.(\hat{Y}_i) = 13.36$. At these values of the independent variables, with $t_{16,0.025} = 2.12$, 95 percent confidence limits for the mean of the LDL and the prediction limits are (126.53, 183.17) and (100.64,

209.06) respectively. These figures are obtained from the *Minitab*. They can be obtained in general from the expressions presented in Appendix A10.2.

### 10.4.3  Multiple correlation, adjusted R² and partial correlation

The fraction of the SST that is attributed to the regression is $R^2 = SSR/SST$, which is the square of the multiple correlation coefficient. It is the square of the correlation of the observed $Y_i$ and the estimator $\hat{Y}_i$. For the regression of Y on the p independent variables, $[(n-p-1)/p]R^2/(1-R^2) = F(p, n-p-1)$, which shows that the *F*-ratio increases as $R^2$ increases.

As the number of independent variables in a regression model is increased, the SSE does not increase, SSR does not decrease and $R^2$ does not decrease. With the averages of the SSR and SST, the *Adjusted R²*, denoted by $\bar{R}^2$, is obtained from

$$\left(1-\bar{R}^2\right) = [SSE/(n-p-1)]/[SST/(n-1)] = [(n-1)/(n-p-1)]\left(1-R^2\right). \quad (10.39)$$

As a result, $\bar{R}^2$ becomes smaller than $R^2$. For the regression of LDL on Age, Weight and Fitness in Example 10.5, $R^2 = (22146.5/29754.2) = 0.74$. Since $(1-\bar{R}_2) = (19/16)(1-0.74)$, $\bar{R}^2 = 0.69$.

For the partial correlation, consider three variables $(X_1, X_2, X_3)$. From a sample of size $n$ observed on these variables, the residuals of the regression of $X_1$ on $X_3$ and of $X_2$ on $X_3$ respectively are

$$e_{1i} = (X_{1i}-\bar{X}_1)-b_{1.3}(X_{3i}-\bar{X}_3)$$

and

$$e_{2i} = (X_{2i}-\bar{X}_2)-b_{2.3}(X_{3i}-\bar{X}_3).$$

In these expressions, $b_{1.3} = S_{13}/S_3^2$ and $b_{2.3} = S_{23}/S_3^2$ are the estimators of the slope coefficients of the regressions of $X_1$ and $X_2$ respectively on $X_3$. Note that

$$S_{13} = \sum_1^n (X_{1i}-\bar{X}_1)(X_{3i}-\bar{X}_3), \quad S_{23} = \sum_1^n (X_{2i}-\bar{X}_2)(X_{3i}-\bar{X}_3) \text{ and } S_3^2 = \sum_1^n (X_{3i}-\bar{X}_3)^2.$$

The *partial correlation coefficient* of $X_1$ and $X_2$ on $X_3$ is the correlation of $e_{1i}$ and $e_{2i}$ and is given by

$$r_{12.3} = \frac{r_{12}-r_{13}r_{23}}{\left(1-r_{13}^2\right)^{1/2}\left(1-r_{23}^2\right)^{1/2}}. \quad (10.40)$$

These residuals are obtained from regressing $X_1$ and $X_2$ separately on $X_3$, that is adjusting them separately for the effect of $X_3$.

If $(X_1, X_2)$ are positively correlated and their correlations with $X_3$ are both positive or negative, $r_{12.3}$ will be smaller than $r_{12}$. For an illustration, representing (LDL, Weight, Age) by $(X_1, X_2, X_3)$, from the correlations in Table T10.1 (c), $r_{12} = 0.85$, $r_{13} = 0.74$ and $r_{23} = 0.74$. From (10.40), $r_{12.3} = (0.85-0.74^2)/(1-0.74^2)^{1/2}$ $(1-0.74^2)^{1/2} = 0.67$. Adjusting for age, the correlation of LDL and weight has reduced from 0.85 to 0.67.

If $(X_1, X_2)$ are negatively correlated, $X_1$ negatively correlated but $X_2$ is positively correlated with $X_3$, $r_{12.3}$ will be larger than $r_{12}$. From Table 10.1(c), With $(X_1, X_2, X_3)$ representing (HDL, Weight, Age), $r_{12} = -0.70$, $r_{13} = -0.57$ and $r_{23} = 0.74$. From (10.40), $r_{12.3} = -0.50$. Adjusting for age, the correlation of HDL and Weight has increased from –0.70 to –0.50.

## 10.4.4   Effect of including two or more independent variables and the partial F-test

As seen in Examples 10.1 and 10.2, the slope coefficient of the regression of LDL on weight is significantly different from zero with the $p$-value of $2.67 \times 10^{-6}$. As will be seen in Exercise 10.3, the slope coefficient of the regression of LDL on age is also significantly different from zero with the $p$-value of 0.00017. This is the result of the high correlations of 0.85 and 0.74 of weight and age with the LDL. However, for the regression in Examples 10.3 and 10.4 of LDL on age and weight together, the slope coefficient for weight is highly significant at the $p$-value of 0.002, but that of age is barely significant with the large $p$-value of 0.183. This result is the consequence of the high correlation of 0.74 of weight and age. In summary, the effect of weight on LDL after including age is highly significant, but the effect of age on LDL after including weight in the regression is not significant.

The effect of including each of the independent variables in a multiple regression equation can be examined through the $t$-tests. The effect of including two or more independent variables together can be examined through the *partial F-test* as described below. The model for the regression of $Y$ on $(p+q)$ independent variables is

$$Y_i = \beta_0 + \beta_1 X_{1i} + \ldots + \beta_p X_{p,i} + \beta_{p+1} X_{p+1,i} + \ldots + \beta_{p+q} X_{p+q,i} + \varepsilon_i. \tag{10.41}$$

To examine whether the last $q$ independent variables contribute significantly to the regression, the null hypothesis is specified as $H_0 : \beta_{p+1} = \ldots = \beta_{p+q} = 0$ with the alternative hypothesis that at least one of these q regression coefficients is non-zero.

For the above model, SSR $(p+q)$ and SSE $(p+q)$ are the regression and residual sums of squares with $(p+q)$ and $[n - 1 - (p+q)]$ d.f. respectively, and $\hat{\sigma}^2 = SSE(p+q)/[n-1-(p+q)]$ with $[n-1-(p+q)]$ d.f. is unbiased for $\sigma^2$. Under the null hypothesis, the regression and residual sums of squares become $SSR(p)$ and $SSE(p)$ with $p$ and $(n-1-p)$ d.f. respectively. The Test Statistic for the above hypothesis is given by the partial $F$-test

$$F[q, n-1-(p+q)] = \frac{[SSE(p) - SSE(p+q)]/q}{\hat{\sigma}^2}. \tag{10.42}$$

The numerator of this expression in the square brackets is the decrease of the SSE from the addition of the $q$ independent variables. It is the same as the increase of the SSR from their addition to the model.

*Example 10.7*   Continuing with Examples 10.1 and 10.5, it can be examined whether the addition of age $(X_1)$ and fitness $(X_3)$ to the regression has any significant effect after including weight $(X_2)$. The null hypothesis now becomes $H_0 : \beta_1 = \beta_3 = 0$ *versus* the alternative that at least one of these regression coefficients is different from zero. The test for this hypothesis is not provided by the individual tests for $H_0 : \beta_1 = 0$ and $H_0 : \beta_3 = 0$, unless the sample correlation of $X_1$ and $X_3$ is zero. The following procedure, *the partial F-test*, leads to the decision regarding the above hypothesis.

From Example 10.5 for the regression of *LDL* $(Y)$ on $(X_1, X_2, X_3)$, $SSR = 22146.5$ with 3 d.f., $SSE = 7607.7$ with 16 d.f. and $\hat{\sigma}^2 = 7607.7/16 = 475.5$. From Example 10.1 for the regression of *LDL* $(Y)$ on $X_2$, $SSR = 21266.93$ with 1d.f. and $SSE = 8487.27$ with 18 d.f.

Decrease of the *SSE* by adding $(X_1, X_3)$ to the model is $(8487.27 - 7607.70) = 879.57$ with $(18 - 16) = 2$ d.f., which is the same as the increase of $(22146.50 - 21266.93) = 879.57$ for the SSR. From (10.42), the test statistic for the above hypothesis $H_0 : \beta_1 = \beta_3 = 0$ becomes $F(2,16) = (879.57/2)/475.5 = 0.93$, with the *p*-value of 0.41. With high *p*-value, this hypothesis is not rejected. Including age and fitness to the regression after weight has only an insignificant effect.

## 10.4.5    Equality of two or more series of regressions

Consider the two independent series or groups of regressions of $Y$ on $(X_1, X_2, ..., X_p)$,

$$Y_i = \beta_0 + \beta_1 X_{1i} + ... + \beta_p X_{pi} + \varepsilon_i,$$
$$i = (1, 2, ..., n_1), \tag{10.43a}$$

and

$$Y_i = \beta_0' + \beta_1' X_{1i} + ... + \beta_p' X_{pi} + \varepsilon_i, \tag{10.43b}$$

$i = (1, 2, ..., n_2)$, with $E(\varepsilon_i | X_{1i}, ..., X_{pi}) = 0$ and $V(\varepsilon_i | X_{1i}, ..., X_{pi}) = \sigma^2$ in each case.

The residual sums of squares for these separate regressions has $(n_1 - p - 1)$ and $(n_2 - p - 1)$ d.f. The corresponding residual mean squares are unbiased for $\sigma^2$. The pooled residual sum of squares SSE(S) from these separate regressions has $(n - 2p - 2)$ d.f, where $n = (n_1 + n_2)$, and $\hat{\sigma}^2 = SSE(S)/(n - 2p - 2)$ is an unbiased estimator of $\sigma^2$. With the null hypothesis of equality of the two regressions, that is, $H_0 : \beta_0 = \beta_0', ..., \beta_p = \beta_p'$, the residual sum of squares SSE(C) from the combined sample of the n units has $(n - p - 1)$ d.f. From the difference of the residual sums of squares with $[(n - p - 1) - (n - 2p - 2)] = (p + 1)$ d.f, the test statistic for this hypothesis is given by

$$F(p + 1, n - 2p - 2) = [SSE(C) - SSE(S)]/\hat{\sigma}^2. \tag{10.44}$$

Tests for the equality of a subset of the regression coefficients of the two series can be similarly developed. All these types of tests can be extended to more than two series or groups. For the hypothesis of the equality of the coefficients of a single variable, for instance, $H_0 : \beta_1 = \beta_1'$, the test statistic is given by

$$t_{n-2p-2} = \frac{\hat{\beta}_1 - \hat{\beta}_1'}{S.E.(\hat{\beta}_1 - \hat{\beta}_1').} \tag{10.45}$$

Following the notation in Appendix A10.2, the estimate $v(\hat{\beta}_1 - \hat{\beta}_1')$ of the variance of $(\hat{\beta}_1 - \hat{\beta}_1')$ is given by $(C_{11} + C_{11}')\hat{\sigma}^2$, and S.E. $(\hat{\beta}_1 - \hat{\beta}_1')$ is obtained from the square root of this variance.

For the case of the regressions for two groups with intercepts of $Y$ on a single independent variable $X$, $\hat{\sigma}^2$ is obtained with $(n - 4)$ d.f by pooling the SSEs from the two regressions. The variance of $(\hat{\beta}_1 - \hat{\beta}_1')$ is given by

$$\hat{\sigma}^2 \{ [1/\sum_1^{n_1} (X_{1i} - \bar{X}_1)^2] + [1/\sum_1^{n_2} (X_{2i} - \bar{X}_2)^2] \}$$ and S.E. $(\hat{\beta}_1 - \hat{\beta}_1')$ is obtained from the square root of this variance. The test statistic for the equality of the two slope coefficients is given by $t_{n-4} = (\hat{\beta}_1 - \hat{\beta}_1') / S.E.(\hat{\beta}_1 - \hat{\beta}_1')$.

*Example 10.8*    The weights and LDLs of two groups of adults of samples of sizes $n_1 = 9$ and $n_2 = 11$ are presented in Table T10.2. The regressions of the LDL (Y) on weight (X) and the ANOVA tables for the two groups and the combined sample of $n = 20$ adults are as follows. Standard errors of the estimates of the coefficients appear in parentheses.

Estimates and ANOVA for the Separate and Combined Regressions of *LDL(Y)* on weight (X).

**Group 1**

$\hat{Y} = -89.09 + 1.49\, X$
$(86.07)\quad(0.62)$

| Source | d.f | SS | MS | F |
|---|---|---|---|---|
| Regression | 1 | 535.01 | 535.01 | 5.88 |
| Residual | 7 | 637.21 | 91.03 | |
| Total | 8 | 1172.22 | | |

**Group 2**

$\hat{Y} = 3.31 + 0.80\, X$
$(33.83)\ (0.21)$

| Source | d.f | SS | MS | F |
|---|---|---|---|---|
| Regression | 1 | 385.26 | 385.26 | 14.6 |
| Residual | 9 | 237.47 | 26.39 | |
| Total | 10 | 622.73 | | |

**Groups 1 and 2 combined**

$\hat{Y} = 22.44 + 0.69\, X$
$(20.33)\quad(0.13)$

| Source | d.f | SS | MS | F |
|---|---|---|---|---|
| Regression | 1 | 1566.5 | 1566.5 | 26.44 |
| Residual | 18 | 1066.3 | 59.2 | |
| Total | 19 | 2632.8 | | |

The separate regressions as well as the combined regression are significant with the $p$-values of 5 percent or smaller. From the Residual SS of the two groups, $SSE(S) = 637.21 + 237.47 = 874.68$ with $(7+9) = 16$ d.f. and $\hat{\sigma}^2 = (874.68/16) =$ 54.67. For the combined regression, $SSE(C) = 1066.3$ with 18 d.f. The $F$-ratio for the equality of the regressions becomes $F(2,16) = [(1066.3 - 874.68)/2]/$ $54.67 = 1.75$ with the $p$-value of 0.21, which is large. As a result, the hypothesis of the equality of the regressions for the two groups is not rejected. The difference among the slopes as well as the intercepts is not significant.

From Table T10.2, $\sum_{1}^{9}(x_{1i} - \bar{x}_1)^2 = 240$ and $\sum_{1}^{11}(x_{2i} - \bar{x}_2)^2 = 606.9$. The sample variance of the difference of the estimates of the two slope coefficients is $[(54.67/240) + (54.67/606.9)] = 0.3179$, and the S.E. of the difference of the estimates becomes 0.56. As a result, the statistic for the hypothesis of equality of the two slope coefficients becomes $t_{16} = (1.49 - 0.80)/0.56 = 1.23$, with the $p$-value of 0.24. The difference between the two slope coefficients is insignificant. This is the test for the equality of the slope coefficients irrespective of whether the two intercepts are equal or not.

## 10.5    Indicator variables

Regressions for two or more series or groups can be conveniently fitted by including *indicator or dummy variables as* the independent variables. They can also be used to fit the regressions with conditions such as the equality of some the coefficients of two or more groups. They are described below for two groups for the commonly occurring situations, which can be extended to more groups.

### 10.5.1    Separate regressions

In Example 10.8 of Section 10.4.5, the separate regressions of $LDL(Y)$ on weight $(X)$ for two groups with sample sizes $n_1 = 9$ and $n_2 = 11$ were obtained. For the two regressions, consider the model

$$Y = \beta_0 + \beta_1 X + \beta_2 d + \beta_3(dX) + \varepsilon, \qquad (10.46)$$

where the dummy variable d takes the value of one (1) for the first group and zero (0) for the second group. The intercept and slope for the first group are $(\beta_0 + \beta_2)$ and $(\beta_1 + \beta_3)$. The intercept and slope for the second group are $(\beta_0, \beta_1)$. The difference of the intercept coefficients is $\beta_2$, and for the slope coefficients it is $\beta_3$.

With the independent variables $(X, d)$ and the sample of size $n = (n_1 + n_2) = (9 + 11) = 20$, the estimate of the regression equation and the ANOVA are as follows:

$$\hat{Y} = 3.31 + 0.80X - 92.40(d) + 0.70(dX).$$

$$(48.7) \quad (0.30) \quad (82.6) \quad (0.56)$$

ANOVA Table for the regression of LDL on weight for the two groups with a dummy variable.

| Source | d.f | SS | MS | F | p-value |
|---|---|---|---|---|---|
| Regression | 3 | 1758.12 | 586.04 | 10.72 | 0.0004 |
| Residual | 16 | 874.68 | 54.67 | | |
| Total | 19 | 2632.80 | | | |

With $d = 1$, the intercept and slope for the first group are $(3.31 - 92.40) = -89.09$ and $(0.80 + 0.70) = 1.50$, and the estimate of the regression equation becomes

$$\hat{Y}_i = -89.09 + 1.50X_i,$$

$i = (1, 2, ..., 9)$. With $d = 0$, the intercept and slope for the second group are 3.31 and 0.80, and the estimate of the regression equation becomes

$$\hat{Y}_i = 3.31 + 0.80X_i,$$

$i = (10, 11, ..., 20)$. The pooled residual sum of squares $(637.21 + 237.47) = 874.68$ with $(7 + 9) = 16$ d.f. obtained in Example 10.8 for the separate regressions is the same as the above residual sum of squares.

The hypothesis of equality of the slopes of the two regressions becomes the same as $H_0 : \beta_3 = 0$. From the above results, the Test Statistic for this hypothesis becomes $t_{16} = (0.70/0.56) = 1.25$ with the $p$-value of 0.24, suggesting that the two slopes are not significantly different. For this hypothesis, $t_{16} = 1.23$ from Example 10.8 in section 10.4.5. The difference in the values of these $t$-statistics is due to the rounding-off of the decimals. Similarly, the hypothesis of equality of the two intercepts is the same as $H_0 : \beta_2 = 0$. The test statistic for this hypothesis is $t_{16} = -(92.4/82.6) = -1.12$ with the $p$-value of 0.28. The difference between the two intercepts is insignificant.

## 10.5.2   Regressions with equal slopes

To fit the above regressions for the two groups or series with equal slopes, the model becomes

$$Y = \beta_0 + \beta_1 X + \beta_2 d + \varepsilon. \tag{10.47}$$

With $d = 1$, the regression equation for the first group becomes $Y = (\beta_0 + \beta_2) + \beta_1 X + \varepsilon$. With $d = 0$, it becomes $Y = \beta_0 + \beta_1 X + \varepsilon$ for the second group.

For the regression equation $Y = \beta_0 + \beta_1 X + \beta_2 d + \varepsilon$ with $d = 1$ for the first group and $d = 0$ for the second, the intercept and slope for the first and second groups become $(\beta_0 + \beta_2, \beta_1)$ and $(\beta_0, \beta_1)$ respectively. With the observations in Table T10.2, the estimate for the regression and the ANOVA are as follows:

$$\hat{Y} = -28.67 + 0.99\,X + 9.28d$$

$$(41.87) \quad (0.26) \quad (6.70)$$

ANOVA Table.

| Source | d.f | SS | MS | F | p-value |
|--------|-----|------|------|------|---------|
| Regression | 2 | 1674.73 | 8373.6 | 14.86 | 0.0013 |
| Residual | 17 | 958.07 | 56.36 | | |
| Total | 19 | 2632.80 | | | |

The estimate of the common slope coefficient is 0.99 with the S.E. of 0.26, with $t_{17} = (0.99/0.26) = 3.81$ and the $p$-value of 0.0014. The common slope is significantly different from zero. For both the groups, LDL significantly depends on the weight. The estimates of the regressions for the first and second groups are

1. $\hat{Y} = -19.39 + 0.99\,X$

and

2. $\hat{Y} = -28.67 + 0.99\,X.$

The statistic for the equality of the intercepts, that is $H_0 : \beta_2 = 0$, becomes $t_{17} = (9.28/6.70) = 1.39$ with the $p$-value of 0.18. The difference between the two intercepts is not significant.

## 10.5.3    Regressions with the same intercepts

For the regressions of LDL on weight for the two groups with the same intercept, consider the model

$$Y = \beta_0 + \beta_1 X + \beta_2 (dX) + \varepsilon. \qquad (10.48)$$

With $d = 1$, the regression equation for the first group becomes $Y = \beta_0 + (\beta_1 + \beta_2)X + \varepsilon$. With $d = 0$, the equation for the second group becomes $Y = \beta_0 + \beta_1 X + \varepsilon$.

From the samples in Table T10.2, The estimate for the regression and the ANOVA are as follows:

$$\hat{Y} = -28.81 + 0.995X + 0.068(dX).$$
$$(39.62) \quad (0.24) \quad (0.045)$$

The statistic for the hypothesis of equality of the two slopes, that is, $H_0 : \beta_2 = 0$, is $t_{17} = (0.068/0.045) = 1.51$ with the $p$-value of 0.15. The slopes are not significantly different.

With $d = 1$, the estimate of the regression for the first group becomes

$$\hat{Y} = -28.81 + 1.063X.$$

With $d = 0$, the regression for the second group becomes

$$\hat{Y} = -28.81 + 0.995\,X.$$

Table 10.6   Estimators for the regression through the origin.

| $V(\varepsilon_i\|X_i)$ | $\hat{\beta}$ | $\hat{\sigma}^2$ | $v(\hat{\beta})$ |
|---|---|---|---|
| $\sigma^2$ | $\sum_1^n X_i Y_i / \sum_1^n X_i^2$ | $\sum_1^n (Y_i - \hat{\beta}X_i)^2/(n-1)$ | $\hat{\sigma}^2 / \sum_1^n X_i^2$ |
| $\sigma^2 X_i$ | $\sum_1^n Y_i / \sum_1^n X_i$ | $\sum_1^n [(Y_i-\hat{\beta}X_i)^2/X_i]/(n-1)$ | $\hat{\sigma}^2 / \sum_1^n X_i$ |
| $\sigma^2 X_i^2$ | $\left[\sum_1^n (Y_i/X_i)\right]/n$ | $\sum_1^n [(Y_i-\hat{\beta}X_i)^2/X_i^2]/(n-1)$ | $\hat{\sigma}^2 / n$ |

## 10.6   Regression through the origin

When the intercept is set to zero, the regression equation in (10.3) for $Y$ on $X$ becomes

$$Y_i = \beta X_i + \varepsilon_i, \tag{10.49}$$

$i=(1,2,\dots,n)$, with $E(\varepsilon_i|X_i)=0$ and $V(\varepsilon_i|X_i)=\sigma^2$. This model represents the cases where the dependent variable $Y_i$ is zero at the beginning or threshold value of the independent variable $X_i$. In some situations, $V(\varepsilon_i|X_i)$ can be proportional to $X_i$ or $X_i^2$. For instance, SBPs ($Y_i$) may increase with age $X_i$ and their variation at each value of the age can be proportional to $X_i$ or $X_i^2$. For some cases, $V(\varepsilon_i|X_i)$ may take a specified form. The Least Squares Estimators of the slope coefficient and $\sigma^2$ are presented in Table 10.6 for $V(\varepsilon_i|X_i)=\sigma^2$, $\sigma^2 X_i$ or $\sigma^2 X_i^2$.

For each of these three cases, the d.f. for $\hat{\sigma}^2$ are $(n-1)$. The S.E. of $\hat{\beta}$ is obtained from $\sqrt{v(\hat{\beta})}$. For the hypothesis $H_0:\beta=0$, the test statistic is given by $t_{n-1}=\hat{\beta}/\sqrt{v(\hat{\beta})}$. The $(1-\alpha)$ percent confidence limits for $\beta$ are obtained from $\hat{\beta} \pm t_{n-1,\alpha/2}\sqrt{v(\hat{\beta})}$.

*Example 10.9*   Personal health care expenditures in the United States for nine time periods covering (1960–2010) are presented in Table T10.4. For the regression of Private Health Insurance ($Y$) on Per capita Expenditure ($X$),the following results are obtained for the model in (10.3) with the intercept and $V(\varepsilon_i|X_i)=\sigma^2$.

| Coefficient | Estimate | S.E. | $t_7$ | $p$-value |
|---|---|---|---|---|
| Intercept | −91.07 | 36.85 | −2.47 | 0.043 |
| Slope | 0.245 | 0.00785 | 31.21 | $8.95 \times 10^{-9}$ |

The null hypothesis $H_0:\beta_1=0$ is rejected with the very small $p$-value. The personal insurance amount significantly depends on the per capita income as expected.

The estimate of the intercept coefficient $\alpha$ is $-91.07$ with the sample S.E. of 36.85. The null hypothesis $H_0$: $\beta_0 = 0$ for the intercept is also rejected with the p-value of 0.043.

Although, the above test for the intercept shows that it is not zero, we may consider the regression through the origin with the model in (10.49) with $V(\varepsilon_i|X_i) = \sigma^2$. In this case, $\hat{\beta} = 0.23$, $\hat{\sigma}^2 = 6857.0$, and S.E.$(\hat{\beta}) = 0.00588$. As a result, $t_8 = (0.23/0.00588) = 39.12$ with a very small $p$-value. The amount spent for insurance by individuals depends significantly on their personal healthcare expenditure.

## 10.7   Estimation of trends

Physicians periodically examine blood pressures, lipid levels and similar health-related characteristics of the patients. National and international organizations like the CDC record the annual health related information of the public. The *Growth Charts* of children present heights, weights and BMIs of (2–20)-year-old boys and girls. Ogden et al. (2006, 2010), for instance, examined the obesity trends among children and adults in the United States. The linear or nonlinear trends of the response variable $(Y)$ over the years or time periods, the independent variable $(X)$, can be estimated through the regression models.

*Example 10.10   Trends of adult obesity.* The percentages $(Y)$ of the overweight (including obese, BMI $\geq 25$) of persons, 20–74 years, in the United States over seven periods during 1960–2010 are presented in Table T10.3. The time periods are coded as $(X)$. The regression for the percentage $(Y)$ of the overweight males and females over the years is

$$\hat{Y} = 42.4 + 0.524X.$$
$$(1.47)\ \ (0.045)$$

The S.E.s of the coefficients appear in the parentheses. The t-statistic for the slope coefficient is $(0.524/0.045) = 11.53$ with 5 d.f. and a very small p-value. The overweight percentages have increased significantly over the 50 years from 1960 to 2010.

For another illustration, Coloson et al. (2009) analyzed the trend for the sleeping positions of newborn infants from the responses of approximately 1,000 interviews each year in the 48 contiguous States in the United States. The *supine* position which reduces the risk of the *Sudden Infant Death Syndrome* (SIDS) *increased* from 1993 to 2000. The average percentages for the supine position from their Figure 1 for the eight years 1993–2000 approximately are (20, 25, 34, 31, 51, 47, 54, 59), and it is close to 64 percent after that period. The linear trend estimate of the average percentage $(Y)$ over the eight years, $X = (1, 2, \ldots, 8)$, is $\hat{Y} = 14.57 + 5.68X$ with the S.E.s of 3.40 and 0.67 for the intercept and slope coefficients. The test statistic for the slope is $t_6 = (5.68/0.67) = 8.48$ with a very small $p$-value. The increase of the trend for the supine position during the eight years is highly significant.

In some situations, the trend can follow a polynomial with the second and higher degree terms for the independent variable. The multiple regression model in (10.34) can be employed to estimate the coefficients of such a model.

*Example 10.11    Linear and nonlinear trends.* The healthcare expenditure (Y, billions $) for all persons in the United States for the nine periods (X) of the 50 years, 1960–2010, is presented in Table T10.4. Results of the different regressions of Y on X are as follows:

1. Regression through the origin. $\hat{Y} = 37.3X$, with the S.E. of 3.142 for the slope coefficient and $t_8 = 11.86$. The regression is highly significant.

2. The linear regression estimate is $\hat{Y} = -389.2 + 46.55X$, with the estimated S.E. of 5.84 for the slope coefficient. The test statistic for $H_0 : \beta_1 = 0$ is $t_7 = (46.55/5.84) = 7.97$ with a very small $p$-value. The 50-year increased trend of the expenditure is highly significant.

3. The observations suggest that a second-degree polynomial for the trend of the expenditures may be suitable. For the Multiple Regression Model in (10.18) with $(X_1, X_2) = (X, X^2)$, the estimate of $E(Y|X) = \beta_0 + \beta_1 X + \beta_2 X^2$ becomes $\hat{Y} = 64.66 - 17.71X + 1.20X^2$. From the ANOVA Table, the test statistic for the significance of the regression, that is, $H_0 : \beta_1 = \beta_2 = 0$, is $F(2, 6) = 1003.73$, with a very small $p$-value. This result suggests that the second-degree polynomial can be used for predicting the healthcare expenditure. This estimate for the regression and Figure 10.2 are obtained from the *Minitab*.

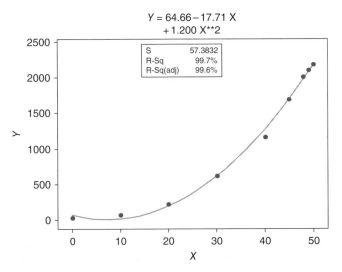

*Figure 10.2    Expenditure for all persons in the United States over the nine periods from 1960 to 2010.*

## 10.8    Logistic regression and the odds ratio

The response, success and failure, of a treatment can be represented by the random variable $Y$ taking the values of one (1) and zero (0) respectively, with the probabilities $P(Y=1)=p$ and $P(Y=0)=(1-p)$. The expected value and variance of $Y$ are $p$ and $p(1-p)$. It is frequently of interest to relate this expected value of the response to one or more discrete or continuous predictors. With a single predictor $X$, this relationship may be considered to be of the form $p=\beta_0+\beta_1 x$ of a linear regression equation. However, $0 \le p \le 1$ and the right-hand side of this equation can take both positive and negative values.

The *logit* of $p$ is the natural logarithm $ln[p/(1-p)]$ and it can take both positive and negative values. For the linear *logistic regression*,

$$\text{logit}(p)=\beta_0+\beta_1 x \qquad (10.50)$$

is considered. From this model,

$$p=\frac{e^{\beta_0+\beta_1 x}}{1+e^{\beta_0+\beta_1 x}}=\frac{1}{1+e^{-(\beta_0+\beta_1 x)}}. \qquad (10.51)$$

This equation relating p to a continuous predictor $X$ becomes *S-shaped*, as shown in Figure 10.3. For some applications, the above type of model with more predictors and covariates is considered. Software programs are available for estimating the regression coefficients of the model through the *Maximum Likelihood* procedure. Estimation of the odds and odds ratio for $Y$ obtained from (10.51) is considered in the following subsections; MINITAB is used for the illustrations. For the case of the dichotomous predictor, the odds ratio can be estimated from the 2x2 contingency table.

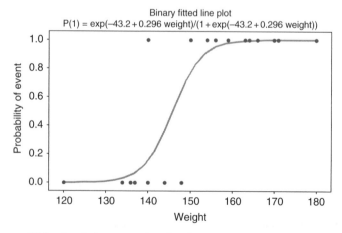

*Figure 10.3    Logistic regression for the increase of LDL with weight.*

## 10.8.1   A single continuous predictor

At the value of $x$ for the predictor, logit $p(x) = \beta_0 + \beta_1 x$. At $(x+1)$, logit $p(x+1) = \beta_0 + \beta_1(x+1)$. With this model,

$$\text{logit } p(x+1) - \text{logit } p(x) = \ln\left[\frac{p(x+1)}{1-p(x+1)} \Big/ \frac{p(x)}{1-p(x)}\right] = \beta_1 \qquad (10.52a)$$

and the odds ratio for the response $Y$ becomes

$$OR = \frac{p(x+1)}{1-p(x+1)} \Big/ \frac{p(x)}{1-p(x)} = e^{\beta_1}. \qquad (10.52b)$$

Thus, for a one-unit change in the predictor $X$, the odds ratio for the response $Y$ becomes $e^{\beta_1}$. With the estimate $\hat{\beta}_1$, the estimate for the odds ratio is obtained from $e^{\hat{\beta}_1}$ and its $(1-\alpha)$ percent confidence limits from $e^{\hat{\beta}_1 \pm z_{\alpha/2} S.E.(\hat{\beta}_1)}$. Similarly, the estimate for the odds ratio of the response becomes $e^{d\beta_1}$ when the predictor changes from $x$ to $(x+d)$, and its confidence limits become $e^{d[\hat{\beta}_1 \pm z_{\alpha/2} S.E.(\hat{\beta}_1)]}$.

For the population with the 20 sample units in Table T10.1(a), consider LDL ($Y$) for the response variable with weight ($X$) as the predictor. With $Y = (1, 0)$ for LDL $\geq$ 100 and LDL $<$ 100 respectively, the estimates for the logistic regression for $Y$ are as follows.

| Coefficient | Estimate | S.E. | $z$ | $p$-value | OR | 95% Conf. lts for (OR) |
|---|---|---|---|---|---|---|
| Intercept | −43.23 | 19.95 | −2.17 | 0.03 | | |
| Weight | 0.296 | 0.136 | 2.17 | 0.03 | 1.34 | 1.03, 1.76 |

There is a 34 percent increase in the odds ratio for each additional pound of weight, with the 95 percent confidence limits of $(3, 76)$ percent. For an addition of five pounds of weight, the odds ratio becomes $5(1.34) = 6.7$ with the 95 percent confidence limits $5(1.03) = 5.15$ and $5(1.76) = 8.8$.

## 10.8.2   Two continuous predictors

With the predictors $(X_1, X_2)$, for the response Y,

$$\text{logit } p(x_1, x_2) = \beta_0 + \beta_1 x_1 + \beta_2 x_2. \qquad (10.53)$$

When the predictor $X_1$ increases from $x_1$ to $(x_1 + 1)$ at a fixed value of $x_2$ for the second predictor,

$$\text{logit } p(x_1 + 1, x_2) = \beta_0 + \beta_1(x_1 + 1) + \beta_2 x_2. \qquad (10.54a)$$

Now,

$$\text{logit}\, p(x_1 + 1, x_2) - \text{logit}\, p(x_1, x_2)$$

$$= ln \left[ \frac{p(x_1 + 1, x_2)}{1 - p(x_1 + 1, x_2)} \Big/ \frac{p(x_1, x_2)}{1 - p(x_1, x_2)} \right] = \beta_1. \qquad (10.54b)$$

Thus, the odds ratio of $Y$ for one unit change in $X_1$ is $e^{\beta_1}$. Similarly, its odds ratio for one unit change in $X_2$ becomes $e^{\beta_2}$. With the estimates $\hat{\beta}_1$ and $\hat{\beta}_2$ for the slope coefficients, the odds ratios are obtained from $e^{\hat{\beta}_1}$ and $e^{\hat{\beta}_2}$. The $(1 - \alpha)$ percent confidence limits for the odds ratios become $e^{\hat{\beta}_1 \pm z_{\alpha/2} S.E.(\hat{\beta}_1)}$ and $e^{\hat{\beta}_2 \pm z_{\alpha/2} S.E.(\hat{\beta}_2)}$. For more than two predictors, odds ratio are found similarly from the multiple regression of the logit.

As an illustration, consider $Y = (1, 0)$ for $LDL \geq 100$ and $LDL < 100$ and the predictors age and weight, $(X_1, X_2)$. The following estimates are obtained from the logistic regression of $Y$ on these two predictors.

| Coefficient | Estimate | S.E. | $z$ | $p$-value | OR | 95% confidence limits for OR |
|---|---|---|---|---|---|---|
| Intercept | −40.33 | 22.10 | −1.83 | 0.068 | | |
| Age | 0.057 | 0.218 | 0.26 | 0.796 | 1.06 | 0.69, 1.62 |
| Weight | 0.263 | 0.179 | 1.47 | 0.141 | 1.30 | 0.92, 1.85 |

The odds for LDL exceeding 100 are 6 percent for each additional year. They are 30 percent for each pound of increase of the weight.

## 10.8.3   A single dichotomous predictor

For the response, as before consider $Y = 1$ and $Y = 0$ when $LDL \geq 100$ and $LDL < 100$. For the predictor, consider $X = (1, 0)$ for the age at least 40 and less than 40. The outcomes for the sample of the $n = 20$ units in Table T10.1(a) can be presented in the following $2 \times 2$ Contingency Table.

| | $X = 1$ | $X = 0$ | Total |
|---|---|---|---|
| $Y = 1$ | $a = 10$ | $b = 3$ | $(a + b) = 13$ |
| $Y = 0$ | $c = 1$ | $d = 6$ | $(c + d) = 7$ |
| Total | $(a + c) = 11$ | $(b + d) = 9$ | $n = 20$ |

The probabilities for $Y = 1$ and $Y = 0$ at $X = 1$ are $a/(a + c)$ and $c/(a + c)$ with the odds $(a/c)$. Similarly, the odds at $X = 0$ are $(b/d)$. The odds ratio becomes $(a/c)/(b/d) = (ad/bc) = 20$.

From (10.50), $ln$(odds) are given by $(\beta_0 + \beta_1)$ and $\beta_0$ at $X = (1, 0)$. As a result, $ln\ (OR) = \beta_1$ and $(OR) = e^{\beta_1}$. From the observations in the above contingency table, $(\hat{\beta}_0 + \hat{\beta}_1) = ln(10/1) = 2.303$ and $\hat{\beta}_0 = ln(3/6) = -0.693$. From these figures, $ln\left(\widehat{OR}\right) = \hat{\beta}_1 = 2.996$ and $\left(\widehat{OR}\right) = e^{2.996} = 20$, same as above found directly. As shown in (6.15), $v\left[ln\left(\widehat{OR}\right)\right] = (1/a + 1/b + 1/c + 1/d) = 1.6$ and $S.E.\left[ln\left(\widehat{OR}\right)\right] = 1.265$. The 95 percent confidence limits for $ln\left(\widehat{OR}\right)$ are $[2.996 - 1.96(1.265)] = 0.5166$ and $[2.996 + 1.96(1.265)] = 5.475$. Now, the confidence limits for the odds ratio are given by $e^{0.5166} = 1.68$ and $e^{5.475} = 238.65$.

For the dichotomous predictor, the following results from the MINITAB coincide with the above estimates obtained from the contingency table.

| Coefficient | Estimate | S.E. | $z$ | $p$-value | OR | 95% conf.lts for (OR) |
|---|---|---|---|---|---|---|
| Intercept | –0.69 | 0.71 | –0.98 | 0.327 | | |
| Age $\geq$ 40 | 2.996 | 1.26 | 2.37 | 0.018 | 20 | 1.68, 238.65 |

## 10.9    Weighted Least Squares (WLS) estimator

For the regression model in (10.3) with one independent variable and later for the models with two or more independent variables, it was assumed that $V(\varepsilon_i|X_i) = \sigma^2$, same at each $X_i$, $i = (1, 2, ..., n)$. In practice, this variance may be unequal and can take the form of $\sigma_i^2 = \sigma^2/W_i$, where $W_i$ is known. With the transformation of (10.3) as

$$W_i^{1/2}Y_i = \beta_0 W_i^{1/2} + \beta_1 W_i^{1/2}X_i + \delta_i, \tag{10.55}$$

where $\delta_i = W_i^{1/2}\varepsilon_i$, $E(\delta_i|X_i) = 0$ and $V(\delta_i|X_i) = \sigma^2$. The estimators $(\hat{\beta}_0, \hat{\beta}_1)$ of the intercept and slope coefficients are obtained by minimizing $\sum_1^n W_i(Y_i - \beta_0 - \beta_1 X_i)^2$ with respect to $(\beta_0, \beta_1)$. The estimator

$$\hat{\sigma}^2 = \sum_1^n W_i\left(Y_i - \hat{\beta}_0 - \hat{\beta}_1 X_i\right)^2/(n-2) \tag{10.56}$$

is unbiased for $\sigma^2$. When the variances of $\varepsilon_i$ are unequal, similar transformation is made for the models in (10.18) and (10.34) with two or more independent variables. The WLS estimators are also known as the *Generalized Least Square* (GLS) estimators.

If $V(\varepsilon_i) = \sigma_i^2 = \sigma^2/W_i$ for the model in (10.49) for the regression through the origin, minimizing $\sum_1^n W_i(Y_i - \beta X_i)^2$, the estimator for the slope coefficient becomes

$$\hat{\beta} = \sum_{1}^{n} W_i X_i Y_i / \sum_{1}^{n} W_i X_i^2. \tag{10.57}$$

If $\sigma_i^2 = \sigma^2$, $\hat{\beta} = \sum_{1}^{n} X_i Y_i / \sum_{1}^{n} X_i^2$. For some applications, the variance $\sigma_i^2$ was found to

be proportional to $X_i$ of the form $\sigma^2 X_i$. In this case, $\hat{\beta} = (\sum_{1}^{n} Y_i / \sum_{1}^{n} X_i) = (\bar{Y}/\bar{X})$, which

is the ratio of the two sample means. If $\sigma_i^2$ is proportional to $X_i^2$ of the form $\sigma^2 X_i^2$, the

estimator in (10.57) becomes $\hat{\beta} = (1/n) \sum_{1}^{n} (Y_i / X_i)$, average of the ratios. The unbi-

ased estimator of the variance of $\sigma^2$ is given by

$$\hat{\sigma}^2 = \sum_{1}^{n} W_i (Y_i - \hat{\beta} X_i)^2 / (n-1). \tag{10.58}$$

These results were presented earlier in Table 10.6

## 10.10   Correlation

As described in Appendix A10.1 and Section (10.2.3), the square of the correlation of
the observed $Y_i$ and the estimates $\hat{Y}_i$ of the regression of $Y$ on $X$ is the same as $r^2$, square
of the sample correlation coefficient $r = S_{xy}/S_x S_y$ of $(x_i, y_i)$, $i = (1, 2, \ldots, n)$. The multiple and partial correlation coefficients of the regression of a dependent variable Y on
two or more independent variables are described in Sections 10.4.3. The multiple correlation coefficient $R$ is the correlation of the dependent variable $Y$ and the estimator $\hat{Y}$
obtained from its linear regression on two or more independent variables. The partial
correlation coefficient of two variables is the correlation of the residuals of their
regressions on one or more independent variables.

Besides the above correlation coefficients in regression analysis, two random
variables $(X, Y)$ can be mutually related. Physical characteristics as well as mental
abilities of growing children tend to be related. Natural phenomena like the atmos-
pheric temperature, precipitation, humidity and rainfall are related in general. This
type of relationship between $(X, Y)$ is defined by the population correlation coefficient

$$\rho = \frac{\sigma_{xy}}{\sigma_x \sigma_y} = \frac{Cov(X,Y)}{\sqrt{V(X)V(Y)}}, \tag{10.59}$$

$(-1 \leq \rho \leq 1)$. If the two variables are perfectly correlated, $\rho = 1$, and $\rho = -1$ if they are
perfectly negatively correlated. From the observations $(X_i, Y_i)$, $i = (1, 2, \ldots, n)$, of a
sample of $n$ units, an estimator of $\rho$ is given by the sample correlation coefficient $r = S_{xy}/S_x S_y$.

The population correlation coefficients of three random variables can be repre-
sented by $\rho_{12}, \rho_{13}$ and $\rho_{23}$. With the subscripts (1, 2, 3) for (age, weight, fitness)

respectively, as presented in Table T10.1(c), the estimates from the sample of 20 units are $r_{12} = 0.74$, $r_{13} = -0.82$ and $r_{23} = -0.42$. Although age and weight are positively correlated, fitness is negatively correlated with both age and weight, as can be expected!

In the following sections, tests of hypotheses and confidence limits related to the population correlation coefficient of two random variables $(X, Y)$ are presented. They are assumed to follow the *bivariate normal distribution* described in Section 4.6.with means $(\mu_x, \mu_y)$, variances $\left(\sigma_x^2, \sigma_y^2\right)$ and correlation $\rho_{xy} = (\sigma_{xy}/\sigma_x\sigma_y)$, where $\sigma_{xy}$ is the covariance of $X$ and $Y$.

For the case of three or more random variables $(X_1, X_2, ..., X_k)$, the correlation between two of the variables conditional on the remaining, the partial correlation, can be considered. The correlation $\rho_{12.3}$ of the first two variables conditional on the third is an example. The sample estimate $r_{12.3}$ of this correlation takes the same form as (10.40).

### 10.10.1    Test of the hypothesis that two random variables are uncorrelated

For the population correlation coefficient $\rho$, consider the null hypothesis $H_0 : \rho = 0$ *versus* the alternative $H_1 : \rho \neq 0$. With its estimator r obtained from a sample of $n$ units, the test statistic is given by

$$t_{n-2} = \frac{r-0}{[(1-r^2)/(n-2)]^{1/2}}. \qquad (10.60)$$

It is the same as the statistic for $H_0 : \beta_1 = 0$ *versus* $H_0 : \beta_1 = 0$ presented in Table 10.2 for the linear regression model in (10.3). Note that $t_{n-2}^2 = (SSR/1)/[SSE/(n-2)]$ follows the $F$-distribution $F(1, n - 2)$.

For the illustrations in this and the following two sections and for Exercises 10.11–10.13, the subscripts $(1, 2, 3)$ are used for (age, weight and fitness). The sample correlations in Table 10.1(c) are employed for the tests of hypotheses and confidence limits.

As an illustration, for age and weight, consider $H_0 : \rho_{12} = 0$ *versus* $H_1 : \rho_{12} \neq 0$. From Table 10.1(c), $t_{18} = (0.74-0)/(0.025)^{1/2} = 4.68$. The null hypothesis is rejected with the $p$-value of 0.0002 or smaller.

### 10.10.2    Test of the hypothesis that the correlation coefficient takes a specified value

Fisher (1915) shows that $z = (1/2)ln[(1+r)/(1-r)]$ approximately follows the normal distribution with mean $E(z) = (1/2)ln[(1 +\rho)/(1 -\rho)]$ and variance $V(z) = 1/(n-3)$. Now, $Z = [z-E(z)](n-3)^{1/2}$ follows the standard normal distribution with zero mean and unit standard deviation.

As an example, to test $H_0 : \rho_{12} = 0.5$ *versus* $\rho_{12} \neq 0.5$ for the correlation of age and weight, $z = (1/2)ln[(1 + 0.74)/(1 - 0.74)] = 0.9505$, and $E(z) = (1/2)$ $ln[(1 + 0.5)/(1 - 0.5)] = 0.5493$. Now, $Z = (0.9505 - 0.5493)(17)^{1/2} = 1.65$, with the p-value of 0.10. Hence, the null hypothesis is not rejected with a significance level of 10 percent or higher.

### 10.10.3    Confidence limits for the correlation coefficient

Following Fisher's (1915) approximation, $P\left\{ -z_{\alpha/2} \leq [z - E(z)](n-3)^{1/2} \leq z_{\alpha/2} \right\} = (1 - \alpha)$. From this result, $(1 - \alpha)$ percent confidence limits for $E(z)$ are obtained from $z \pm z_{\alpha/2}/(n-3)^{1/2}$. Expressing these limits as $C_l$ and $C_u$, confidence limits for $\rho$ are given by $(e^{2c_l} - 1)/(e^{2c_l} + 1)$ and $(e^{2c_u} - 1)/(e^{2c_u} + 1)$.

Following the above two sections, 95 percent confidence limits for $E(z)$ are $C_l = \left[ 0.9505 - 1.96/(17)^{1/2} \right] = 0.4751$, and $C_u = \left[ 0.9505 + 1.96/(17)^{1/2} \right] = 1.4259$. Now, from the above expressions, confidence limits for $\rho_{12}$, the correlation of age and weight, become (0.44, 0.89).

Using the *EXCEL* program, $z$ is obtained from *Fisher*, and the confidence limits for $\rho$ are obtained from $z \pm z_{\alpha/2}/(n-3)^{1/2}$ through *Fisherinv*.

## 10.11    Further topics in regression

In Section 10.2, the regression of $Y$ on $X$ was considered to be linear, and $V(\varepsilon_i | X_i)$ was assumed to be the same at each $X_i$. The validity of these assumptions and other aspects like regression with missing observations are examined in this section. The observations of $X_i$ or $Y_i$ outside the acceptable range of the values are known as the *outliers*, and they are excluded from estimating the regression coefficients. Predictions of $Y_i$ at the values of $X_i$ outside the acceptable range can lead to misleading inferences.

### 10.11.1    Linearity of the regression model and the lack of fit test

The null hypothesis that $E(Y|X_i)$ depends linearly on $X_i$ is specified by the model in (10.3). The regression equation with $n_i$ ($>1$) values of $Y$ at $X_i$ becomes

$$Y_{ij} = \beta_0 + \beta_1 X_i + \varepsilon_{ij}, \tag{10.61}$$

$i = (1, \ 2, \dots, k)$ and $j = (1, \ 2, \ \dots, \ n_i)$ with the assumptions $E(\varepsilon_{ij} | X_i) = 0$ and $V(\varepsilon_{ij} | X_i) = \sigma^2$.

With $n = \sum_1^k n_i$, $\bar{X} = \sum_1^k n_i X_i / n$, $\bar{Y}_i = \sum_1^{n_i} Y_{ij}/n_i$, and $\bar{Y} = \sum_1^k \sum_1^{n_i} Y_{ij}/n = \sum_1^k n_i \bar{Y}_i / n$, the Least Squares estimators for $\beta_0$, $\beta_1$ and $E(Y_{ij} | X_i)$ are given by

$$\hat{\beta}_0 = \bar{Y} - \hat{\beta}_1 \bar{X},$$

$$\hat{\beta}_1 = \sum_{1}^{k} \sum_{1}^{n_i} (X_i - \bar{X})(Y_{ij} - \bar{Y}) / \sum_{1}^{k} n_i (X_i - \bar{X})^2$$

and

$$\hat{Y}_{ij} = \hat{\beta}_0 + \hat{\beta} X_i. \tag{10.62}$$

The residual sum of squares with $(n-2)$ d.f can be expressed as

$$SSE = \sum_{1}^{k} \sum_{1}^{n_i} (Y_{ij} - \hat{Y}_{ij})^2 = \sum_{1}^{k} \sum_{1}^{n_i} (Y_{ij} - \bar{Y}_i)^2 + \sum_{1}^{k} \sum_{1}^{n_i} (\bar{Y}_i - \hat{Y}_{ij})^2 \tag{10.63}$$

The right hand side expressions are the Pure Error sum of squares SSP and the Lack of Fit sum of squares SSL with $(n-k)$ and $(k-2)$ d.f. respectively, provided $n_i > 1$, $i = (1, 2,..., n)$. For the above null hypothesis of the linearity of the model, the test statistic, is given by

$$F = [SSL/(k-2)]/[SSP/(n-k)], \tag{10.64}$$

which follows the $F$-distribution with $(k-2)$ and $(n-k)$ d.f.

The Regression SS is $SSR = \hat{\beta}_1^2 \sum_{1}^{n} n_i (X_i - \bar{X})^2$. The test for the significance of the regression, that is, for $H_0 : \beta_1 = 0$, is given by $F = [(SSR/1)/SSE/(n-2)]$, which follows the $F$-distribution with one and $(n-2)$ d.f., which in turn is the same as $t^2$ with $(n-2)$ d.f.

For an illustration, consider the weights ($Y$ in kg) of the sample of 20-year-old boys in Table 1.1 grouped into four classes of sizes $n_i = (4, 5, 6, 5)$ with the average heights $X_i = (165, 172.2, 175.83, 184.4)$ cm and the corresponding weights (54, 55, 58, 59), (60, 62, 63, 66, 68), (72, 75, 75, 78, 80, 82) and (84, 86, 88, 95, 102). The estimate of $E(Y_{ij}|X_i)$ becomes

$$\hat{Y}_{ij} = -253.5 + 1.86 X_i$$

$$(29.06) \quad (0.166)$$

with the S.E.s in the parentheses. The ANOVA for the regression is as follows:

Regression of weights on heights in Table 1.1 and the Lack of fit test.

| Source | d.f. | SS | MS | F | p-value |
|---|---|---|---|---|---|
| Regression | 1 | 3128.7 | 3128.7 | 126.52 | 0.000 |
| Residual | 18 | 445.1 | 24.7 | | |
| Lack of fit | 2 | 99.3 | 49.7 | 2.3 | 0.133 |
| Pure Error | 16 | 345.8 | 21.6 | | |
| Total | 19 | 3573.8 | | | |

The Lack of fit is not significant. The above hypothesis of the linearity of the regression model is not rejected. The linear regression of weights on heights is highly significant. The above figures are obtained from the *Minitab*.

If only $k' < k$ of the X values with $n_i > 1$ contribute to SSP and SSL, the degrees of freedom for these two sums of squares will be $\sum_1^{k'} (n_i - 1)$ and $[(n-2) - \sum_1^{k'} (n_i - 1)]$ respectively. They remain as $(n-1)$ for the Total SS and $(n-2)$ for the SSE.

## 10.11.2   The assumption that $V(\varepsilon_i | X_i) = \sigma^2$, same at each $X_i$

The estimator $\hat{Y}_i$ can be expressed as

$$\hat{Y}_i = c_{i1} Y_1 + c_{i2} Y_2 + \ldots + c_{in} Y_n \tag{10.65}$$

where $c_{ij} = (1/n) + (X_i - \bar{X})(X_j - \bar{X}) / \sum_1^n (X_i - \bar{X})^2$. From (10.3) and (10.65), we find that the variances and covariances of the observed residuals $e_i = (Y_i - \hat{Y}_i)$, $i = (1, 2, \ldots, n)$ depend on the variances and covariances of $\varepsilon_i$. The above equality of the variances of $\varepsilon_i$ can be examined from the variances of $e_i$ in different ranges of $X_i$. If the variances $\sigma_i^2$ at $X_i$ are found to be unequal, the Weighted Least square procedure of Section 10.9 can be employed for the estimation of the regression coefficients and prediction of the dependent variable. Section 10.6 presents estimation for the regression through the origin when $\sigma_i^2$ is proportional to $X_i$ or $X_i^2$.

## 10.11.3   Missing observations

For the multiple regression of Y on the independent variables $(X_1, X_2, \ldots, X_p)$, consider the case where all the observations on the n sample units are available for the independent variables but only on $n_1$ units for Y. Yates (1933) considers

$$\phi = \sum_1^{n_1} (Y_i - \beta_0 - \beta_1 X_{1i} - \ldots - \beta_p X_{pi})^2 + \sum_{n_1+1}^n (Y_i - \beta_0 - \beta_1 X_{1i} - \ldots - \beta_p X_{pi})^2. \tag{10.66}$$

The first and second expressions on the right-hand side contain the $n_1$ responding and $n_2 = (n - n_1)$ nonresponding units. Along with the $(p+1)$ regression coefficients, the $n_2$ missing values of $Y_i$ are also considered to be the *parameters*. The estimates of the $(n_2 + p + 1)$ parameters are obtained by minimizing (10.66). The estimates for the $(p+1)$ regression coefficients are the same as the Least Squares estimates $(\hat{\beta}_0, \hat{\beta}_1, \ldots, \hat{\beta}_p)$ obtained by minimizing the first expression. The estimates for the $n_2$ missing values of $Y_i$ in the second expression become

$$\hat{Y}_i = \hat{\beta}_0 + \hat{\beta}_1 X_{1i} + \hat{\beta}_2 X_{2i} + \ldots + \hat{\beta}_p X_{pi}, \tag{10.67}$$

$i = (n_1 + 1, \ldots, n)$. Substituting $(\hat{\beta}_0, \hat{\beta}_1, \ldots, \hat{\beta}_p)$ and these $n_2$ estimates in (10.66), the estimate of $\sigma^2$ becomes

$$\hat{\sigma}^2 = \frac{\sum_{1}^{n_1}\left(Y_i - \hat{\beta}_0 - \hat{\beta}_1 X_{1i} - \ldots - \hat{\beta}_p X_{pi}\right)^2}{n - (n_2 + p + 1)} \tag{10.68}$$

The degrees of freedom in the denominator is the same as $(n_1 - p - 1)$. This estimate for $\sigma^2$ is the same as the estimate obtained from the regression of $Y$ on $(X_1, X_2, \ldots, Xp)$ with the $n_1$ responding units. Little and Rubin (2014) illustrate some of the modifications and extensions appeared in the literature.

For the linear regression of $Y$ on $X$, consider the case where the observations on $X$ are available for all the $n$ units of the sample but only on $n_1$ units for $Y$. From the estimate of the regression with the $n_1$ pairs $(X_i, Y_i)$, the $n_2$ missing values of $Y$ can be predicted. This method can be extended if some of the responses on $X$ are not available. In an iterative procedure, the missing $Y_i$ are predicted from the regression of $Y$ on $X$ and the missing $X_i$ in turn from the regression of $X$ on $Y$.

### 10.11.4 Transformation of the regression model

In some applications, the model relating $Y$ and $X$ may take, for instance, the nonlinear form $E(Y|X_i) = \beta_0 e^{\beta_1 X_i}$. Transforming the model, $\log_e E(Y|X_i) = \log_e \beta_0 + \beta_1 X_i$. The Least squares estimates of $\beta_1$ and $\log_e \beta_0$ and $E(Y|X_i)$ are obtained from the regression of $\log_e Y_i$ on $X_i$. Estimate of $\beta_0$ is obtained from exponentiating the estimate of $\log_e \beta_0$.

### 10.11.5 Errors of measurements of $(X_i, Y_i)$

One or both the predictor and the dependent variable may be measured with errors. The sample observations $(X_i, Y_i)$, $i = (1, 2, \ldots, n)$, may be of the form $U_i = (X_i + \delta_i)$ and $V_i = (Y_i + \eta_i)$. The errors $(\delta_i, \eta_i)$ are considered to be independent random variables with zero expectations and variances $\sigma_\delta^2$ and $\sigma_\eta^2$ respectively. The regression model for $V_i$ on $U_i$ is

$$V_i = \beta_0 + \beta_1 U_i + \varepsilon_i. \tag{10.69}$$

The Least Squares estimators of $\beta_1$ and $\beta_o$ are

$$b_1 = \sum_{1}^{n}(U_i - \bar{U})(V_i - \bar{V}) / \sum_{1}^{n}(U_i - \bar{U})^2$$

and

$$b_0 = \bar{V} - b_1 \bar{U}, \tag{10.70}$$

where $\bar{U} = \sum_{1}^{n} U_i / n$ and $\bar{V} = \sum_{1}^{n} V_i / n$. As $n$ becomes large, $b_1$ approaches $\sigma_{XY} / (\sigma_X^2 + \sigma_\delta^2)$, which is an underestimate of $\beta_1 = \sigma_{XY} / \sigma_X^2$. In these expressions, $\sigma_X^2$ and

$\sigma_{XY}$ are the variance of $X$ and covariance of $(X, Y)$ respectively. Thus, errors in the predictor should be avoided.

# Exercises

Sample observations from Table T10.1(a–c) are used for Exercises 10.10–10.14. Age, weight and Fitness are denoted by the subscripts (1, 2, 3).

**10.1.** Following Examples 10.1 and 10.2 for the regression of LDL $(Y)$ on weight $(X)$, (a) estimate $E(Y|X=165)$ and find its $S.E.$, (b) find the 95 percent confidence limits for $E(Y|X=165)$ and the prediction limits for $Y$ at $X=165$.

**10.2.** Following Examples (10.1) and (10.2) for the regression of LDL$(Y)$ on weight $(X)$, test the null hypothesis (a) $\beta_1 = 2$ *versus* the alternative that $\beta_1 \neq 2$ and (b) $\beta_1 = 3$ *versus* the alternative $\beta_1 \neq 3$.

**10.3.** From the 20 sample observations in Table T10.1(a), (a) fit the regression of LDL $(Y)$ on age $(X_1)$, (b) test for the significance of the regression, (c) find the 95 percent confidence limits for the intercept, slope and for $E(Y|X_1 = 75)$, and (d) the prediction intervals for the LDL for a 65-year-old individual.

**10.4.** With the 20 sample observations in Table T10.1(a), (a) fit the regression of HDL$(Y)$ on age $(X_1)$, (b) test the significance of the regression and (c) find the 95 percent confidence and prediction intervals for HDL at $X_1 = 75$.

**10.5.** With the 20 sample observations in Table T10.1(a), (a) fit the regression of HDL$(Y)$ on weight $(X_2)$, (b) test the significance of the regression and (c) find the 95 percent confidence and prediction intervals for HDL at $X_2 = 150$ and 165.

**10.6.** From the sample of 20 units in Table T10.1(a), fit the regression of HDL $(Y)$ on age $(X_1)$, weight $(X_2)$ and fitness $(X_3)$. (1) Test for the significance of the regression. (2) Test for the significance of the three regression coefficients. (3) Find the 95 percent confidence limits and prediction interval at $X_1 = 70$, $X_2 = 170$ and $X_3 = 90$.

**10.7.** (a) From the obesity percentages for the males and females presented in Table T10.3, estimate the regression equations for the overweight percentages over the years and test for their significance. (b) Test for the difference of the rates of increase of the obesity for males and females.

**10.8.** From the figures in Table T10.4 for healthcare expenditure, examine the second-degree polynomial trend for the per capita expenditure and private insurance.

**10.9.** The following per capita Medicare expenditures in the United States ($Y$ in 2006 U.S. dollars) for the 15 years $(X)$, 1992–2006, are obtained from the graphical presentation of Fisher et al. (2009). (a) Fit the trend line for the expenditure, test for the significance of the regression, and find the confidence limits for the intercept and slope coefficients. (b) Find the confidence and prediction intervals for the expenditure in 2020.

| Year | Expenditure ($1,000) | Year | Expenditure ($1,000) | Year | Expenditure ($1,000) |
|------|----------------------|------|----------------------|------|----------------------|
| 1 | 5.0 | 6 | 6.9 | 11 | 7.1 |
| 2 | 5.1 | 7 | 6.8 | 12 | 7.8 |
| 3 | 5.9 | 8 | 6.9 | 13 | 8.0 |
| 4 | 6.1 | 9 | 6.8 | 14 | 8.1 |
| 5 | 6.5 | 10 | 7.0 | 15 | 8.1 |

**10.10.** For the dependent variable, consider $Y = (1, 0)$ if HDL $\leq 40$ and HDL $> 40$ respectively. Find the odds ratio for $Y$ with (a) age, (b) weight and (c) age and weight as the predictors.

**10.11.** From the sample information in Table T10.1(c) test the hypothesis that weight and fitness are not correlated.

**10.12.** Test the hypothesis (a) $H_0 : \rho_{12} = 0.3$ *versus* $H_1 : \rho_{12} \neq 0.3$, (b) $H_0 : \rho_{13} = -0.4$ *versus* $H_1 : \rho_{13} \neq -0.4$, and (c) $H_0 : \rho_{13} = -0.6$ versus $H_1 : \rho_{13} \neq -0.6$

**10.13.** Find the 95 percent confidence limits for $\rho_{13}$.

**10.14.** Find the 95 percent confidence limits for $\rho_{12}$ if $r_{12}$ was found to be 0.26 from a sample of $n = 20$ units.

# Appendix A10

## A10.1  Square of the correlation of $Y_i$ and $\hat{Y}_i$

From (10.7), $\text{Cov}(Y_i, \hat{Y}_i) = \hat{\beta}_1 S_{xy}$, and $V(\hat{Y}_i) = \hat{\beta}_1^2 S_x^2$. Since $V(Y_i) = S_y^2$, square of the correlation of $Y_i$ and $\hat{Y}_i$ becomes $\hat{\beta}_1^2 S_{xy}^2 / (\hat{\beta}_1^2 S_x^2) S_y^2 = r^2$.

## A10.2  Multiple regression

The mean in (10.32) can be expressed as $E(Y|X) = X\beta$, where $Y$ is the $n$-vector of observations, $\beta$ is the $(p + 1)$ – vector of the regression coefficients, and $X$ is an $n \times (p + 1)$ matrix. Corresponding to (10.33), the dispersion matrix of $Y$ becomes $\sigma^2 I$, where $I$ is the identity matrix with ones in the diagonal and zeros in the off-diagonal.

The Multiple Regression equation in (10.34) can be expressed as $Y = X\beta + \varepsilon$, where $Y$ is the $n$-vector of observations. The expected value of the $n$-vector of the random errors $\varepsilon$ is zero, and its dispersion matrix becomes $\sigma^2 I$. For the Least Squares estimation, minimization of $(Y - X\beta)'(Y - X\beta)$, which is the same as (10.35), results in the *normal equations* $X'X\beta = X'Y$. They can be expressed as

$$\sum_{1}^{n}\left(Y_i-\hat{\beta}_0-\hat{\beta}_1 X_{1i}-\hat{\beta}_2 X_{2i}-\ldots-\hat{\beta}_p X_{pi}\right)=0,$$

$$\sum_{1}^{n}\left(Y_i-\hat{\beta}_0-\hat{\beta}_1 X_{1i}-\hat{\beta}_2 X_{2i}-\ldots-\hat{\beta}_p X_{pi}\right)X_{1i}=0,$$

$$\sum_{1}^{n}\left(Y_i-\hat{\beta}_0-\hat{\beta}_1 X_{1i}-\hat{\beta}_2 X_{2i}-\ldots-\hat{\beta}_p X_{pi}\right)X_{2i}=0,$$

$$\cdots\cdots\cdots\cdots\cdots\cdots\cdots\cdots\cdots\cdots\cdots\cdots\cdots\cdots\cdots\cdots\cdots\cdots$$

$$\sum_{1}^{n}\left(Y_i-\hat{\beta}_0-\hat{\beta}_1 X_{1i}-\hat{\beta}_2 X_{2i}-\ldots\hat{\beta}_p X_{pi}\right)X_{2i}=0.$$

The estimators for the regression coefficients are given by $\hat{\beta}=(X'X)^{-1}X'Y$. They are *unbiased* for $\beta$ with dispersion matrix $\sigma^2(X'X)^{-1}$. From this matrix, the variances and covariances of these estimators can be expressed as $\sigma^2 C_{kl}$, $(k,l)=(0,1,\ldots,p)$. From the first normal equation, the estimator of the intercept becomes $\hat{\beta}_0=\bar{Y}-\hat{\beta}_1\bar{X}_1-\hat{\beta}_2\bar{X}_2-\ldots-\hat{\beta}_p\bar{X}_p$.

The estimator for the mean in (10.32) becomes $\hat{Y}=X\hat{\beta}$. It is unbiased and its variance-covariance matrix is given by $\sigma^2 X(X'X)^{-1}X'$. The unbiased estimator for the expected value $E\left(Y|X_{1i},X_{2i},\ldots,X_{pi}\right)$ is given by

$$\begin{aligned}\hat{Y}_i&=\hat{\beta}_0+\hat{\beta}_1 X_{1i}+\hat{\beta}_2 X_{2i}+\ldots+\hat{\beta}_p X_{pi}\\&=\bar{Y}+\hat{\beta}_1 x_{1i}+\hat{\beta}_2 x_{2i}+\ldots+\hat{\beta}_p x_{pi},\end{aligned}\tag{A10.1}$$

where $x_{1i}=(X_{1i}-\bar{X}_1),x_{2i}=(X_{2i}-\bar{X}_2),\ldots,x_{pi}=\left(X_{pi}-\bar{X}_p\right)$. The variance of this estimator can be expressed as

$$V\left(\hat{Y}_i\right)=\sigma^2\left(1/n+C_{11}+C_{22}+\ldots+C_{pp}+2C_{12}+\ldots\right)\tag{A10.2}$$

The predictor $\hat{Y}_{new}$ for new values of the independent variables is obtained from (A10.1). With the expression in (A10.2) for $V(\hat{Y}_{new})$, the variance of the predictor becomes $\sigma^2+V\left(\hat{Y}_{new}\right)$.

The $n$-vector $e=\left(Y-\hat{Y}\right)$ of the residuals is uncorrelated with $\hat{Y}$. An unbiased estimator of $\sigma^2$ is given by

$$\hat{\sigma}^2=e'e/(n-p-1)=\left(Y-X\hat{\beta}\right)'\left(Y-X\hat{\beta}\right)/(n-p-1)=\sum_{1}^{n}\left(Y_i-\hat{Y}_i\right)^2/(n-p-1).$$

$$\tag{A10.3}$$

The estimates $v(\hat{\beta}_0), v(\hat{\beta}_1), v(\hat{\beta}_2), \ldots, v(\hat{\beta}_{p-1})$ for the variances of the regression coefficients, their covariances, and $v(\hat{Y}_i)$ for the variance in (A10.2) are obtained by substituting $\hat{\sigma}^2$ for $\sigma^2$.

## A10.3  Expression for SSR in (10.38)

The SSR can be expressed as

$$\left[\hat{\beta}_1^2 \sum_1^n x_{1i}^2 + \hat{\beta}_2^2 \sum_1^n x_{2i}^2 + \ldots + 2\hat{\beta}_1\hat{\beta}_2 \sum_1^n x_{1i}x_{2i} + \ldots\right] = \left[\hat{\beta}_1 \sum_1^n x_{1i}y_i + \hat{\beta}_2 \sum_1^n x_{2i}y_i + \ldots\right],$$

where $y_i = (Y_i - \bar{Y})$, $x_{1i} = (X_{1i} - \bar{X}_1)$ and $x_{2i} = (X_{2i} - \bar{X}_2)$.

# 11

# Analysis of variance and covariance: Designs of experiments

## 11.1 Introduction

Clinical experiments are conducted to evaluate the differences among the effectiveness of medical treatments. For the sake of comparisons, one or more controls or placebos are included in some of these experiments. Examining the interactions between the treatments and assessing the influence of concomitant factors on the responses or outcomes of the treatments also become important in a number of the experiments.

The treatments in an experiment and the affecting factors are arranged in the one-way, two-way and extended types of classifications. The Analysis of Variance (ANOVA) procedures are employed for the statistical evaluations of the effects of the treatments and the related factors from the observed responses of a clinically designed experiment. They are also extensively employed for the statistical inferences in case-control, cohort, retrospective and observational studies.

The Completely Randomized design, Randomized Blocks, one-way, two-way cross – classifications, interaction in a two-way classification, Analysis of Variance and Analysis of Covariance techniques and related topics are presented in the following sections with illustrations. Balanced and unbalanced One-Way Random Effects models are presented in Sections 11.3, 11.4 and 11.6, and also in Chapter 12. Rao (1997) comprehensively presents the different estimation and inference procedures for the fixed, random and mixed effects models of practical interest.

*Statistical Methodologies with Medical Applications*, First Edition. Poduri S.R.S. Rao.
© 2017 John Wiley & Sons, Ltd. Published 2017 by John Wiley & Sons, Ltd.

## 11.2    One-way classification: Balanced design

In this design, k treatments are independently and randomly assigned to m units each. The responses to the treatments are represented by the model

$$y_{ij} = \mu_i + \varepsilon_{ij}$$
$$= \mu + \alpha_i + \varepsilon_{ij},$$

(11.1)

$i = (1, 2, \ldots, k)$ and $j = (1, 2, \ldots, m)$. The expectation and variance of the response $y_{ij}$ to the $i$th treatment are denoted by $\mu_i$ and $\sigma^2$ respectively. The variance is assumed to be the same for all the $k$ treatments, but it can be different in general. Denoting the overall mean by $\mu$, $\alpha_i = (\mu_i - \mu)$ is the *effect* of the $i$th treatment. It can be expressed as the deviation of $\mu_i$ from a constant instead of the overall mean. For the case of an experiment conducted to evaluate $k$ specified means, (11.1) is known as the *fixed-effects* model. The expectation and variance of the random error $\varepsilon_{ij}$ are zero and $\sigma^2$. The random errors $\varepsilon_{ij}$ are assumed to be uncorrelated for each treatment and between the treatments. They are assumed to follow independent normal distributions with zero means and variance $\sigma^2$. The above model also represents $m$ sample observations from each of $k$ populations or groups with means $\mu_i$ and the same variance $\sigma^2$.

The mean of the $m$ units of the $i$th treatment and the overall mean of the $n = km$ units of the $k$ treatments respectively are $\bar{y}_i = \sum_{j=1}^{m} y_{ij}/m$ and $\bar{y} = \sum_{i=1}^{k}\sum_{j=1}^{m} y_{ij}/n = \sum_{i=1}^{k} \bar{y}_i/k$. Minimization of $\phi = \sum_{ij} (y_{ij} - \mu - \alpha_i)^2$ with respect to $(\mu, \alpha_i)$ with the condition $\sum_i \alpha_i = 0$ results in the estimators $\hat{\mu} = \bar{y}$ and $\hat{\alpha}_i = (\bar{y}_i - \bar{y})$.

The null hypothesis of the equality of the $k$ treatment means is

$$H_0 : \mu_1 = \mu_2 = \ldots = \mu_k.$$

(11.2)

If $\mu$ is the overall mean, this null hypothesis is the same as

$$H_0 : \alpha_1 = \alpha_2 = \ldots = \alpha_k = 0,$$

(11.3)

that is, $\alpha_i = 0$, $i = (1, 2, \ldots, k)$. The alternative hypothesis is that at least one of the treatment effects differs from the rest.

The variation of the $n$ observations from the overall mean can be expressed as

$$\sum_{i=1}^{k}\sum_{j=1}^{m} (y_{ij} - \bar{y})^2 = m\sum_{i=1}^{k} (\bar{y}_i - \bar{y})^2 + \sum_{i=1}^{k}\sum_{j=1}^{m} (y_{ij} - \bar{y}_i)^2.$$

(11.4)

The first term on the right-hand side is the variation among the $k$ means, and the second term is the dispersion of the m units within the treatments. This decomposition is formally expressed as

$$\text{Total } SS = \text{Between } SS + \text{Within } SS = S_B + S_W \tag{11.5}$$

Dividing by the respective d.f., the Between and Within Mean Squares are given by $M_B = S_B/(k-1)$ and $M_W = S_W/(n-k)$. The sample variance of the $i$th group $s_i^2 = \sum_1^m (y_{ij} - \bar{y}_i)^2/(m-1)$ is unbiased for $\sigma^2$. As a result, the Within Mean Square $M_W$, which is the same as the pooled sample variance $s^2 = \sum_1^k s_i^2/k$, is unbiased for $\sigma^2$.

From (11.1), the expected value of the Between Mean Square becomes

$$E(M_B) = \sigma^2 + m \sum_{i=1}^k \alpha_i^2/(k-1), \tag{11.6}$$

which exceeds $\sigma^2$ when $H_0$ in (11.3) for the treatment effects is not valid. The ratio $[M_B/E(M_B)]/[M_W/E(M_W)]$ follows the $F$-distribution with $(k-1)$ and $(n-k)$ d.f. If the null hypothesis is valid, $E(M_B) = E(M_W)$. The test statistic for this null hypothesis is given by

$$F = M_B/M_W, \tag{11.7}$$

which follows the $F$-distribution with $(k-1)$ and $(n-k)$ d.f. The different Sums of Squares (SS) and, Mean Squares (MS) and the F – ratio are presented in Table 11.1.

*Example 11.1*   With the sample observations in Table T11.2, the ANOVA for the null hypothesis of the equality of the means of the systolic blood pressures (SBPs) of the three adult groups before the exercise program is as follows.

ANOVA for the SBPs before the exercise program.

| Source | d.f. | SS | MS | F | $p$-value |
|--------|------|------|------|------|---------|
| Between groups | 2 | 403.8 | 201.9 | 3.440 | .047 |
| Within groups | 27 | 1582.5 | 58.61 | | |
| Total | 29 | 1986.3 | | | |

Table 11.1   ANOVA for the equality of the treatment effects. One-way classification.

| Source | d.f | SS | MS | F |
|--------|------|------|------|------|
| Between | $k-1$ | $S_B$ | $M_B = S_B/(k-1)$ | $M_B/M_W$ |
| Within | $(n-k)$ | $S_W$ | $\hat{\sigma}^2 = M_W = S_W/(n-k)$ | |
| Total | $(n-1)$ | $S_B + S_W$ | | |

The estimate of $\sigma^2$ is $\hat{\sigma}^2 = 58.61$. At a significance level of 4.7 percent or higher, the difference between the means of the SBPs of the three groups before the exercise program is significant.

A simple method for finding the Total, Between and Within Sums of Squares is as follows: The totals of the SBPs of the three groups are (1424, 1400, 1487). The grand total of the $n = 30$ observations is $G = 4311$ and the Correction Factor becomes $C.F. = (G^2/n) = 619490.7$. Now, Total $SS = [\sum_{ij} y_{ij}^2 - C.F.] = (621477 - C.F.) =$

1986.3, Between $SS = \left[\left(1424^2 + 1400^2 + 1487^2\right)/10 - C.F.\right] = 403.8$. By subtraction, Within $SS = 1986.3 - 403.8 = 1582.5$.

## 11.3   One-way random effects model: Balanced design

For this design, the means $\mu_i$, $i = (1,2,\ldots,k)$, for the k groups or treatments are considered to be a random sample from a population with $E(\mu_i) = \mu$ and $V(\mu_i) = \sigma_\alpha^2$. As in the case of the *fixed effects*, the model for the sample observations is given by

$$y_{ij} = \mu_i + \varepsilon_{ij}$$
$$= \mu + \alpha_i + \varepsilon_{ij},$$

(11.8)

$i = (1,2,\ldots,k)$ and $j = (1,2,\ldots,m)$, where $\alpha_i = (\mu_i - \mu)$ is the **random effect** of the ith treatment. The assumptions for the error $\varepsilon_{ij}$ are the same as in Section 11.2. It is assumed that the random effect $\alpha_i$ is uncorrelated with $\varepsilon_{ij}$, and $\alpha_i$ and $\alpha_{i'}'$ $(i \neq i')$ are uncorrelated. When $\mu_i$ follows the normal distribution with expectation and variance as above, the *random effect* $\alpha_i = (\mu_i - \mu)$ follows the normal distribution with zero mean and variance $\sigma_\alpha^2$. Now, $y_{ij}$ follows the normal distribution with mean $\mu$ and variance $(\sigma_\alpha^2 + \sigma^2)$. Further, $Cov(y_{ij}, y_{ij'}) = \sigma_\alpha^2$, $(j \neq j') = (1,2,\ldots,m)$.

## 11.4   Inference for the variance components and the mean

For both the fixed and random effects models in (11.1) and (11.8), $E(M_W) = \sigma^2$. The test statistic for $H_0 : \sigma^2 = \sigma_0^2$ is given by

$$U = (n-k)s^2/\sigma_0^2 = (n-k)M_w/\sigma_0^2,$$

(11.9)

which follows the chisquare distribution with $(n - k)$ d.f. The $(1-\alpha)$ percent confidence limits for $\sigma^2$ are obtained from $(n-k)s^2/b$ and $(n-k)s^2/a$, where $(a,b)$ are the lower and upper $(1-\alpha)$ percentiles of this distribution.

From (11.4) and (11.8), $E(M_B) = m\sigma_\alpha^2 + \sigma^2$. An unbiased estimator of $\sigma_\alpha^2$ is given by

$$\hat{\sigma}_\alpha^2 = (M_B - M_W)/m. \tag{11.10}$$

If this expression takes a negative value, zero or a small positive quantity may be substituted for the estimate. The variance of this estimator and its unbiased estimator are given by

$$V(\hat{\sigma}_\alpha^2) = [2/(k-1)](\sigma_\alpha^2 + \sigma^2/m)^2 + 2\sigma^4/(n-k)m^2 \tag{11.11}$$

and

$$v(\hat{\sigma}_\alpha^2) = [2/(k+1)] \left[ \sum_i (\bar{y}_i - \bar{y})^2/(k-1) \right]^2 + 2\hat{\sigma}^4/(n-k+2)m^2 \tag{11.12}$$

$$= \frac{2}{k+1}\left(\frac{M_B}{m}\right)^2 + \frac{2}{n-k+2}\left(\frac{M_W}{m}\right)^2.$$

As in the case of the fixed effects model, $[M_B/E(M_B)]/[M_W/E(M_W)]$ follows the $F$-distribution with $(k-1)$ and $(n-k)$ d.f. The test statistic for the hypothesis $H_0 : \sigma_\alpha^2 = 0$ is given by

$$F = M_B/M_W \tag{11.13}$$

which follows the $F$-distribution with $(k-1)$ and $(n-k)$ d.f. This statistic is the same as the $F$-ratio in (11.7) for testing the equality of the k treatment effects. An estimate of $R = \sigma_\alpha^2/\sigma^2$ is given by $(M_B - M_W)/mM_W$. The $(1-\alpha)$ percent confidence limits for this ratio are obtained from

$$\frac{1}{m}\left(\frac{F}{F_u} - 1\right) \leq R \leq \frac{1}{m}\left(\frac{F}{F_l} - 1\right). \tag{11.14}$$

In this expression, $F_u$ and $F_l$ are the $(1-\alpha)$ percentiles of the above F-distribution. The overall sample mean $\bar{y} = \sum_i \bar{y}_i/k$ is unbiased for $\mu$ with variance

$$V(\bar{y}) = (\sigma_\alpha^2 + \sigma^2/m)/k \tag{11.15}$$

and estimator of variance

$$v(\bar{y}) = \sum_i (\bar{y}_i - \bar{y})^2/k(k-1). \tag{11.16}$$

With $S.E.(\bar{y}) = \sqrt{v(\bar{y})}$, the test statistic for $H_0 : \mu = \mu_0$ is given by

$$t_{k-1} = (\bar{y} - \mu_0)/S.E.(\bar{y}), \tag{11.17}$$

which follows the t-distribution with $(k-1)$ d.f. The $(1-\alpha)$ percent confidence limits for $\mu$ are obtained from $\bar{y} \pm t_{k-1,\alpha/2} S.E.(\bar{y})$.

*Example 11.2*   With the random effects model for the SBPs in Example 11.1, $\hat{\sigma}_\alpha^2 = (201.9-58.61)/10 = 14.33$. From (11.12), $v(\hat{\sigma}_\alpha^2) = 206.19$ and $S.E.(\hat{\sigma}_\alpha^2) = 14.36$.

The estimate for $\mu$ is $\bar{y} = (142.4+140.0+148.7)/3 = 143.7$. From (11.16) $v(\bar{y}) = (40.38/6) = 6.73$ and $S.E.(\bar{y}) = 2.59$. With $t_{2,0.025} = 4.303$, the lower and upper confidence limits for $\mu$ are $143.7-4.303(2.59) = 132.56$ and $143.7+4.303(2.59) = 154.46$.

# 11.5   One-way classification: Unbalanced design and fixed effects

In general, the sample sizes $n_i$ for the $k$ treatments are unequal and the model for the responses becomes

$$y_{ij} = \mu_i + \varepsilon_{ij}$$
$$= \mu + \alpha_i + \varepsilon_{ij},$$

$$(11.18)$$

$i = (1,2,\ldots,k)$ and $j = (1,2,\ldots,n_i)$. The effect of the $i$th treatment is denoted by $\alpha_i = (\mu_i - \mu)$. The mean of the responses of the $n_i$ units for the $i$th treatment and the overall mean of the $n = \sum_1^k n_i$ units of all the $k$ treatments respectively are $\bar{y}_i = \sum_1^{n_i} y_{ij}/n_i$ and $\bar{y} = \sum_1^k \sum_1^{n_i} y_{ij}/n = \sum_1^k n_i \bar{y}_i/n$. Minimization of $\phi = \sum_{ij}(y_{ij}-\mu-\alpha_i)^2$ with respect to $(\mu, \alpha_i)$ with the condition $\sum_i n_i \alpha_i = 0$ results in the estimators $\hat{\mu} = \bar{y}$ and $\hat{\alpha}_i = (\bar{y}_i - \bar{y})$. The Total Sum of Squares of all the n observations can be decomposed as

$$\sum_1^k \sum_1^{n_i}(y_{ij}-\bar{y})^2 = \sum_1^k n_i(\bar{y}_i-\bar{y})^2 + \sum_1^k \sum_1^{n_i}(y_{ij}-\bar{y}_i)^2.$$

$$(11.19)$$

As in the balanced case, the left-hand-side expression is the Total SS with $(n-1)$ d.f. The right-hand-side expressions are the Between SS and Within SS, $S_B$ and $S_W$, with $(k-1)$ and $(n-k)$ d.f. respectively.

For the $i$th treatment, $s_i^2 = \sum_1^{n_i}(y_{ij}-\bar{y}_i)^2/(n_i-1)$ is an unbiased estimator of $\sigma^2$.

Since the variances for the $k$ treatments are the same, the pooled sample variance

$\hat{\sigma}^2 = s^2 = \sum_{1}^{k}(n_i-1)s_i^2/(n-k)$, which is the Within Mean Square $M_W = S_W/(n-k)$, is unbiased for $\sigma^2$. The Between Mean Square is $M_B = S_B/(k-1)$. From (11.19),

$$E(M_B) = \sigma^2 + \sum_{1}^{k} n_i \alpha_i^2/(k-1).$$ (11.20)

The null hypothesis for the equality of the means of the $k$ treatments is

$$H_0 : \mu_1 = \mu_2 = \ldots = \mu_k.$$ (11.21)

With the treatment effects $\alpha_i = (\mu_i - \mu)$, $i = (1,2,\ldots,k)$, this hypothesis is the same as

$$H_0 : \alpha_1 = \alpha_2 = \ldots \alpha_k = 0.$$ (11.22)

The test statistic for this hypothesis is given by

$$F = M_B/M_W,$$ (11.23)

which follows the $F$-distribution with $(k-1, n-k)$ d.f. The ANOVA table for this hypothesis is the same as Table 11.1 with the corresponding expressions in (11.19) for $S_B$ and $S_W$.

*Example 11.3*  Age and weight of a total of $n = 30$ adults classified into $k = 3$ groups of sizes $n_1 = 9$, $n_2 = 13$ and $n_3 = 8$, of 30–49, 50–69 and $\geq 70$ years of age are presented in Table T11.3. Their systolic blood pressures (SBPs in mmHg) before and after an exercise program appear in Table T11.4. The ANOVA to test the differences among the means of the SBPs of the three groups before the exercise program is as follows:

ANOVA for the means of the SBPs before the program.

| Source | d.f. | SS | MS | F | $p$-value |
|---|---|---|---|---|---|
| Between | 2 | 1133.5 | 566.7 | 15.13 | $3.9 \times 10^{-5}$ |
| Within | 27 | 1011.5 | 37.5 | | |
| Total | 29 | 2145 | | | |

The estimate of $\sigma^2$ is $\hat{\sigma}^2 = 37.5$. The $F$-ratio of 15.13 with (2, 27) d.f. and the small $p$-value suggest that the difference among the means of the SBPs for the three groups is highly significant.

## 11.6 Unbalanced one-way classification: Random effects

As in Section 11.3, the means $\mu_i$, $i = (1, 2, ...., k)$, for the k groups or treatments are considered to be a random sample from a population with mean $E(\mu_i) = \mu$ and variance $V(\mu_i) = \sigma_\alpha^2$. Samples of sizes $n_i$ are selected from the k groups. The model is the same as (11.18) with the random effects $\alpha_i$. The expressions for sums of squares $(S_B, S_W)$ are the same as presented in (11.19), and the mean squares are given by $M_B = S_B/(k-1)$ and $M_W = S_W/(n-k)$. From the expressions for these mean squares, $E(M_W) = \sigma^2$ and

$$E(M_B) = \frac{\sum\limits_{1}^{k} n_i(n-n_i)}{n(k-1)} \sigma_\alpha^2 + \sigma^2. \tag{11.24}$$

An unbiased estimator of $\sigma_\alpha^2$ is given by

$$\hat{\sigma}_\alpha^2 = (M_B - M_W)/m_0, \tag{11.25}$$

where $m_0 = \sum\limits_{i} n_i(n-n_i)/n(k-1)$. Its variance as given by Rao (1997) is presented in Appendix A11.1. The minimum variance unbiased estimator of $\mu$ is the Weighted Least Squares (WLS) estimator

$$\bar{y}_W = \sum\limits_{i} W_i \bar{y}_i/W, \tag{11.26}$$

where $V_i = V(\bar{y}_i) = (\sigma_\alpha^2 + \sigma^2/n_i)$, $W_i = 1/V_i$ and $W = \sum\limits_{i} W_i$. Its variance becomes

$$V(\bar{y}_w) = 1/W. \tag{11.27}$$

The test statistic for the hypothesis $H_0 : \sigma_\alpha^2 = 0$ is $F = M_B/M_W$ which follows the F-distribution with $(k-1, n-k)$ d.f. This statistic is the same as (11.23) for testing the equality of the k treatment effects. Approximate $(1-\alpha)$ percent confidence limits for the ratio $R = \sigma_\alpha^2/\sigma^2$ are obtained from

$$\frac{1}{m_0}\left(\frac{F}{F_u} - 1\right) \leq R \leq \frac{1}{m_0}\left(\frac{F}{F_l} - 1\right), \tag{11.28}$$

where $(F_l, F_u)$ are the $(1-\alpha)$ percentage point of the above F-distribution.

*Example 11.4*   SBPs before the exercise program: Table T11.4. As presented above, $m_0 = 9.77$ or approximately 10. The means for the three groups are (132.22, 142.62, 148.13). From (11.25) and Example 11.3, $\hat{\sigma}_\alpha^2 = (566.7 - 37.5)/10 = 52.92$. With the estimates of $(\sigma_\alpha^2, \sigma^2)$, the estimates of $V_i$ are $v_1 = (52.92 + 37.5/9) = 57.09$, $v_2 = (52.92 + 37.5/13) = 55.80$ and $v_3 = (52.92 + 37.5/8) = 57.61$. The estimates of $W_i$ are $w_1 = 1/57.09 = 0.0175$, $w_2 = 1/55.80 = 0.0179$ and $w_3 = 1/57.61 = 0.0174$. The estimate of $W$ is $w = (0.0175 + 0.0179 + 0.0174) = 0.0528$. With these weights, $\bar{y}_W = 140.99$, $v(\bar{y}_w) = 1/0.0528 = 18.94$ and $S.E.(\bar{y}_w) = 4.35$.

## 11.7   Intraclass correlation

In biological, genetic, medical and similar studies, it is of interest to examine the relationship between all pairs of members of the same class, cluster, family, group or species. The intraclass correlation is a measure of this relationship. With the subscript $i = (1, 2, ..,k)$ for the class and $(j \neq j') = (1, 2, ..., m)$ for the members of the same class, this correlation of $y_{ij}$ and $y_{ij'}$ is defined as

$$\rho = \frac{Cov(y_{ij}, y_{ij'})}{\sqrt{V(y_{ij})V(y_{ij'})}}. \tag{11.29}$$

With the model in (11.8) for $y_{ij}$ and the assumptions for $\alpha_i$ and $\varepsilon_{ij}$, $V(y_{ij}) = V(y_{ij'}) = \sigma_\alpha^2 + \sigma^2$ and $Cov(y_{ij}, y_{ij'}) = \sigma_\alpha^2$. This correlation can be expressed as

$$\rho = \frac{\sigma_\alpha^2}{\sigma_\alpha^2 + \sigma^2}. \tag{11.30}$$

As in the case of the correlation coefficient between two random variables, $0 \leq \rho \leq 1$. With the estimates for $(\sigma^2, \sigma_\alpha^2)$ in Section (11. 4), an estimator for $\rho$ is given by

$$\hat{\rho} = \frac{(M_B - M_W)}{M_B + (m-1)M_W} = \frac{F-1}{F + (m-1)}. \tag{11.31}$$

where $F = M_B/M_W$. This estimator increases as the Within Mean Square $M_W$ increases. The $(1-\alpha)$ percent confidence limits for $\rho$ are given by

$$\frac{F - F_u}{F + (m-1)F_u} \leq \rho \leq \frac{F - F_l}{F + (m-1)F_l}, \tag{11.32}$$

where $(F_l, F_u)$ are the $(1-\alpha)$ percentiles of the F-distribution with $(k-1, n-k)$ d.f.

As an illustration, for the SBPs in Examples 11.1 and 11.2, $\hat{\rho} = 14.33/(14.33 + 58.61) = 0.196$ from (11.30) with the estimates of $(\sigma^2, \sigma_\alpha^2)$. The same result is obtained from (11.31) with $F = 3.44$. For $(1-\alpha) = 0.95$, $F_l(2,27) = 0.025$ and $F_u(2,27) = 4.242$. From (11.32), the upper limit for $\rho$ becomes $(3.44 - 0.025)/[3.44 + 9(0.025)] = 0.93$. The lower limit becomes negative and it is set to zero.

For the unbalanced random effects model described in Section 11.6, an estimate for $\rho$ and its approximate confidence limits can be obtained from (11.31) and (11.32) by replacing m with $m_0$. For the SBPs before the exercise program in Example 11.4, 95 percent confidence limits for $\rho$ are $(15.13-4.242)/[15.13+9(4.242)] = 0.204$ and $(15.13 - 0.025)/[15.13 + 9(0.025)] = 0.984$.

# 11.8    Analysis of covariance: The balanced design

The Analysis of Covariance combines the ANOVA and regression methods for the inferences related to the treatment effects. In this approach, the responses are adjusted for the covariates or concomitant variables. These variables can be of the quantitative type such as age, weight or the initial responses before the treatments are applied. They can also be of the qualitative type, for instance, related to family history. In some experiments, both types of covariates are used for evaluating the treatment effects. Comparisons among the means and treatment effects can be performed with increased precisions if the responses are adjusted for the covariates. The model with one covariate is considered in the following sections.

## 11.8.1    The model and least squares estimation

It was found in Example 11.1 that the difference among the means of the SBPs of the three groups was significant. The SBPs ($y_{ij}$) of the individuals may be related to their weights ($x_{ij}$). It would be of interest to examine the differences among the means of the SBPs after their adjustment for the weights. For a linear relationship of these variables, the Analysis of Covariance model is

$$y_{ij} = \mu_i + \beta\left(x_{ij} - \bar{x}\right) + \varepsilon_{ij}$$
$$= \mu + \alpha_i + \beta\left(x_{ij} - \bar{x}\right) + \varepsilon_{ij},$$

(11.33)

$i = (1,2,\ldots,k)$ and $j = (1,2,\ldots,m)$ can be considered. In this expression, $\bar{x} = \sum_{i=1}^{k}\sum_{j=1}^{m} x_{ij}/n = \sum_{i=1}^{k} \bar{x}_i/k$ is the overall mean of the covariate for all the $k$ treatments.

As in the case of the ANOVA model in (11.1), $\alpha_i$ is the effect of the $i$th treatment or group, and the random error $\varepsilon_{ij}$ is assumed to follow the normal distribution with zero mean and variance $\sigma^2$. This model represents the regressions of $y_{ij}$ on $x_{ij}$ for the $k$ treatments with the same slope $\beta$ but different intercepts $\mu_i - \beta\bar{x}$. The Least Squares Estimators of the slope, mean of the $i$th treatment and the difference of the effects of the $i$th and $j$th treatments are obtained by minimizing

$$\phi = \sum_{i=1}^{k}\sum_{j=1}^{m} \left[y_{ij} - \mu_i - \beta\left(x_{ij} - \bar{x}\right)\right]^2$$

(11.34)

with respect to $\beta$ and $\mu_i$. This minimization results in the estimators

$$\hat{\beta} = \sum_{i=1}^{k}\sum_{j=1}^{m}(x_{ij}-\bar{x}_i)(y_{ij}-\bar{y}_i) \bigg/ \sum_{i=1}^{k}\sum_{j=1}^{m}(x_{ij}-\bar{x}_i)^2, \tag{11.35}$$

$$\hat{\mu}_i = \bar{y}_i - \hat{\beta}(\bar{x}_i - \bar{x}) \tag{11.36}$$

and

$$(\hat{\alpha}_i - \hat{\alpha}_j) = (\hat{\mu}_i - \hat{\mu}_j) = (\bar{y}_i - \bar{y}_j) - \hat{\beta}(\bar{x}_i - \bar{x}_j). \tag{11.37}$$

The Total, Between and Within Sum of Squares (SS) and Sum of Products (SP) of the covariate $x_{ij}$ and response $y_{ij}$, ($Txx$, $Tyy$, $Txy$; $Bxx$, $Byy$, $Bxy$; $Wxx$, $Wyy$, $Wxy$) are presented in Appendix A 11.2 for unequal sample sizes $n_i$ for the treatments. For the balanced design, they are obtained with $n_i = m$ for all the $k$ groups or treatments. The estimator $\hat{\beta}$ in (11.35) for the slope is the same as $W_{xy}/W_{xx}$ and the Regression SS becomes $\hat{\beta}^2 W_{xx} = W_{xy}^2/W_{xx}$. With the above estimators, from (11.34),

$$\text{Error } SS = W_{y.x} = W_{yy} - W_{xy}^2/W_{xx} \tag{11.38}$$

with $(n - k - 1)$ d.f., and

$$\hat{\sigma}^2 = W_{y.x}/(n-k-1) \tag{11.39}$$

is unbiased for $\sigma^2$. Note that $W_{yy}$ and the Regression SS have $(n - k)$ and 1 d.f. respectively.

The estimators in (11.35)–(11.37) are unbiased respectively for the slope $\beta$, the mean $\mu_i$, and difference of the treatment effects $(\alpha_i - \alpha_j)$. Their variances are given by

$$V(\hat{\beta}) = \sigma^2/W_{xx}, \tag{11.40}$$

$$V(\hat{\mu}_i) = \sigma^2\left[\frac{1}{m} + \frac{(\bar{x}_i - \bar{x})^2}{W_{xx}}\right] \tag{11.41}$$

and

$$V(\hat{\alpha}_i - \hat{\alpha}_j) = \sigma^2\left[\frac{2}{m} + \frac{(\bar{x}_i - \bar{x}_j)^2}{W_{xx}}\right]. \tag{11.42}$$

The estimates of these variances $v(\hat{\beta})$, $v(\hat{\mu}_i)$ and $v(\hat{\alpha}_i - \hat{\alpha}_j)$ are obtained by replacing $\sigma^2$ with $\hat{\sigma}^2$ in (11.39). For the tests of hypotheses and confidence limits related to the above parameters, S.E.s are obtained from the square roots of these estimates of the variances.

## 11.8.2   Tests of hypotheses for the slope coefficient and equality of the means

The null hypothesis to examine whether the response $y_{ij}$ significantly depends on the covariate $x_{ij}$ is $H_0 : \beta = 0$. The statistic for this hypothesis is given by

$$t_{n-k-1} = \hat{\beta} / \sqrt{\hat{\sigma}^2 / W_{xx}} \qquad (11.43)$$

which follows the t-distribution with $(n - k - 1)$ d.f. The square of this statistic becomes

$$F(1, n-k-1) = \left( W_{xy}^2 / W_{xx} \right) / \hat{\sigma}^2 \qquad (11.44)$$

which follows the $F$-distribution with one (1) and $(n-k-1)$ d.f.

The null hypothesis that all the means are the same, that is, $H_0 : \mu_i = \mu$, for $i = (1,2,\ldots,k)$, is the same as $H_0 : \alpha_i = 0$, for $i = (1,2,\ldots,k)$. Minimizing (11.34) under this hypothesis, the estimators for the slope coefficient becomes

$$\hat{\beta} = \sum_{i=1}^{k} \sum_{j=1}^{m} (x_{ij} - \bar{x})(y_{ij} - \bar{y}) / \sum_{1=1}^{k} \sum_{j=1}^{m} (x_{ij} - \bar{x})^2 = T_{xy}/T_{xx}. \qquad (11.45)$$

From this minimization,

$$\text{Regression SS} = \hat{\beta}^2 T_{xx} = T_{xy}^2 / T_{xx}$$

with 1 d.f. and

$$\text{Error SS} = T_{y.x} = T_{yy} - T_{xy}^2 / T_{xx} \qquad (11.46)$$

with $[(n - 1) - 1] = (n - 2)$ d.f.

From (11.38) and (11.46), the addition to the Error SS due to this hypothesis of equality of the treatment effects is $(T_{y.x} - W_{y.x})$ with $[(n-2) - (n-k-1)] = (k-1)$ d.f. The test statistic for the above hypothesis of the equality of the treatment effects is given by

$$F(k-1, n-k-1) = \frac{(T_{y.x} - W_{y.x})/(k-1)}{\hat{\sigma}^2}, \qquad (11.47)$$

which follows the $F$-distribution with $(k-1)$ and $(n-k-1)$ d.f. The sums of squares and cross-products for this hypothesis are summarized in Table 11.2.

*Example 11.5*   The weights (x) and SBPs (y) before the exercise program for three groups with samples of size $m = 10$ from each group are presented in Tables T11.1 and T11.2. The SS and SP for x and y are given below.

Table 11.2   Sums of Squares and Cross Products for the Analysis of Covariance.

| Source | d.f | $x$ | $y$ | $xy$ | SS and d.f. under $H_0 : \alpha_i = 0$ | |
|---|---|---|---|---|---|---|
| Between | $k-1$ | $B_{xx}$ | $B_{yy}$ | $B_{xy}$ | | |
| Within | $n-k$ | $W_{xx}$ | $W_{yy}$ | $W_{xy}$ | $W_{y.x} = W_{yy} - W_{xy}^2/W_{xx}$ | $n-k-1$ |
| Total | $n-1$ | $T_{xx}$ | $T_{yy}$ | $T_{xy}$ | $T_{y.x} = T_{yy} - T_{xy}^2/T_{xx}$ | $n-2$ |

$\hat{\sigma}^2 = W_{y.x}/(n-k-1)$. $\qquad\qquad\qquad F(k-1,n-k-1) = \left(T_{y.x} - W_{y.x}\right)/\hat{\sigma}^2$

| Source | d.f. | $x$ | $y$ | $xy$ |
|---|---|---|---|---|
| Between | 2 | 1192.47 | 403.8 | 263.6 |
| Within | 27 | 331.00 | 1582.5 | 385.6 |
| Total | 29 | 1523.47 | 1986.3 | 649.2 |

The estimate for the slope is $\hat{\beta} = \left(W_{xy}/W_{xx}\right) = (385.6/331) = 1.165$. The Regression SS and Residual SS respectively are $\left(W_{xy}^2/W_{xx}\right) = \left(385.6^2/331\right) = 449.21$ and $W_{y.x} = 1582.5 - 449.21 = 1133.29$, and $\hat{\sigma}^2 = (1133.29/26) = 43.59$. The test statistic for $H_0 : \beta = 0$ becomes $F(1, 26) = (449.21/43.59) = 10.31$ with the $p$-value of 0.0035, indicating that weight has a significant effect on the SBP.

To test the hypothesis that the Means of the SBPs for the three groups are the same, $T_{y.x} = 1986.3 - 649.2^2/1523.47 = 1709.65$, and the test statistic becomes $F(2, 26) = [(1709.65 - 1133.29)/2]/43.59 = 6.61$ with the $p$-value of 0.0048. With this small $p$-value, the difference between the means of the three groups is highly significant. It was found in Example 11.1 that without adjusting for the weights, the difference between the means of the SBPs for the three groups is barely significant at the 4.7 percent level.

### 11.8.3   Confidence limits for the adjusted means and their differences

For the means $\mu_i$, $(1-\alpha)$ percent confidence limits are obtained from $\hat{\mu}_i \pm t_{n-k-1, \alpha/2} \sqrt{v(\hat{\mu}_i)}$. For the difference of the effects of two treatments, they are obtained from

$$\left(\hat{\alpha}_i - \hat{\alpha}_j\right) \pm t_{n-k-1, \alpha/2} \sqrt{v\left(\hat{\alpha}_i - \hat{\alpha}_j\right)}.$$

*Example 11.6*   For the three groups, the means of the SBPs before the exercise program, adjusted and unadjusted for the weights, S.E.s of the estimates and 95 percent confidence limits for $\mu_i$ obtained from Tables T11.1, T11.2 and Example 11.5 with

$t_{26,0.025} = 2.056$ are as follows. The average weights for the three groups are (158.3, 170.5, 172.6) lbs, and the overall mean is $\bar{x} = 167.13$. From Example 11.5, $\hat{\sigma}^2 = 43.59$. The S.E.s of $\hat{\mu}_i$ obtained from (11.41) with this estimate for $\sigma^2$ and the ranks of the estimates of $\hat{\mu}_i$ appear in the parentheses. Adjusting the SBPs for the weights has altered the means of the highest and the next highest means.

| $\bar{y}_i$ | $\hat{\mu}_i$ | Confidence limits for $\mu_i$ |
|---|---|---|
| 142.4 (2) | 152.69 (1) (3.82) | 144.84, 160.54 |
| 140.0 (3) | 136.07 (3) (2.42) | 131.09, 141.05 |
| 148.7 (1) | 142.33 (2) (2.88) | 136.41, 148.25 |

The estimate for the difference of the adjusted effects of the first two groups is $(152.69 - 136.07) = 16.62$. From (11.42), its estimated variance and S.E. become $43.59\left[(2/10) + (158.3-170.5)^2/331\right] = 28.32$ and 5.32. With $t_{26,0.025} = 2.056$, the 95 percent confidence limits for the difference of the two adjusted means are $16.62 - 2.056(5.32) = 5.68$ and $16.62 + 2.056(5.32) = 27.56$.

## 11.9  Analysis of covariance: Unbalanced design

All the expressions in this section for the unbalanced design are analogous to the ones in Section 11.8 for the case of the balanced design.

With unequal sample sizes $n_{ij}$ for the $k$ treatments, the model in (11.33) becomes

$$y_{ij} = \mu_i + \beta\left(x_{ij} - \bar{x}\right) + \varepsilon_{ij}$$
$$= \mu + \alpha_i + \beta\left(x_{ij} - \bar{x}\right) + \varepsilon_{ij}, \tag{11.48}$$

$i = (1,2,\ldots,k)$ and $j = (1,2,\ldots,n_i)$, where $n = \sum_1^k n_i$ and $\bar{x} = \sum_1^k \sum_1^{n_i} x_{ij}/n$.

The Least Squares Estimators of the slope, mean of the $i$th treatment and the difference of the effects of the $i$th and $j$th treatments are obtained by minimizing

$$\phi = \sum_1^k \sum_1^{n_i} \left[y_{ij} - \mu_i - \beta\left(x_{ij} - \bar{x}\right)\right]^2. \tag{11.49}$$

These estimators become

$$\hat{\beta} = \sum_1^k \sum_1^{n_i} \left( x_{ij} - \bar{x}_i \right) \left( y_{ij} - \bar{y}_i \right) / \sum_1^k \sum_1^{n_i} \left( x_{ij} - \bar{x}_i \right)^2, \tag{11.50}$$

$$\hat{\mu}_i = \bar{y}_i - \hat{\beta}(\bar{x}_i - \bar{x}) \tag{11.51}$$

and

$$\left( \hat{\alpha}_i - \hat{\alpha}_j \right) = \left( \bar{y}_i - \bar{y}_j \right) - \hat{\beta} \left( \bar{x}_i - \bar{x}_j \right). \tag{11.52}$$

In these expressions $(\bar{x}_i, \bar{y}_i)$ are the means of the k treatments. These three estimators are respectively unbiased for $\beta, \mu_i$ and $\left( \mu_i - \mu_j \right) = \left( \alpha_i - \alpha_j \right)$. Their variances take the same form as (11.40), (11.41) and (11.42) except that $(1/m)$ in (11.41) is replaced by $(1/n_i)$ and $(2/m)$ in (11.42) by $(1/n_i + 1/n_j)$.

The Total, Between and Within Sum of Squares (SS) and Sum of Products (SP) of the covariate $x_{ij}$ and response $y_{ij}$, $(T_{xx}, T_{yy}, T_{xy}; B_{xx}, B_{yy}, B_{xy}; W_{xx}, W_{yy}, W_{xy})$ are presented in Appendix (A 11.2). The estimator in (11.50) for the slope is the same as $W_{xy}/W_{xx}$ and the Regression SS becomes $\hat{\beta}^2 W_{xx} = W_{xy}^2/W_{xx}$. With the above estimators, from (11.49),

$$\text{Error SS} = W_{y.x} = W_{yy} - W_{xy}^2/W_{xx} \tag{11.53}$$

with $(n - k - 1)$ d.f., and $\hat{\sigma}^2 = W_{y.x}/(n-k-1)$ is unbiased for $\sigma^2$. For testing $H_0 : \beta = 0$, the statistic $F = \left( W_{xy}^2/W_{xx} \right)/\hat{\sigma}^2$ follows the F-distribution with $(1, n - k - 1)$ d.f.

The null hypothesis that all the means are equal, that is $H_0 : \mu_i = \mu$, for i = (1,2,...,k), is the same as $H_0 : \alpha_i = 0$, for $i = (1, 2, ..., k)$. Minimizing (11.49) when this null hypothesis is valid, the estimator for the slope becomes

$$\hat{\beta} = \sum_1^k \sum_1^{n_i} \left( x_{ij} - \bar{x} \right) \left( y_{ij} - \bar{y} \right) / \sum_1^k \sum_1^{n_i} \left( x_{ij} - \bar{x} \right)^2 = T_{xy}/T_{xx}. \tag{11.54}$$

Now, the Regression SS is $\hat{\beta}^2 T_{xx} = T_{xy}^2/T_{xx}$ with 1 d.f. and

$$\text{Error SS} = T_{y.x} = T_{yy} - T_{xy}^2/T_{xx} \tag{11.55}$$

with $(n - 2)$ d.f.

The test statistic for the above hypothesis of the equality of the treatment effects is given by

$$F(k-1, n-k-1) = \frac{(T_{y.x} - W_{y.x})/(k-1)}{\hat{\sigma}^2}, \tag{11.56}$$

which follows the F-distribution with $(k - 1, n - k - 1)$ d.f.

*Example 11.7*    For samples of sizes (9, 13, 8) of three adult groups, age and weight are presented in Table T11.3 and the SBPs before and after an exercise program in Table T11.4. The average weights of the three groups are (164.56, 173.15, 174.25) lbs. For the SBPs ($y_{ij}$) before the exercise program, consider the differences among the means for the three age groups with weight as the covariate ($x_{ij}$). The SS and SP for these variables are given below. From these results,

| Source | d.f. | $x$ | $y$ | $xy$ |
|---|---|---|---|---|
| Between | 2 | 518.05 | 1133.46 | 739.29 |
| Within | 27 | 865.54 | 1011.51 | 555.55 |
| Total | 29 | 1383.59 | 2144.97 | 1294.75 |

$\hat{\beta} = (555.55/865.54) = 0.6419$, Regression SS $= (555.55)^2/865.54 = 356.58$, Error SS $= W_{y.x} = (1011.51 - 356.58) = 654.93$ and $\hat{\sigma}^2 = (654.93/26) = 25.19$.

Test for $H_0 : \beta = 0$

$F_{1,26} = (356.58/25.19) = 14.16$ with the $p$-value of 0.0009, suggesting that the SBP significantly depends on weight.

Test for $H_0 : \mu_1 = \mu_2 = \ldots = \mu_k$

$T_{y.x} = (2144.97 - 1294.75^2/1383.59) = 933.35$.

$F_{2,26} = [(933.35 - 654.93)/2]/25.19 = 5.53$ with the $p$-value of 0.01 suggesting that after adjusting for weight the difference among the means of the SBPs for the three age groups is significantly different.

## 11.9.1    Confidence limits for the adjusted means and the differences of the treatment effects

Variances of the estimates of the means and their differences are obtained as described above, and the standard errors are obtained from their square roots. For specified probability $(1 - \alpha)$, confidence limits for the means and their differences are obtained from $\hat{\mu}_i \pm t_{\alpha/2, n-k-1} S.E.(\hat{\mu}_i)$ and $(\hat{\mu}_i - \hat{\mu}_{i'}) \pm t_{\alpha/2, n-k-1} S.E.(\hat{\mu}_i - \hat{\mu}_{i'}), (i \neq i') = (1, 2, \ldots, k)$.

*Example 11.8*    From Tables T11.3 and T11.4 and Example 11.7, $\bar{x} = 170.65$, $W_{xx} = 865.54$, $\hat{\beta} = 0.6419$ and $\hat{\sigma}^2 = 25.19$. The sample sizes, estimates and 95 percent confidence limits for the adjusted means for the SBPs before the exercise program are as follows. The S.E.s and ranks of the means appear in the parentheses.

| Sample size : $n_i$ | $\bar{y}_i$ | $\hat{\mu}_i$ | Confidence limits |
|---|---|---|---|
| 9 | 132.22 (3) | 136.13 (3) (1.97) | 132.08, 140.18 |
| 13 | 142.62 (2) | 141.02 (2) (1.46) | 138.02, 144.02 |
| 8 | 148.13 (1) | 145.82 (1) (1.88) | 141.96, 149.69 |

As seen in the above section, the SBPs do not significantly depend on weights. This is one reason that the ranks of the adjusted means have not changed in spite of the difference of the average weights.

The difference of the highest and lowest estimated means is $(145.82 - 136.13) = 9.69$, with the estimate of variance $25.19\left[(1/8 + 1/9) + (174.25 - 164.56)^2 / 865.54\right] = 8.68$ and S.E. of 2.95. With $t_{26, 0.025} = 2.056$, 95 percent confidence limits for the difference of these two adjusted means become $(3.62, 15.76)$.

## 11.10   Randomized blocks

The effects of a set of treatments on lipid levels can be examined through the one-way ANOVA procedure by administering each of the treatments randomly to individuals – for instance, in different age groups. In the Analysis of Covariance procedure, the treatment effects are examined after adjusting their responses to the age of the individuals. In the Randomized Blocks design, the treatments being examined are administered randomly to the individuals in each of the age groups. In this two-way classification, the age groups are the blocks, and the individuals become the experimental units. The differences among the treatment effects are examined after eliminating the effect of the differences among the averages of the age. Similarly, the differences between the means of the age are examined after eliminating the effect of the differences among the treatment effects. To test the differences among the treatment effects with increased precision, the individuals in each age group should be close to each other in health-related characteristics but differ from the other groups.

The model for the responses $y_{ij}$ of $t$ treatments in $b$ blocks is

$$y_{ij} = \mu + \beta_i + \tau_j + \varepsilon_{ij}, \tag{11.57}$$

$i = (1,2,\ldots,b)$ and $j = (1,2,\ldots,t)$. The effects of the blocks and treatments are denoted by $\beta_i$ and $\tau_j$, and the overall mean or effect by $\mu$. The random error $\varepsilon_{ij}$ is assumed to follow the normal distribution with zero mean and variance $\sigma^2$. The means of the blocks and treatments are $\bar{y}_{i.} = \sum_{j=1}^{t} y_{ij}/t$ and $\bar{y}_{.j} = \sum_{i=1}^{b} y_{ij}/b$, and the overall mean is $\bar{y} = \sum_{1}^{b} \sum_{1}^{t} y_{ij}/bt$. Minimization of $\phi = \sum_{ij}(y_{ij} - \mu - \beta_i - \tau_j)^2$ with respect to $(\mu, \beta_i, \tau_j)$ with the conditions $\sum_i \beta_i = 0$ and $\sum_j \tau_j = 0$ results in the estimators $\hat{\mu} = \bar{y}$, $\hat{\beta}_i = (\bar{y}_{i.} - \bar{y})$ and $\hat{\tau}_j = (\bar{y}_{.j} - \bar{y})$.

The total number of observations is $n = bt$. The Total SS can be expressed as

$$\sum_{1}^{b} \sum_{1}^{t} (y_{ij} - \bar{y})^2 = t \sum_{1}^{b} (\bar{y}_{i.} - \bar{y})^2 + b \sum_{1}^{t} (\bar{y}_{.j} - \bar{y})^2 + \sum_{1}^{b} \sum_{1}^{t} (y_{ij} - \bar{y}_{i.} - \bar{y}_{.j} + \bar{y})^2. \tag{11.58}$$

Table 11.3   Expected values of the mean squares. Randomized blocks design.

| Source | d.f. | MS | E(MS) |
|---|---|---|---|
| Blocks | $(b-1)$ | $M_B$ | $\sigma^2 + t \sum_{i=1}^{b} \beta_i^2 / (b-1)$ |
| Treatments | $(t-1)$ | $M_T$ | $\sigma^2 + b \sum_{j=1}^{t} \tau_j^2 / (t-1)$ |
| Error | $(b-1)(t-1)$ | $M_E$ | $\sigma^2$ |

The right-hand side expressions respectively are the Between Blocks SS ($S_B$), Between Treatments SS ($S_T$), and Error SS ($S_E$). The degrees of freedom for these SS are $(b-1)$, $(t-1)$, and $(b-1)(t-1)$ respectively. The Blocks, Treatments and the Residual or Error Mean Squares are obtained from $M_B = S_B/(b-1)$, $M_T = S_T/(t-1)$ and $M_E = S_E/(b-1)(t-1)$. The expected values of the Mean Squares are presented in Table 11.3.

The Error Mean Square $M_E$ is unbiased for $\sigma^2$. The null hypothesis that there is no difference among the effects of the b blocks is

$$H_0 : \beta_1 = \beta_2 = \ldots = \beta_b = 0. \tag{11.59}$$

The expected value of $M_B$ becomes the same as $\sigma^2$ when this hypothesis is valid. The test statistic for this null hypothesis is given by $F = M_B/M_E$, which follows the $F$-distribution with $(b-1)$ and $(b-1)(t-1)$ d.f. The null hypothesis of the equality of the t treatment effects is

$$H_0 : \tau_1 = \tau_2 = \ldots = \tau_t = 0. \tag{11.60}$$

The test statistic for this hypothesis is $F = M_T/M_E$, which follows the $F$-distribution with $(t-1)$ and $(b-1)(t-1)$ d.f.

*Example 11.9*   Four treatments ($t_1, t_2, t_3, t_4$) and a *control* treatment ($t_0$) are *randomly* assigned to five patients in each of four age groups, blocks ($b_1, b_2, b_3, b_4$). Assignment of the treatments and the lipid levels (LDL, HDL) after administering the treatments are presented in Table 11.4. The ANOVA for the LDLs is presented below.

ANOVA for the LDLs in Table 11.4.

| Source | d.f. | SS | MS | F | p-value |
|---|---|---|---|---|---|
| Age groups | 3 | 1204.95 | 401.65 | 6.87 | 0.006 |
| Treatments | 4 | 310.2 | 77.55 | 1.33 | 0.31 |
| Error | 12 | 701.8 | 58.48 | | |
| Total | 19 | 2216.95 | | | |

Table 11.4   Lipid levels (LDL, HDL) of four age groups after administering four treatments and a control. Randomized blocks design.

| Age groups | $t_4$ | $t_1$ | $t_0$ | $t_3$ | $t_2$ |
|---|---|---|---|---|---|
| $b_1$ | 60, 35 | 90, 40 | 75, 45 | 65, 50 | 70, 42 |
| | $t_1$ | $t_3$ | $t_4$ | $t_0$ | $t_2$ |
| $b_2$ | 80, 45 | 80, 45 | 75, 45 | 75, 30 | 75, 45 |
| | $t_1$ | $t_4$ | $t_0$ | $t_2$ | $t_3$ |
| $b_3$ | 84, 35 | 90, 40 | 70, 35 | 95, 30 | 82, 42 |
| | $t_0$ | $t_1$ | $t_4$ | $t_3$ | $t_2$ |
| $b_4$ | 88, 30 | 100, 30 | 95, 38 | 90, 36 | 90, 32 |

Estimate of $\sigma^2$ is $\hat{\sigma}^2 = 58.48$. The difference among the means of the age groups is significant at the 1 percent level or smaller, but the difference between the treatment effects is not significant even at the 5 percent level.

### 11.10.1   Randomized blocks: Random and mixed effects models

As seen above, the Randomized Blocks experiment is a two-way classification with blocks and treatments as the two factors. In some experiments and investigations, either the blocks or treatments or both are considered to be random.

For the case of the blocks *random* but treatments *fixed*, (11.57) becomes the *mixed effects* model, with $E(\beta_i) = 0$, $V(\beta_i) = \sigma_\beta^2$ and $Cov(\beta_i, \beta_{i'}) = 0$ for $(i \neq i')$. The expected value of the Between Mean Square $M_B$ in Table (11.3) becomes $\sigma^2 + t\sigma_\beta^2$. For this case, the test of hypothesis for the blocks becomes $H_0 : \sigma_\beta^2 = 0$. The test statistic for this hypothesis remains the same as $F = M_B/M_E$, which follows the $F$-distribution with $[(b-1), (t-1)(b-1)]$ d.f.

For the case of the treatments *random* but blocks *fixed*, (11.57) becomes the *mixed effects* model, with $E(\tau_j) = 0$, $V(\tau_j) = \sigma_\tau^2$ and $Cov(\tau_j, \tau_{j'}) = 0$ for $(j \neq j')$. The expected value of the Between Mean Square $M_T$ in Table (11.3) becomes $\sigma^2 + b\sigma_\tau^2$. For this case, the test of hypothesis for the treatments becomes $H_0 : \sigma_\tau^2 = 0$. The test statistic for this hypothesis remains the same as $F = M_T/M_E$, which follows the $F$-distribution with $[(t-1), (t-1)(b-1)]$ d.f.

## 11.11   Repeated measures design

In some clinical experiments, diagnostic measurements are repeated on the patients at different time intervals or under different conditions. The observations for each patient become correlated and the model becomes the same as (11.57) with the patients as blocks as in Section 11.10. The hypothesis of equality of the effects of the treatments, the time intervals, is the same as (11.60). The test statistic for this hypothesis is $F = M_T/M_E$, which follows the $F$-distribution with $[(t-1), (t-1)(b-1)]$ d.f. The patient effect $\beta_i$ is considered random with $E(\beta_i) = 0$ and $V(\beta_i) = \sigma_\beta^2$. The test statistic for the hypothesis $H_0 : \sigma_\beta^2 = 0$ becomes $F = M_B/M_E$, which follows the F-distribution with $[(b-1), (t-1)(b-1)]$ d.f.

*Example 11.10* The SBPs and DBPs (diastolic blood pressures) of three patients repeated over four time intervals are presented in Table 11.5. The ANOVA for the SBPs is presented below.

ANOVA for the SBPs in Table 11.5.

| Source | d.f | SS | MS | F | $p$-value |
|---|---|---|---|---|---|
| Patients | 2 | 218 | 109 | 7.85 | 0.021 |
| Treatments | 3 | 130.67 | 43.56 | 3.14 | 0.108 |
| Error | 6 | 83.33 | 13.89 | | |
| Total | 11 | 432 | | | |

The estimate of $\sigma^2$ is 13.89. The difference between the effects of the treatments is not significant. The hypothesis $H_0 : \sigma_\beta^2 = 0$ is rejected at the $p$-value of 0.021.

In the Crossover designs, treatments are sequentially assigned to the experimental units. In the longitudinal studies, observations on the treatments become available over periods of time. The observations of these types of experiments with repeated measures are analyzed through suitable models.

Table 11.5    SBPs (top) and DBPs (bottom) of three patients observed over four time intervals. Repeated measures.

| | | Time intervals (Treatments) | | | |
|---|---|---|---|---|---|
| | | 1 | 2 | 3 | 4 |
| | 1 | 160 | 160 | 150 | 148 |
| | | 90 | 86 | 92 | 84 |
| Patients | 2 | 158 | 160 | 156 | 148 |
| | | 100 | 90 | 88 | 80 |
| | 3 | 144 | 148 | 146 | 146 |
| | | 92 | 82 | 84 | 80 |

SBPs: Block (patient) means: 154.5, 155.5, 146.0.
Treatment means: 154, 156, 150.67, 147.33.
Mean and variance of the 12 observations: (152, 39.27).
DBPs: Block (patient) means: 88.0, 89.5, 84.5.
Treatment means: 94, 86, 88, 81.33.
Mean and variance of the 12 observations: (87.33, 34.42).

## 11.12    Latin squares

The Randomized Blocks design described in Section (11.10) is a two-way classifica-tion. In the illustration considered, differences between the treatments are analyzed after adjusting for the differences among the age groups. In the Latin Square design, differences between $t$ treatments are examined after adjusting for the differences of two factors, each at $t$ levels. In this design, each treatment appears at each level of the two factors. The design for $t = 4$ treatments (A, B, C, D) with four levels each of a row and column factor takes the following form. Other cyclical arrangements of the treatments are possible.

|     |   | Column |   |   |   |
| --- | --- | --- | --- | --- | --- |
|     |   | 1 | 2 | 3 | 4 |
|     | 1 | A | B | C | D |
| Row | 2 | B | C | D | A |
|     | 3 | C | D | A | B |
|     | 4 | D | A | B | C |

### 11.12.1    The model and analysis

The model for this experiment is

$$y_{ijk} = \mu + \alpha_i + \beta_j + \gamma_k + \varepsilon_{ijk}, \tag{11.61}$$

for $(i, j, k) = (1, 2, \ldots, t)$. The row, column and treatment effects are respectively represented by $(\alpha_i, \beta_j, \gamma_k)$ with $\sum_i \alpha_i = 0$, $\sum_j \beta_j = 0$ and $\sum_k \gamma_k = 0$. The overall mean of the rows, columns and treatments is denoted by $\mu$. The expectation of the random error $\varepsilon_{ijk}$ is zero, and its variance is assumed to be $\sigma^2$. The hypotheses of inter-est are

$$H_0 : \alpha_1 = \alpha_2 = \ldots = \alpha_t = 0,$$
$$H_0 : \beta_1 = \beta_2 = \ldots = \beta_t = 0$$

and

$$H_0 : \gamma_1 = \gamma_2 = \ldots = \gamma_t = 0. \tag{11.62}$$

The row, column and treatment totals of the observations are $r_i = \sum_{jk} y_{ijk}$, $c_j = \sum_{ik} y_{ijk}$ and $t_k = \sum_{ij} y_{ijk}$. The corresponding means are $\bar{y}_{i..} = r_i/t$, $\bar{y}_{.j.} = c_j/t$ and

$\bar{y}_{..k} = t_k/t$. The overall total and mean respectively are $G = \sum_{ijk} y_{ijk}$ and $\bar{y} = G/t^2$. The Row, Column and Treatment SS each with $(t-1)$ d.f. are

$$S_R = t \sum_i (\bar{y}_{i..} - \bar{y})^2 = \sum_i r_i^2/t - C.F,$$

$$S_C = t \sum_j (\bar{y}_{.j.} - \bar{y})^2 = \sum_j c_j^2/t - C.F$$

and

$$S_T = t \sum_k (\bar{y}_{..k} - \bar{y})^2 = \sum_k t_k^2 - C.F, \qquad (11.63)$$

where the "Correction Factor" $C.F = G^2/t^2$. The Total SS is $\sum_{ijk} (y_{ijk} - \bar{y})^2$. The Error SS with $[(t^2 - 1) - 3(t-1)] = (t-1)(t-2)$ d.f. is given by

$$S_E = \sum_{ijk} (y_{ijk} - \bar{y})^2 - S_R - S_C - S_T. \qquad (11.64)$$

The row, column and treatment mean squares are $M_R = S_R/(t-1)$, $M_C = S_C/(t-1)$ and $M_T = S_T/(t-1)$. The error mean square $M_E = S_E/(t-1)(t-2)$ is unbiased for $\sigma^2$. The test statistics for the three hypotheses in (11.62) are given by the $F$-ratios $M_R/M_E$, $M_C/M_E$ and $M_T/M_E$, each with $(t-1)$ and $(t-1)(t-2)$ d.f.

*Example 11.11* For four treatments (A, B, C, D) with the above arrangement, the percent decrease of the SBP for patients of four age groups and four levels of hypertension are presented in Table 11.6. The ANOVA for the reduction of the SBPs follows.

The totals and means of the four treatments (A, B, C, D) are (100, 70, 65, 45) and (25, 17.5, 16.25, 11.25). The total of the 16 observations is 280 and C.F. $= 280^2/16 = 4900$.

Table 11.6 Percentage decrease of the SBP Latin Square design.

|  |  | Mild | Moderate | High | Very high | Total | Mean |
|---|---|---|---|---|---|---|---|
|  | 50–60 | 15 | 15 | 10 | 10 | 50 | 12.50 |
| Age | 60–65 | 15 | 15 | 10 | 25 | 65 | 16.25 |
|  | 65–75 | 20 | 10 | 30 | 20 | 80 | 20.00 |
|  | >75 | 15 | 30 | 20 | 20 | 85 | 21.25 |
| Total |  | 65 | 70 | 70 | 75 |  |  |
| Mean |  | 16.25 | 17.5 | 17.5 | 18.75 |  |  |

ANOVA for the hypotheses in (11.62).

| Source | d.f. | SS | MS | F | p-value |
|---|---|---|---|---|---|
| Rows | 3 | 187.5 | 62.5 | 5.60 | 0.036 |
| Columns | 3 | 12.5 | 4.17 | 0.46 | 0.720 |
| Treatments | 3 | 387.5 | 129.17 | 12.40 | 0.006 |
| Error | 6 | 62.5 | 10.42 | | |
| Total | 15 | 650 | | | |

The estimate of $\sigma^2$ is 10.42. The difference between the treatment effects for reducing the SBPs is highly significant. The difference between the age groups for the reduction is also significant, but not for the reduction between the hypertension levels.

## 11.13   Cross-over design

In this design, treatments are sequentially assigned more than once to the patients or experimental units. A Latin Square design for $t = 3$ treatments (A, B, C) for three levels of the SBP (rows) assigned to $t = 3$ patients initially (columns 1–3) and at the second time (columns 4–6) takes the form of the following Crossover design:

Crossover design for three treatments.

| SBP levels | Patients | | | | | |
|---|---|---|---|---|---|---|
| | 1 | 2 | 3 | 4 | 5 | 6 |
| 1 | A | B | C | A | B | C |
| 2 | B | C | A | B | C | A |
| 3 | C | A | B | C | A | B |

The model for this design is

$$y_{ijk} = \mu + \alpha_i + \beta_j + \gamma_k + \delta_{l(i)} + \varepsilon_{ijkl} \qquad (11.65)$$

$i = (1, 2, \ldots, t)$ rows, $j = (1, 2, \ldots, t)$ columns, $k = (1, 2, \ldots, t)$ treatments and $l = (1, 2, \ldots, m)$ for the assignment of the patients. The percentage reduction for three levels of the SBP for three treatments is presented in Table 11.7.

Table 11.7   Reduction of the SBP for three treatments. Cross-over design.

| | | 1 | 2 | 3 | 4 | 5 | 6 | Total |
|---|---|---|---|---|---|---|---|---|
| | 1 | 15 | 10 | 10 | 20 | 10 | 5 | 70 |
| SBP levels | 2 | 5 | 20 | 20 | 10 | 10 | 15 | 80 |
| | 3 | 10 | 25 | 25 | 5 | 20 | 10 | 95 |
| Total | | 30 | 55 | 55 | 35 | 40 | 30 | 245 |

*Example 11.12*   For the observations in Table 11.7, the number of assignments of the three treatments to each of the three patients are $m = 2$. The overall total for the $t^2 m = 18$ observations is $G = 245$ and $C.F = 245^2/18 = 3334.72$. Totals of the treatments $(A, B, C)$ are $(115, 70, 60)$. Totals of the $t = 3$ columns of the $m = 2$ assignments are $(65, 95, 85)$. The different $SS$ are as follows:

---

Total $SS = (15^2 + \ldots + 10^2) - C.F = 740.28$ with $(t^2 m - 1) = 17$ d.f.

Rows $SS = (70^2 + 80^2 + 95^2)/(3 \times 2) - C.F = 52.78$ with $(t - 1) = 2$ d.f.

Column $SS = (30^2 + \ldots + 30^2)/3 - C.F. = 223.61$ with $(tm - 1) = 5$ d.f.

Column SS for the $m = 2$ assignments together is $(65^2 + 95^2 + 85^2)/6 - C.F. = 77.78$ with $(t - 1) = 2$ d.f.

Patients in Columns SS is $(223.61 - 77.78) = 145.83$ with $(tm - 1) - (t - 1) = t(m - 1) = 3$ d.f.

Treatment $SS = (115^2 + 70^2 + 60^2)/(3 \times 2) - C.F. = 286.11$ with $(t - 1) = 2$ d.f

Residual SS $= (740.28 - 52.78 - 223.61 - 286.11) = 177.78$ with $(t^2 m - 1) - (t - 1) - (tm - 1) - (t - 1) = (t - 1)(tm - 2) = 8$ d.f. These results are summarized below.

---

ANOVA for the Cross-over design for the treatments of the SBPs.

| Source | d.f | SS | MS | F | $p$-value |
|---|---|---|---|---|---|
| SBP levels (rows) | 2 | 52.78 | 29.39 | 1.32 | 0.32 |
| Patients (Columns) | 5 | 223.61 | 44.72 | 2.01 | 0.18 |
| Patients (Columns) of the two assignments | 2 | 77.78 | 38.89 | 1.75 | 0.23 |
| Patients in the two assignments | 3 | 145.83 | 48.61 | 2.19 | 0.17 |
| Treatments | 2 | 286.11 | 143.06 | 6.44 | 0.022 |
| Residual | 8 | 177.77 | 22.22 | | |
| Total | 17 | 740.28 | | | |

The estimate of $\sigma^2$ is 22.22. The difference between the treatment effects is significant with the $p$-value of 0.022. The difference of the effects of the patients or the SBP levels is not significant at the nominal 5 percent or lower level.

Louis et al. (1986) review the cross-over designs employed for different types of medical problems, and describe the principal factors to be considered for a cross-over design, such as the order of administering the treatments and their carry-over effects.

## 11.14   Two-way cross-classification

The effects of weight and fitness programs on the SBPs of adults, for instance, can be examined through this type of classification. The SBPs of one or more of the adults are observed for each combination of the weight and fitness factors, the row and column classifications. Similarly, the effects of weight and diet on hypertension or lipid levels can be studied through a cross-classification. In some studies and experiments, there can be an *interaction* between these factors. This type of design is *balanced* if the same number of units are observed for each combination of the row **x** column classification; otherwise it is *unbalanced*. In some experiments, the effects of more than two factors and their interactions are examined. In the mixed effects models, some of the factors are considered to be fixed and the remaining random.

The balanced design consists of m observations in each of the rc cells formed by r rows and c columns. The observations in the $(ij)$th cell are represented by the model

$$y_{ijk} = \mu_{ij} + \varepsilon_{ijk}$$

$$= \mu + (\mu_{i.} - \mu) + (\mu_{.j} - \mu) + (\mu_{ij} - \mu_{i.} - \mu_{.j} + \mu) + \varepsilon_{ijk} \qquad (11.66)$$

$$= \mu + \alpha_i + \beta_j + \gamma_{ij} + \varepsilon_{ijk},$$

$i = (1, 2, ..., r)$, $j = (1, 2, ..., c)$ and $k = (1, 2, ..., m)$. The overall mean is denoted by $\mu = \sum_i \sum_j \mu_{ij}/rc$. The mean of the $i$th row and its effect are $\mu_{i.} = \sum_j \mu_{ij}/c$ and $\alpha_i = \mu_{i.} - \mu$. Similarly, $\mu_{.j} = \sum_i \mu_{ij}/r$ and $\beta_j = \mu_{.j} - \mu$ are the mean and effect of the $j$th column. In some designs, the row and column effects may be related: for instance, effects of weight and diets. A definition for the lack of interaction of these effects is that the (1) difference between the means of any two rows is the same for each column, and (2) difference between the means of any two columns is the same for each row. From the first statement, $\left[ (\mu_{ij} - \mu_{i'j}) - (\mu_{ij'} - \mu_{i'j'}) \right] = 0$ for $i \neq i$ and $j \neq j'$. Averaging this expression over $(i', j')$, $\gamma_{ij} = (\mu_{ij} - \mu_{i.} - \mu_{.j} + \mu) = 0$, where $\gamma_{ij}$ is the *interaction* between the row and column effects.

## 11.14.1   Additive model: Balanced design

If there is no interaction between the row and column effects, the observations in the $(ij)$ cell can be represented by the additive model

$$y_{ijk} = \mu_{ij} + \varepsilon_{ijk}$$

$$= \mu + (\mu_{i.} - \mu) + (\mu_{.j} - \mu) + \varepsilon_{ijk} \qquad (11.67)$$

$$= \mu + \alpha_i + \beta_j + \varepsilon_{ijk},$$

$i = (1, 2, ..., r)$, $j = (1, 2, ..., c)$ and $k = (1, 2, ..., m)$. The row and column effects are $\alpha_i = \mu_{i.} - \mu$ and $\beta_j = \mu_{.j} - \mu$. The total sample size becomes $n = rcm$. The mean of the kth cell, $i$th row and $j$th column respectively are $\bar{y}_{ij.} = \sum_k y_{ijk}/m$, $\bar{y}_{i..} = \sum_{jk} y_{ijk}/cm$ and

$\bar{y}_{.j.} = \sum_{ik} y_{ijk}/rm$. The overall sample mean is $\bar{y} = \sum_{ijk} y_{ijk}/n = \sum_{ij} \bar{y}_{ij.}/rc = \sum_i \bar{y}_{i..}/r =$

$\sum_j \bar{y}_{.j.}/c$. Minimization of

$$\phi = \sum_{ijk} \left(y_{ijk} - \mu - \alpha_i - \beta_j\right)^2 \tag{11.68}$$

with respect to $(\mu, \alpha_i, \beta_j)$ with the conditions $\sum_i \alpha_i = 0$ and $\sum_j \beta_j = 0$, results in the

estimators $\hat{\mu} = \bar{y}$, $\hat{\alpha}_i = (\bar{y}_{i..} - \bar{y})$ and $\hat{\beta}_j = (\bar{y}_{.j.} - \bar{y})$.

The Total SS with $(n - 1)$ d.f. can be expressed as

$$\sum_{ijk} \left(y_{ijk} - \bar{y}\right)^2 = cm \sum_i (\bar{y}_{i..} - \bar{y})^2 + rm \sum_j (\bar{y}_{.j.} - \bar{y})^2 + m \sum_{ij} \left(y_{ijk} - \bar{y}_{i..} - \bar{y}_{.j.} + \bar{y}\right)^2.$$
$$\tag{11.69}$$

The right-hand side expressions respectively are the Row SS, Column SS and Error SS, ($SS_R$, $SS_C$, $SS_E$), with $(r - 1)$, $(c - 1)$ and $(n - r - c + 1)$ d.f. The corresponding mean squares are $M_R = S_R/(r - 1)$, $M_C = S_C/(c - 1)$ and $M_E = S_E/(n - r - c + 1)$, and $\hat{\sigma}^2 = M_E$ is unbiased for $\sigma^2$. The test for the hypothesis of equality of the row effects, that is,

$$H_0 : \alpha_1 = \alpha_2 = \ldots = \alpha_k = 0 \tag{11.70}$$

is given by $F = M_R/\hat{\sigma}^2$, which follows the $F$-distribution with $(r-1)$ and $(n-r-c+1)$ d.f. Similarly, the test for the hypothesis of no difference among the column effects, that is,

$$H_0 : \beta_1 = \beta_2 = \ldots = \beta_c = 0 \tag{11.71}$$

is given by $F = M_C/\hat{\sigma}^2$, which follows the F-distribution with $(c-1)$ and $(n-r-c+1)$ d.f.

*Example 11.13* The SBPs of two adults in each of three weight classifications and three fitness programs are presented in Table 11.8; 120 is subtracted from each figure. The ANOVA is presented below.

ANOVA for the tests of the (weight x fitness) classification.

| Source | d.f. | SS | MS | F | p-value |
|--------|------|------|------|------|---------|
| Weight | 2 | 187.78 | 94.89 | 27.08 | $2.31 \times 10^{-5}$ |
| Fitness | 2 | 301.78 | 150.89 | 43.06 | $1.84 \times 10^{-6}$ |
| Error | 13 | 45.56 | 3.50 | | |
| Total | 17 | 537.11 | | | |

Table 11.8    SBPs for the two-way weight × fitness program classifications.

|  |  | Fitness Program | | | |
|  |  | Walking | Running | Exercise | Mean |
| --- | --- | --- | --- | --- | --- |
| Weight | 150–160 | 20, 20 | 18, 16 | 10, 12 | 16 |
|  | 160–170 | 24, 22 | 14, 16 | 12, 14 | 17 |
|  | >170 | 30, 28 | 20, 26 | 18, 18 | 23.33 |
|  | Mean | 24 | 18.33 | 14 | 18.78 |

For the SBPs, the differences of the effects among the weight classifications as well as the fitness program classifications are highly significant.

## 11.14.2    Two-way cross-classification with interaction: Balanced design

When there is interaction between the row and column effects, the observations in the $rc$ cells are represented by (11.66) with $\sum_i \alpha_i = 0$ and $\sum_j \beta_j = 0$ and $\sum_i \sum_j \gamma_{ij} = 0$.

Minimizing

$$\phi = \sum_{ijk} \left(y_{ijk} - \mu - \alpha_i - \beta_j - \gamma_{ij}\right)^2 \tag{11.72}$$

with these conditions results in the estimators $\hat{\mu} = \bar{y}$, $\hat{\alpha}_i = \left(\bar{y}_{i..} - \bar{y}\right)$ and $\hat{\beta}_j = \left(\bar{y}_{.j.} - \bar{y}\right)$ and $\hat{\gamma}_{ij} = \left(\bar{y}_{ij.} - \bar{y}_{i..} - \bar{y}_{.j.} + \bar{y}\right)$. The Total SS can be expressed as

$$\sum_{ijk} \left(y_{ijk} - \bar{y}\right)^2 = \sum_{ijk} \left(y_{ijk} - \bar{y}_{ij.}\right)^2 + m \sum_{ij} \left(\bar{y}_{ij.} - \bar{y}\right)^2. \tag{11.73}$$

The first expression on the right-hand side is the Within cell sum of squares $S_E$, which is the Error SS with $(n - rc) = rc(m - 1)$ d.f. The error mean square $\hat{\sigma}^2 = M_E = S_E/(n - rc)$ is unbiased for $\sigma^2$. The second expression is the Between cell sum of squares $S_B$ with $(rc - 1)$ d.f. It can be expressed as

$$S_B = cm \sum_i \left(\bar{y}_{i..} - \bar{y}\right)^2 + rm \sum_j \left(\bar{y}_{.j.} - \bar{y}\right)^2 + m \sum_{ij} \left(\bar{y}_{ij.} - \bar{y}_{i..} - \bar{y}_{.j.} + \bar{y}\right)^2 \tag{11.74}$$

The expressions on the right-hand side respectively are sums of squares between rows and between columns and the interaction sums of squares, $(S_R, S_C, S_I)$, with $(r - 1)$, $(c - 1)$ and $(rc - r - c + 1) = (r - 1)(c - 1)$ d.f. The corresponding mean squares are $M_R = S_R/(r - 1)$, $M_C = S_C/(c - 1)$ and $M_I = S_I/(r - 1)(c - 1)$. For the additive model in (11.67), the interaction SS is added to the Error SS. The interaction

SS can be obtained by subtracting the row and column sums of squares from the Between cell sum of squares.

The test statistics for the hypotheses regarding the row, column and interaction effects are as follows:

| Null hypothesis | Test statistic |
|---|---|
| $H_0: \alpha_1 = \alpha_2 = \ldots = \alpha_r = 0$ | $F_{(r-1),\ (n-rc)} = M_R/\hat{\sigma}^2$ |
| $H_0: \beta_1 = \beta_2 = \ldots = \beta_c = 0$ | $F_{(c-1),\ (n-rc)} = M_C/\hat{\sigma}^2$ |
| $H_0: \gamma_{ij} = 0$ | $F_{(r-1)(c-1),\ (n-rc)} = M_I/\hat{\sigma}^2$ |

*Example 11.14*   Consider the data for the SBPs in Table 11.8 with interaction for the (weight **x** fitness) classification. The tests for the two factors and the interaction are as follows.

| Source | d.f. | SS | MS | F | p-value |
|---|---|---|---|---|---|
| Weight | 2 | 189.78 | 94.89 | 28.47 | 0.00013 |
| Fitness | 2 | 301.78 | 150.89 | 45.27 | $2.01 \times 10^{-5}$ |
| Interaction | 4 | 15.56 | 3.89 | 1.17 | 0.39 |
| Error | 9 | 30.00 | 3.33 | | |
| Total | 17 | 537.11 | | | |

For this classification, $\hat{\sigma}^2 = 3.33$. The difference among the effects of the weights as well as among the fitness programs for the SBPs is highly significant, but their interaction is not significant.

For the model without interaction, the Error SS of 45.56 with 13 d.f. in Example 11.13 is the total of the above Interaction SS of 15.56 and the Error SS of 30.00 with $(4+9) = 13$ d.f.

## 11.14.3   Two-way cross-classification: Unbalanced additive model

For several applications, the number of observations $n_{ij}$ in the $(ij)$th cell tend to be unequal in general. The observations for this general case are represented by the model in (11.67) with $k = (1,2,\ldots,n_{ij})$. The sample sizes of the $i$th row and the $j$th column respectively are $n_{i.} = \sum_j n_{ij}$, $n_{.j} = \sum_i n_{ij}$, and the overall sample size becomes $n = \sum_{ij} n_{ij} = \sum_i n_{i.} = \sum_j n_{.j}$. The sample means of the $ij$th cell, $i$th row and $j$th column respectively are $\bar{y}_{ij.} = \sum_k y_{ijk}/n_{ij}, \bar{y}_{i..} = \sum_{jk} y_{ijk}/n_{i.}$ and $\bar{y}_{.j.} = \sum_{ik} y_{ijk}/n_{.j}$.

The overall sample mean becomes $\bar{y} = \sum_{ijk} y_{ijk}/n = \sum_{ij} n_{ij}\bar{y}_{ij.}/n = \sum_{i} n_i\bar{y}_{i.}/n =$ $\sum_{j} n_{.j}\bar{y}_{.j}/n$. Minimization of

$$\varphi = \sum_{ijk} \left( y_{ijk} - \mu - \alpha_i - \beta_j \right)^2 \tag{11.75}$$

with respect to $(\mu, \alpha_i, \beta_j)$ with the conditions $\sum_{i} n_{i.}\alpha_i = 0$ and $\sum_{j} n_{.j}\beta_j = 0$ results in the estimators $\hat{\mu} = \bar{y}$, $\hat{\alpha}_i = (\bar{y}_{i..} - \bar{y})$ and $\hat{\beta}_j = (\bar{y}_{.j.} - \bar{y})$. With these estimators, the Total SS can be expressed as

$$\sum_{ijk} \left( y_{ijk} - \bar{y} \right)^2 = \sum_{ijk} \left( y_{ijk} - \bar{y}_{ij.} \right)^2 + \sum_{ij} \left( \bar{y}_{ij.} - \bar{y} \right)^2$$

$$= \sum_{i} n_{i.} \left( \bar{y}_{i..} - \bar{y} \right)^2 + \sum_{j} n_{.j} \left( \bar{y}_{.j.} - \bar{y} \right)^2 + \sum_{ijk} \left( y_{ijk} - \bar{y}_{i..} - \bar{y}_{.j.} + \bar{y} \right)^2. \tag{11.76}$$

The first two terms on the right-hand side respectively are the unadjusted row and column sums of squares, $S_R$(unadj.) and $S_C$(unadj.) with $(r-1)$ and $(c-1)$ d.f. The last term is the Error SS with $(n-r-c+1)$ d.f.

Unlike in the case of the balanced design in Section 11.14.2, the above estimators for the row and column effects are correlated, and the unadjusted row and column sums of squares are not independent. The tests of hypotheses based on $S_R$(unadj.) and $S_C$(unadj.) lead to misleading conclusions. To circumvent this problem, (11.75) is minimized without the above conditions for the row and column effects. As presented in Rao (1997, pp. 44–51), the estimating equations for the row and column effects are respectively given by

$$n_{i.}\hat{\alpha}_i - \sum_{j} n_{ij}\left( \sum n_{ij}\hat{\alpha}_i/n_{.j} \right) = y_{i..} - \sum n_{ij}(y_{.j.}/n_{.j}) = Q_i \tag{11.77}$$

and

$$n_{.j}\hat{\beta}_j - \sum_{i} n_{ij}\left( \sum n_{ij}\hat{\beta}_j/n_{i.} \right) = y_{.j.} - \sum n_{ij}(y_{i..}/n_{i.}) = Q'_j. \tag{11.78}$$

In these expressions, $y_{i..} = \sum_{jk} y_{ijk}$ and $y_{.j.} = \sum_{ik} y_{ijk}$ are the row and column totals. The adjusted row and column totals are obtained from $Q_i$ and $Q'_j$. From the minimization, the Error SS becomes

$$S_E = \sum_{ijk} \left( y_{ijk} - \bar{y} \right)^2 - \sum_{i} \hat{\alpha}_i Q_i - \sum_{j} n_{.j} \left( \bar{y}_{.j.} - \bar{y} \right)^2 \tag{11.79}$$

$$= \sum_{ijk} \left(y_{ijk}-\bar{y}\right)^2 - \sum_j \hat{\beta}_j Q'_j - \sum_i n_{i\cdot}\left(\bar{y}_{i\cdot\cdot}-\bar{y}\right)^2. \qquad (11.80)$$

In these expressions, $\sum_i \hat{\alpha}_i Q_i$ and $\sum_j \hat{\beta}_j Q'_j$ are the sums of squares due to the rows adjusted for columns and due to the columns adjusted for rows, $S_R(\text{adj.})$ and $S_C(\text{adj.})$ respectively. Notice that

$$S_R(\text{adj.}) + S_C(\text{Unadj.}) = S_R(\text{Unadj.}) + S_C(\text{adj.}). \qquad (11.81)$$

The d.f. for both the unadjusted and adjusted SS due to rows are $(r-1)$, and the d.f. for the unadjusted and adjusted SS due to columns are $(c-1)$. The adjusted row and column mean squares are $M_R(\text{adj.}) = S_R(\text{adj.})/(r-1)$ and $M_C(\text{adj.}) = S_C(\text{adj.})/(c-1)$. The Error mean square is $M_E = S_E/(n-r-c+1)$ with $(n-r-c+1)$ d.f. and it is unbiased for $\sigma^2$.

The ANOVA tests for the equality of the row effects and for the column effects are presented in Table 11.9.

The estimating equations for $\alpha_i$ in (11.77) are linearly dependent. Estimates for $\alpha_i$ can be obtained from these equations with the condition $\sum_i \alpha_i = 0$ or setting one of the $\alpha_i$ s to be zero. Similarly, estimates for $\beta_j$ can be obtained from (11.78) with $\sum_j \beta_j = 0$ or setting one of the $\beta_j$ s to be zero.

*Example 11.15*    Consider the following observations for the SBPs of $n = 20$ adults for the (weight × fitness) classification, which are the same as in Table 11.8 except for the additional observations for the exercise program in the first two weight classes.

|  |  | Fitness | | | | |
|---|---|---|---|---|---|---|
|  |  | Walking | Running | Exercise | $n_{i\cdot\cdot}$ | $y_{i\cdot\cdot}$ |
|  | 150–160 | 20, 20 | 18, 16 | 10, 12, 14 | 7 | 110 |
| Weight | 160–170 | 24, 22 | 14, 16 | 14, 16, 12 | 7 | 118 |
|  | >170 | 30, 28 | 20, 26 | 18, 18 | 6 | 140 |
|  | $n_{\cdot j\cdot}$ | 6 | 6 | 8 |  |  |
|  | $y_{\cdot j\cdot}$ | 144 | 110 | 114 |  |  |

Table 11.9    ANOVA for the row and column effects. Unbalanced two-way Cross classification.

| Source | d.f. | SS | F |
|---|---|---|---|
| Rows | $(r-1)$ | $S_R(\text{adj.})$ | $[S_R(\text{adj.})/(r-1)]/\hat{\sigma}^2$ |
| Columns | $(c-1)$ | $S_C(\text{adj.})$ | $[S_C(\text{adj.})/(c-1)]/\hat{\sigma}^2$ |
| Error | $(r-1)(c-1)$ | $S_E$ |  |

For these observations, Total SS $= 564.3$, $S_R(unadj.) = 213.18$ and $S_C(unadj.) = 325.97$. The adjusted row totals are

$$Q_1 = 110 - [2(144/6) + 2(110/6) + 3(114/8)] = -418/24,$$
$$Q_2 = 118 - [1(144/6) + 2(110/6) + 3(114/8)] = -226/24$$

and

$$Q_3 = 140 - [2(144/6) + 2(110/6) + 2(114/8)] = 644/24.$$

From the three estimating equations in (11.77) for the row effects,

$$109\alpha_1 - 59\alpha_2 - 50\alpha_3 = -418,$$

$$-59\alpha_1 + 109\alpha_2 - 50\alpha_3 = -226$$

and

$$-50\alpha_1 - 50\alpha_2 + 100\alpha_3 = 644.$$

Setting $\alpha_1 = 0$, from the first two equations, $\hat{\alpha}_2 = 400/350$ and $\hat{\alpha}_3 = 2454/350$. With these estimates, $S_R(adj.) = (400/350)(-226/24) + (2454/350)(644/24) = 177.38$. The same value for the adjusted row SS is obtained by setting $\alpha_1$ or $\alpha_2$ to be zero and estimating the remaining row effects.

For the above observations for the SBPs, Total $SS = 564.8$ with 19 d.f., $S_R(adj.) = 177.38$ and $S_C(unadj.) = 325.97$. From (11.79), $S_E = (564.8 - 177.38 - 325.97) = 61.45$ with $(19 - 2 - 2) = 15$ d.f. The adjusted column sum of squares can be found from (11.80). Alternatively, from (11.81), $S_C(adj.) = [S_R(adj.) + S_C(unadj.) - S_R(unadj.)] = (177.38 + 325.97 - 213.18) = 290.17$. The following ANOVA table presents the $F$-ratios for testing the row and column and interaction effects.

ANOVA for the weight x fitness classification without interaction.

| Source | d.f | SS(adj.) | MS | F | p-value |
|---|---|---|---|---|---|
| Weight | 2 | 177.38 | 88.69 | 21.63 | $3.81 \times 10^{-5}$ |
| Fitness | 2 | 290.17 | 145.09 | 35.39 | $2.1 \times 10^{-6}$ |
| Error | 15 | 61.45 | 4.10 | | |
| Total | 19 | 564.80 | | | |

The estimate of $\sigma^2$ is $\hat{\sigma}^2 = 4.10$. The difference of the average SBPs is highly significant among both the weight and fitness classifications.

## 11.14.4    Unbalanced cross-classification with interaction

The model for this case is the same as (11.66), with $k = (1, 2, \ldots, n_{ij})$. The Total SS can be expressed

$$\sum_{ijk} \left( y_{ijk} - \bar{y} \right)^2 = \sum_{ijk} \left( y_{ijk} - \bar{y}_{ij.} \right)^2 + \sum_{ij} \left( \bar{y}_{ij.} - \bar{y} \right)^2 \tag{11.82}$$

The right-hand side expressions are the Within cell and Between cell sums of squares, $S_E$ and $S_B$ with $(n - rc)$ and $(rc - 1)$ d.f. respectively. The Interaction SS with $(r - 1)(c - 1)$ d.f. is obtained from

$$S_I = S_B - S_R(\text{adj.}) - S_C(\text{unadj.}) = S_B - S_R(\text{unadj.}) - S_C(\text{adj.}) \tag{11.83}$$

The estimator of $\sigma^2$ is given by $S_E / (n - rc)$. The ANOVA tests for the equality of the row and column effects and the absence of interaction are presented Table 11.10.

*Example 11.16*    For the observations in Example 11.15 for the SBPs, the tests for the differences among the row and column effects and the lack of interaction are presented below. For this unbalanced model, $S_B = 522.8$ with $(rc - 1) = 8$ d.f., and $S_I = (522.8 - 177.38 - 325.97) = (522.8 - 213.18 - 290.17) = 19.45$ with $(r - 1)(c - 1) = 4$ d.f. The Within cell SS becomes $S_E = (S_T - S_B) = (564.8 - 522.8) = 42.0$ with $(n - rc) = 11$ d.f. The following ANOVA Table presents the $F$-ratios for testing the effects of weight, fitness and their interaction with the adjusted sums of squares.

ANOVA for the SBP with interaction between the weight and fitness classifications.

| Source | d.f. | SS | MS | F | p-value |
|---|---|---|---|---|---|
| Weight | 2 | 177.38 | 88.69 | 23.22 | 0.00011 |
| Fitness | 2 | 290.17 | 145.09 | 37.98 | $1.15 \times 10^{-5}$ |
| Interaction | 4 | 19.45 | 4.86 | 1.27 | 0.34 |
| Error | 11 | 42.0 | 3.82 | | |
| Total | 19 | 564.8 | | | |

Table 11.10    ANOVA for the row and column effects. Unbalanced two-way Cross classification with interaction.

| Source | d.f. | SS | F |
|---|---|---|---|
| Rows | $(r - 1)$ | $S_R(\text{adj.})$ | $[S_R(\text{adj.})/(r - 1)]/\hat{\sigma}^2$ |
| Columns | $(c - 1)$ | $S_C(\text{adj.})$ | $[S_C(\text{adj.})/(c - 1)]/\hat{\sigma}^2$ |
| Interaction | $(r - 1)(c - 1)$ | $S_I$ | $[S_I/(r - 1)(c - 1)]/\hat{\sigma}^2$ |
| Error | $n - rc$ | $S_E$ | |
| Total | $n - 1$ | | |

The estimate of $\sigma^2$ is $\hat{\sigma}^2 = 3.82$. The difference of the effects of the weight and fitness classifications for the SBP are highly significant, but the interaction is not significant.

## 11.14.5   Multiplicative interaction and Tukey's test for nonadditivity

If there is only one observation in each cell, the Within cell SS in (11.73) becomes zero. With the multiplicative effect $\alpha_i \beta_j$ for the interaction, Tukey (1949) considers the model

$$y_{ij} = \mu + \alpha_i + \beta_j + \lambda \alpha_i \beta_j + \varepsilon_{ij} \qquad (11.84)$$

$i = (1, 2, ..., r)$ and $j = (1, 2, ...., c)$. The row and column means and the overall mean are $\bar{y}_{i.} = \sum_j y_{ij}/c$, $\bar{y}_{.j} = \sum_i y_{ij}/r$ and $\bar{y} = \sum_{ij} y_{ij}/n$, where $n = rc$ is the total number of observations. The Total, row and column sums of squares are $S_T = \sum_{ij} (y_{ij} - \bar{y})^2$, $S_R = c \sum_i (\bar{y}_{i.} - \bar{y})^2$ and $S_C = r \sum_j (\bar{y}_{.j} - \bar{y})^2$. The row and column mean squares are $M_R = S_R/(r-1)$ and $M_C = S_C/(c-1)$.

The sum of squares for nonadditivity is given by

$$S_N = \frac{rc \left[ \sum_{ij} (\bar{y}_{i.} - \bar{y})(\bar{y}_{.j} - \bar{y}) y_{ij} \right]^2}{S_R S_C} \qquad (11.85)$$

with (1) d.f. The interaction mean square $M_N$ is the same as $S_N$. The residual or error sum of squares is given by

$$S_E = S_T - S_R - S_C - S_N \qquad (11.86)$$

with $(r-1)(c-1) - 1$ d.f. The error mean square $M_E$ is obtained by dividing $S_E$ with these degrees of freedom, and it is an unbiased estimator of $\sigma^2$.

The test statics for the hypotheses of the equality of the row effects, column effects and lack of interaction respectively are obtained by the $F$-ratios with their mean squares in the numerators and $M_E$ in the denominator. The degrees of freedom for the numerators are $(r-1)$, $(c-1)$ and $(1)$. The degrees of freedom for the denominator are $(r-1)(c-1) - 1$.

## 11.15   Missing observations in the designs of experiments

Some of the observations in a design of an experiment may be missing or excluded. In the classical approach, they are estimated by minimizing the residual sum of squares.

For the one-way unbalanced fixed effects model, the Total SS and Between SS and Within SS in (11.19) can be expressed as

$$\text{Total SS} = \sum_{1}^{k}\sum_{1}^{n_i} y_{ij}^2 - C.F$$

and

$$\text{Between SS} = \left( \frac{T_1^2}{n_1} + \frac{T_2^2}{n_2} + \ldots + \frac{T_k^2}{n_k} \right) - C.F, \tag{11.87}$$

where $T_i$ is the total of the $i$th treatment $G = \sum_{1}^{k}\sum_{1}^{n_i} y_{ij}$ is the grand total of all the observations and C.F. is the *Correction Factor* $G^2/n$. From these expressions the Within SS or Error SS becomes

$$\text{Error SS} = \sum_{1}^{k}\sum_{1}^{n_i} y_{ij}^2 - \left( \frac{T_1^2}{n_1} + \frac{T_2^2}{n_2} + \ldots + \frac{T_k^2}{n_k} \right). \tag{11.88}$$

If the first observation of the first treatment $y_{11}$, for instance, is missing, replace $T_1$ by $(T_1' + y_{11})$.

Now, setting the first derivative of this expression with respect to $y_{11}$ to zero, its estimate becomes $\hat{y}_{11} = T_1'/(n_1 - 1)$. It is the mean of the $(n_1 - 1)$ observations which are not missing. Similarly, the estimate of any missing observation of a treatment is given by the mean of the remaining observations of that treatment which are not missing. Snedecor and Cochran (1967, p. 317) pointed out that the ANOVA for the treatments is performed without any substitutions for the missing observations.

If one observation is missing in a Randomized Block or Latin Square design, Allan and Wishart (1930) suggest estimating it by minimizing the Error SS. For the randomized blocks design in Section 11.10, denote the totals of the blocks and treatments by $(B_1, B_2, \ldots, B_k)$ and $(T_1, T_2, \ldots, T_t)$ respectively. The Correction Factor C.F becomes $G^2/n$ where G is the grand total of the $n = bt$ observations. From (11.58),

$$\text{Error SS} = \left( \sum_{1}^{b}\sum_{1}^{t} y_{ij}^2 - C.F \right) - \left[ (B_1^2 + B_2^2 + \ldots + B_b^2)/t - C.F \right]$$

$$- \left[ (T_1^2 + T_2^2 + \ldots + T_t^2)/b - C.F \right]$$

$$= \sum_{1}^{b}\sum_{1}^{t} y_{ij}^2 - (B_1^2 + B_2^2 + \ldots + B_b^2)/t - (T_1^2 + T_2^2 + \ldots + T_t^2)/b - G^2/bt.$$

$$\tag{11.89}$$

If the observation $y_{11}$ for the first treatment in the first block, for instance, is missing, replace $B_1$, $T_1$ and $G$ by $(B_1' + y_{11})$, $(T_1' + y_{11})$ and $G'$, where $(B_1', T_1', G')$ are the totals of the remaining observations. Setting the first derivative of (11.89) with respect to $y_{11}$ to zero, its estimate becomes

$$\hat{y}_{11} = (bB_1' + tT_1' - G')/(b-1)(t-1). \tag{11.90}$$

Snedecor and Cochran (1967, pp. 316–319) illustrate the ANOVA test for the blocks and treatments with this estimated value of the missing observation.

# Exercises

**11.1.** From the 30 sample observations in Table T11.1, test the hypothesis that the means of the weights for the three groups are the same.

**11.2.** From the sample observations in Table T11.2, test the hypothesis that the means of the SBPs of the three groups after the exercise program are the same.

**11.3.** With the random effects model for the weights of the three groups in Table T11.1, estimate $\sigma_\alpha^2$ and find the 95 percent confidence limits for R.

**11.4.** With the random effects model in Table T11.2 for the SBPs after the exercise program, estimate $\sigma_\alpha^2$ and find the 95 percent confidence limits for R.

**11.5.** With the unequal sample size observations in Table T11.4, test the hypothesis of the equality of the means of the SBPs after the exercise program.

**11.6.** From the sample observations in Table T11.4 for the SBPs after the exercise program, find $\hat{\sigma}_\alpha^2$, $\bar{y}_w$ and $S.E.(\bar{y}_w)$.

**11.7.** With the observations in Tables T11.1 and T11.2 for the three groups with equal sample size $m = 10$, examine whether the means of the SBPs after the exercise program adjusted for weights are significantly different.

**11.8.** From the information in Tables T11.1 and T11.2 and Exercise 11.7, find the estimates and 95 percent confidence limits for the adjusted means of the SBPs of the three groups after the exercise program, and the difference of the means of the first two groups.

**11.9.** Following Example 11.7, with the unequal sample size observations in Tables T11.3 and T11.4, test for the difference of the means of the SBPs of the three age groups after the exercise program, adjusting for the weights.

**11.10.** With the information in Tables T11.3 and T11.4 and the results of Exercise 11.9 for the SBPs after the exercise program, find the estimates and 95 percent confidence limits for the adjusted means and the difference of the means of the first and third groups.

**11.11.** With the results in Table 11.4 for the HDL, test for the differences among the age groups and between the treatments.

**11.12.** For the repeated measurements of the DBPs of the patients in Table 11.5, test the hypothesis $H_0 : \sigma_\beta^2 = 0$.

**11.13.** Reductions of the SBPs for 16 patients in the Latin square arrangement of Example 11.11 are as follows. Test for the differences between the treatments for reducing the SBP. Test for the differences between the age groups and between the hypertension levels for the reduction.

Decrease of the SBP.

| | | Hypertension | | | | | |
| --- | --- | --- | --- | --- | --- | --- | --- |
| | | Mild | Moderate | High | Very high | Total | Mean |
| Age | 50–60 | 25 | 20 | 25 | 30 | 100 | 25 |
| | 60–65 | 20 | 25 | 30 | 20 | 95 | 23.75 |
| | 65–75 | 25 | 20 | 25 | 15 | 85 | 21.25 |
| | >75 | 15 | 10 | 15 | 20 | 60 | 15 |
| Total | | 85 | 75 | 95 | 85 | | |
| Mean | | 21.25 | 18.75 | 23.75 | 21.25 | | |

**11.14.** The DBPs of the 18 adults in Example 11.13 are presented below; 100 is subtracted from each figure. $r = 3$, $c = 3$, $m = 2$. Test for the differences among the weight classifications and the fitness classifications

| | | Walking | Running | Exercise |
| --- | --- | --- | --- | --- |
| | 150–160 | 8, 6 | 10, 10 | 9, 10 |
| Weight | 160–170 | 10, 8 | 8, 8 | 8, 6 |
| | >170 | 16, 14 | 10, 12 | 8, 8 |

**11.15.** Consider the DBPs in Exercise 11.14 for the weight x fitness classification. Test for the effects of the weight, fitness and their interaction.

**11.16.** For the unbalanced design in Example 11.15, the DBPs for the 20 adults are as follows. Examine the effects of the weights and fitness without and with interaction.

|  |  | Walking | Running | Exercise | $n_{i.}$ | $y_{i..}$ |
|---|---|---|---|---|---|---|
|  |  | | Fitness | | | |
| Weight | 150–160 | 10, 8 | 14, 14 | 12, 14, 16 | 7 | 88 |
|  | 160–170 | 10, 8 | 8, 8 | 10, 12, 10 | 7 | 66 |
|  | > 170 | 10, 12 | 12, 14 | 16, 14 | 6 | 78 |
|  | $n_{.j}$ | 6 | 6 | 8 | | |
|  | $y_{.j.}$ | 58 | 70 | 104 | | |

**11.17.** The following percentages of total fatty acids of foods of five types prepared with partially hydrogenated vegetable oils are obtained from the figures presented by Mozaffarian et al. (2006). Two of the foods in the fifth type with extremely low percentages are ignored. Perform the ANOVA and test for the differences in the averages for the five types of foods.

Percent of total fatty acids.

|  | 1 | 2 | 3 | 4 | 5 |
|---|---|---|---|---|---|
|  | 32 | 28 | 22 | 19 | 21 |
|  | 28 | 25 | 11 | 19 | 34 |
|  | 25 | 25 | 18 | 9 | 25 |
|  | 30 | 26 | 15 | | |
|  | 12 | 16 | | | |
|  | 12 | 21 | | | |
|  | 9 | 14 | | | |
| Mean | 21.14 | 22.14 | 16.5 | 15.67 | 26.67 |
| St.dev. | 9.77 | 5.34 | 4.65 | 5.77 | 6.66 |

**11.18.** For the healthcare expenditure in 2006, (1) "Private expenditure on health as a percentage of total expenditure on health" and (2) "Total expenditure on health as a percentage of gross domestic product" are presented by the WHO for 172 countries of five regions. The averages (top) and standard deviations (bottom) obtained from these figures are as follows:

| Region | Number of Countries | Private Expenditure | Total Expenditure |
|---|---|---|---|
| Americas | 35 | 42.76 | 6.83 |
|  | | 13.91 | 2.01 |
| Europe | 53 | 32.75 | 7.35 |
|  | | 16.38 | 1.85 |
| Africa | 46 | 47.48 | 5.27 |
|  | | 19.05 | 2.20 |

| Asia | 11 | 45.93 | 5.49 |
| | | 26.25 | 4.22 |
| South East Asia | 27 | 31.00 | 6.98 |
| | | 24.12 | 3.72 |

(a) Perform the ANOVA for both the private and total expenditures and examine the differences among the averages for the five regions.

(b) Irrespective of the results in (a), examine whether the averages for the private expenditures for Africa and Asia are the same.

(c) Irrespective of the results in (a), examine whether the averages for the total expenditure are the same for Americas and Europe.

# Appendix A11

## A11.1  Variance of $\hat{\sigma}_\alpha^2$ in (11.25) from Rao (1997, p. 20)

$$V(\hat{\sigma}_\alpha^2) = \frac{2n^2}{\left(n^2 - \sum_i n_i^2\right)^2}$$

$$\left[\sum_i n_i^2 \left(1 - 2\frac{n_i}{n}\right) V_i^2 + \left(\sum_i \frac{n_i^2}{n} V_i\right)^2 + \frac{(k-1)^2}{n-k}\sigma^4\right].$$

## A11.2  The total sum of squares ($T_{xx}$, $T_{yy}$) and sum of products ($T_{xy}$) can be expressed as the within and between components as follows:

$$T_{xx} = \sum_1^k \sum_1^{n_i} (x_{ij} - \bar{x})^2 = \sum_1^k \sum_1^{n_i} (x_{ij} - \bar{x}_i)^2 + \sum_1^k n_i (\bar{x}_i - \bar{x})^2 = W_{xx} + B_{xx},$$

$$T_{yy} = \sum_1^k \sum_1^{n_i} (y_{ij} - \bar{y})^2 = \sum_1^k \sum_1^{n_i} (y_{ij} - \bar{y}_i)^2 + \sum_1^k n_i (\bar{y}_i - \bar{y})^2 = W_{yy} + B_{yy}$$

and

$$T_{xy} = \sum_1^k \sum_1^{n_i} (x_{ij} - \bar{x})(y_{ij} - \bar{y}) = \sum_1^k \sum_1^{n_i} (x_{ij} - \bar{x}_i)(y_{ij} - \bar{y}_i) + \sum_1^k n_i (\bar{x}_i - \bar{x})(\bar{y}_i - \bar{y}) = W_{xy} + B_{xy}.$$

# 12

# Meta-analysis

## 12.1 Introduction

To investigate the effects of air pollution, smoking and similar factors or the benefits of low-dose aspirin and statins, estimates obtained from small or large scale studies are combined. Illustrations of four such studies are presented in Section 12.2. Some types of agricultural, biological, medical and scientific experiments are repeated at the same location, laboratory or research center, or replicated a few times at the same location during a specified period of time. Estimates for the means, treatment effects, odds ratios and similar quantities of interest along with their standard errors become available from all the experiments. In some cases, especially medical experiments, estimates and treatment effects adjusted for one or more covariates along with their standard errors are recorded. Meta-analysis for synthesizing the available estimates through the *fixed* and *random* effects models is presented in the following sections.

## 12.2 Illustrations of large-scale studies

*Smoking.* The U.S. Surgeon General's report on Smoking and Health (1964) was the result of the review of more than 7,000 articles on the effects of smoking on lung cancer, heart disease and similar harmful health-related factors. The increase of mortality rate for smokers over nonsmokers was 70 percent. The risk of developing lung cancer for the average smoker was 9 to 10 times the risk for the nonsmoker; it was 20 times for the heavy smoker. Professor William G. Cochran of the Statistics Department of Harvard University was the statistician on the Surgeon General's Committee on Smoking.

 *Statin and LDL cholesterol.* Baignet et al. (2010) performed a meta-analysis of the reduction of LDL from the "more versus less statin regimen" on 39,612

*Statistical Methodologies with Medical Applications*, First Edition. Poduri S.R.S. Rao.
© 2017 John Wiley & Sons, Ltd. Published 2017 by John Wiley & Sons, Ltd.

individuals from five randomized trials and "statin versus control" on 129, 526 individuals in 21 trials. In both the studies, the reduction of LDL per 1.0 mmol/L after one year of treatment was found to be significant.

*Aspirin and cancer reduction.* Rothwell et al. (2011) analyzed the risk of various types of cancer from daily use of aspirin on 23,535 patients from seven clinical trials, and found that aspirin reduced deaths due to cancer. "Benefits increased with duration of treatment and was consistent across the different study populations."

*Air pollution and mortality risk.* From a study of the persons with chronic obstructive pulmonary disease discharged during 14 years in 34 U.S. cities, Zanobetti (2008) found that the risk of mortality was substantially associated with exposure to air pollution.

## 12.3    Fixed effects model for combining the estimates

Consider the reduction of the SBPs (systolic blood pressures) $y_{ij}$, $i = (1, 2, ..., k)$ and $j = (1, 2, ..., n_i)$, for a sample of $n_i$ persons at the $i$th laboratory, location or healthcare center with $E(y_{ij}|i) = \mu_i$ and variance $V(y_{ij}|i) = \sigma_{0i}^2$. The variance of the sample mean $\bar{y}_i = \sum_1^{n_i} y_{ij}/n_i$ is $V(\bar{y}_i) = \sigma_{0i}^2/n_i$. The sample variance $s_{0i}^2$ with $v_i = (n_i - 1)$ d.f. is unbiased for $\sigma_{0i}^2$. The sample variance and S.E. of $\bar{y}_i$ become $v(\bar{y}_i) = s_{0i}^2/n_i$ and $s_{0i}/\sqrt{n_i}$. For simplicity, denote $\bar{y}_i$, $V(\bar{y})$ and $v(\bar{y}_i)$ by $y_i$, $\sigma_i^2$ and $s_i^2$ respectively.

Similarly, the difference $(\bar{y}_{1i} - \bar{y}_{2i})$ of the sample responses of $(n_i, m_i)$ units to two medical treatments or to a medical treatment and a control is unbiased for the difference of their means $(\mu_1 - \mu_2)$ with variance $V(\bar{y}_{1i} - \bar{y}_{2i}) = \sigma_{0i}^2/d_i$, where $d_i = n_i m_i/(n_i + m_i)$. The estimator of this variance is $v(\bar{y}_{1i} - \bar{y}_{2i}) = s_{01}^2/d_i$, and the sample standard error becomes $s_{oi}/\sqrt{d_i}$, where $s_{oi}^2$ is the pooled estimator of $\sigma_{0i}^2$ with $v_i = (n_i + m_i - 2)$ d.f. As before, denote $(\bar{y}_{1i} - \bar{y}_{2i})$ its variance and estimator of variance by $y_i$, $\sigma_i^2$ and $s_i^2$. For the estimation of $(\mu_1 - \mu_2)$, $(y_i, s_i)$, $i = (1,2,...,k)$, become available from each of the $k$ laboratories.

For the difference $y_i$ of two treatment effects in a randomized block experiment with $b$ blocks and $t$ treatments replicated at $k$ locations, the standard error takes the form of $s_i = s_{0i}/\sqrt{d}$. In this expression, $s_{0i}^2$ is the estimator of the variance per observation with $v = (b-1)(t-1)$ d.f. and $d = b/2$. If this experiment is replicated $k$ times at the same location, the variance per observation becomes $s_0^2 = \sum_1^k s_{0i}^2/k$ with $kv$ d.f., and the S.E. of $y_i$ becomes $s_0/\sqrt{d}$.

To combine the above type of estimators at the $k$ locations, the model

$$y_i = \mu_i + \varepsilon_i$$
$$= \mu + \alpha_i + \varepsilon_i.$$

(12.1)

$i = (1, 2, \ldots, k)$, with the overall mean $\mu$ can be considered. The difference of the mean $\mu_i$ at the $i$th location from the overall mean $\mu$ is denoted by the *fixed effect* $\alpha_i$. The random error $\varepsilon_i$ is assumed to follow the normal distribution with mean zero and variance $\sigma_i^2$.

The Weighted Least Squares Estimator for $\mu$ is

$$\bar{y}_W = \sum_1^k W_i y_i / W \tag{12.2}$$

where $W_i = 1/\sigma_i^2$ and $W = \sum_1^k W_i$. With the estimator $s_i^2$ for $\sigma_i^2$, (12.2) becomes

$$\bar{y}_w = \sum_1^k w_i y_i / w \tag{12.3}$$

where $w_i = 1/s_i^2$ and $w = \sum_1^k w_i$. This estimator is approximately unbiased for the overall mean $\mu$ provided the individual means $\mu_i$ do not differ much from $\mu$. An approximate estimator for its variance $V(\bar{y}_w) = E\left[\sum_1^k w_i^2 \sigma_i^2 / w^2\right]$ is given by $v(\bar{y}_w) = 1/w$, and $S.E.(\bar{y}_w)$ is obtained from $1/\sqrt{w}$.

*Example 12.1   Average decreases of the SBPs.* Sample sizes ($n_i$), average decreases ($y_i$) of the SBPs and standard errors ($s_i$) of 15 groups of adults following a medical treatment are presented in Table 12.1; the initial SBPs were in the range (140–160).

Table 12.1   Average decreases of the SBPs after a medical treatment for 15 groups of adults. Means ($y_i$) and standard deviations ($s_i$).

| $n_i$ | $y_i$ | $s_i$ |
|-------|-------|-------|
| 10    | 10    | 2.0   |
| 10    | 15    | 2.0   |
| 10    | 20    | 3.5   |
| 15    | 20    | 3.0   |
| 15    | 15    | 3.5   |
| 15    | 10    | 2.0   |
| 20    | 30    | 4.0   |
| 20    | 25    | 3.0   |
| 20    | 25    | 2.5   |
| 20    | 20    | 4.0   |
| 25    | 15    | 2.0   |
| 25    | 10    | 2.0   |
| 25    | 15    | 3.5   |
| 25    | 20    | 3.0   |
| 25    | 25    | 3.0   |

From these summary figures, $w = 5.59$, $\sum_1^{15} w_i y_i = 96.79$ and $\bar{y}_w = 17.31$. The sample

variance of $\bar{y}_w$ and its S.E. are $(1/w) = 0.1789$ and $0.423$ respectively.

## 12.4    Random effects model for combining the estimates

To combine the above type of estimators, Cochran (1937, 1938, 1954a) and Yates and Cochran (1938) consider $\alpha_i$ in (12.1) to be a random variable following the normal distribution independent of $\varepsilon_i$ with zero expectation and variance $\sigma_\alpha^2$. The estimator

for $\mu$ is the same as (12.2) with the weights $W_i = 1(\sigma_i^2 + \sigma_i^2)$ and $W = \sum_1^k W_i$. This

estimator is unbiased for $\mu$ with variance $V(\bar{y}_w) = 1/W$. Cochran (1937) considers the following approach to estimate the weights. The sample mean and variance

between the k estimators are $\bar{y} = \sum_1^k y_i/k$ and $s_b^2 = \sum_1^k (y_i - \bar{y})^2/(k-1)$. From (12.1),

$E(s_b^2) = \sigma_\alpha^2 + \sum_1^k \sigma_i^2/k$. Since $E(s_i^2) = \sigma_i^2$, an unbiased estimator of $\sigma_\alpha^2$ is given by

$$\hat{\sigma}_\alpha^2 = s_b^2 - s^2 \tag{12.4}$$

where

$s^2 = \sum_1^k s_i^2/k$. The estimators for $W_i$ and $W$ are $w_i = 1/(\hat{\sigma}_\alpha^2 + s_i^2)$ and $w = \sum_i^k w_i$.

The estimator for $\mu$ now is obtained from (12.3) with these weights.

If the number of locations or centers $k$ and the degrees of freedom $v_i$ for $s_i^2$ are large, the bias of $w_i$ and $w$ to estimate $W_i$ and $W$ and the resulting bias of $\bar{y}_w$ to estimate $\mu$ can be expected to be small. In such a case, $V(\bar{y}_w)$ will be close to $1/W$ and can be estimated by $1/w$.

From the sample means and variances in Table 12.1, $\bar{y} = 18.33$, $s^2 = (131/15) = 8.73$, $s_b^2 = 38.10$, and $\hat{\sigma}_\alpha^2 = (38.10 - 8.73) = 29.37$. With $w_i = 1/(\hat{\sigma}_\alpha^2 + s_i^2)$, $w = 0.3984$. The estimate of $\mu$ becomes $\bar{y}_w = (7.15/0.3984) = 17.95$ with the estimated variance $v(\bar{y}_w) = (1/0.3984) = 2.51$ and S.E. of $1.58$.

If $\sigma_i^2$ do not vary much and they are all close to a common value $\sigma^2$, $\bar{y}_w$ in (12.2)

becomes the same as the *unweighted mean* $\bar{y} = \sum_1^k y_i/k$. Its variance and estimator of

variance become $V(\bar{y}) = (\sigma_\alpha^2 + \sigma^2)/k$ and $v(\bar{y}) = s_b^2/k$. If $\sigma_\alpha^2$ is large relative to each $\sigma_i^2$, $\bar{y}_w$ will be close $\bar{y}$ with this variance and estimator of variance. For the above example, the unweighted mean is $\bar{y} = 18.33$ with the estimate of variance $s_b^2 = (38.1/15) = 2.54$ and S.E. $(\bar{y}) = 1.59$. Since $\hat{\sigma}_\alpha^2$ is larger than each of the variances $s_i^2$, there is very little difference between the estimated standard errors of $\bar{y}_w$ and $\bar{y}$.

## 12.5    Alternative estimators for $\sigma_\alpha^2$

An alternative estimator for this variance component was suggested by DerSimonian and Laird (1986) for the case of known $\sigma_i^2$. The final estimators for $\sigma_\alpha^2$ and $\mu$ are obtained by replacing $\sigma_i^2$ with $s_i^2$. With $W_{0i} = 1/\sigma_i^2$, $W_0 = \sum_1^k W_{0i}$ and $\bar{y}_{W0} = \sum_1^k W_{0i} y_i / W_0$, from (12.1),

$$E\left[\sum_1^k W_{0i}(y_i - \bar{y}_{W0})^2\right] = \left(W_0 - \sum_1^k W_{0i}^2 / W_0\right)\sigma_\alpha^2 + (k-1) \qquad (12.5)$$

As a result, an unbiased estimator of $\sigma_\alpha^2$ is given by

$$\hat{\sigma}_{\alpha 0}^2 = \frac{\displaystyle\sum_1^k W_{0i}(y_i - \bar{y}_{W0})^2 - (k-1)}{W_0 - \displaystyle\sum_1^k W_{0i}^2 / W_0}. \qquad (12.6)$$

This estimator is set to zero if the numerator becomes negative. For the estimate of this variance component, $W_{0i}$ is replaced by $1/s_i^2$ The estimator for $\mu$ now is given by

$$\bar{y}_r = \sum_1^k r_{0i} y_i / r_0 \qquad (12.7)$$

where $r_{0i} = 1/\left(\hat{\sigma}_{\alpha 0}^2 + s_i^2\right)$ and $r_0 = \sum_1^k r_{0i}$. If the number of centers $k$ and the degrees of freedom $v_i$ for $s_i^2$ are large, the bias of this estimator becomes small. In such a case, its variance $V(\bar{y}_r)$ will be close to $1/W$ and can be estimated from $1/r_0$.

For the SBPs in Example 12.1, replacing $W_{0i}$ by $1/s_i^2$, $\hat{\sigma}_{\alpha 0}^2 = (76.56 - 14)/2.04 = 30.67$ from (12.6). With $r_{0i} = 1/\left(\hat{\sigma}_{\alpha 0}^2 + s_i^2\right)$, $r_0 = 0.395$ and $\bar{y}_r = (6.91/0.395) = 17.49$, $v(\bar{y}_r) = (1/r_0) = 2.53$ and $S.E.(\bar{y}_r) = 1.59$. These estimates (30.67, 17.49, 1.59) for $\sigma_\alpha^2$ and $\mu$ and the S.E. of the estimator of $\mu$ do not differ much from the corresponding values (29.37, 17.95, 1.58) found for the procedure in the previous section.

## 12.6    Tests of hypotheses and confidence limits for the variance components

Since $E\left(s_b^2\right) = \sigma_\alpha^2 + \sum_1^k \sigma_i^2 / k$ and $E(s^2) = \sum_1^k \sigma_i^2 / k$

$$F = \frac{s_b^2}{s^2} \qquad (12.8)$$

can be considered for testing the hypothesis $H_0 : \sigma_\alpha^2 = 0$. From Satterthwaite's (1946) approximation presented in Appendix A.12, $s_b^2$ and $s^2$ follow independent Chisquare distributions with $f_1$ and $f_2$ degrees of freedom respectively, where

$$f_1 = (k-1)^2 s^4 / \left[ (k-2) \sum_1^k s_i^4/k + s^4 \right]$$

and

$$f_2 = \left( \sum_1^k s_i^2 \right)^2 \bigg/ \sum_1^k (s_i^4/v_i). \tag{12.9}$$

The ratio of the variances in (12.8) follows the $F$-distribution with $(f_1, f_2)$ degrees of freedom.

If $\sigma_i^2$ are all equal to $\sigma^2$, it is estimated from $s^2 = \sum_1^k v_i s_i^2/v$, where $v = \sum_1^k v_i$. In this case, (12.8) follows the $F$-distribution with $(k-1, v)$ d.f.

The $(1-\alpha)$ percent confidence limits for the ratio $R = \sigma_\alpha^2 / \left( \sum_1^k \sigma_i^2/k \right)$ are obtained from

$$\frac{F}{F_u} - 1 \leq R \leq \frac{F}{F_l} - 1 \tag{12.10}$$

In this expression, $(F_l, F_u)$ are the lower and upper percentage points of the above F-distribution.

For the SBPs in Example 12.1, $f_1 = 12$ and $f_2 = 201$ approximately. From (12.8), $F = (38.10/8.73) = 4.36$ with a very small p-value. The variance component $\sigma_\alpha^2$ is significantly larger than zero.

When $(1-\alpha) = 0.95$, the lower and upper percentiles of the F-distribution with (12, 201) d.f. are $(F_l, F_u) = (0.362, 2.01)$. From (12.10), 95 percent confidence limits for R become $[(4.36/2.01) - 1] = 1.17$ and $(4.36/0.362) - 1 = 11.04$.

## Exercises

**12.1.** The weights of the 15 groups of adults in Example 12.1 were initially in the range. of (170–190) lbs. The averages and S.E.s of the decreases in weights resulting from a prescribed diet were as follows. Find the estimates for $\sigma_\alpha^2$ and $\mu$ and the S.E.s of the estimate of $\mu$ through the procedures in Sections 12.4 and 12.5.

Averages of the decreases in weights and the S.E.s.

| $y_i$ | $s_i$ | $y_i$ | $s_i$ | $y_i$ | $s_i$ |
|---|---|---|---|---|---|
| 10 | 2.0 | 15 | 3.0 | 20 | 4.0 |
| 10 | 2.0 | 15 | 3.5 | 25 | 2.5 |
| 10 | 2.5 | 20 | 3.0 | 25 | 3.0 |
| 10 | 2.5 | 20 | 2.5 | 25 | 2.5 |
| 15 | 3.0 | 20 | 2.0 | 25 | 3.0 |

**12.2.** For the weight reductions in Exercise 12.1, test the hypothesis $H_0 : \sigma_\alpha^2 = 0$ and find 95 percent confidence limits for R.

**12.3.** Consider the model in 12.1 with random effects for the SBPs before and after the exercise program presented in Table T11.4. Denoting the sample means and its variances by $(y_i, s_i^2)$, find estimates of the variance components from (12.4) and the corresponding estimates for the overall means. Compare the S.E.s of these estimates and the unweighted means.

**12.4.** Five treatments $(t = 5)$, including the standard treatment and a placebo, for (LDL, HDL) were randomly administered to $b = 4$ age groups (blocks) in $k = 6$ medical institutions. For the LDL, the estimates of the residual mean squares with $(b-1)(t-1) = 12\,d.f.$ at each institution were $\hat{\sigma}_i^2 = (48, 52, 58, 60, 52, 68)$. The differences of the effect of the standard treatment and the control were $y_i = (12, 12, -4, 6, 10, -6)$. For the differences, find the estimate of the variance component from (12.4) and the corresponding estimate for their overall mean. Compare the standard errors of this estimate and the unweighted mean.

# Appendix A12

Approximation to the distribution of a linear combination of independent Chisquare variables.

Consider the linear combination $M = \sum_{1}^{k} a_i M_i$, where $M_i$ are mean squares with

$f_i M_i/E(M_i)$ following independent Chisquare distributions with $f_i$ degrees of freedom and $a_i$ are constants. Satterthwaite (1946) approximates $f\,M/E(M)$ with the Chisquare distribution with $f$ d.f. Since its variance is equal to $2f$, $f^2 V(M)/E^2(M) = 2f$ and hence $V(M) = 2E^2(M)/f$.

However, $V(M) = \sum_{1}^{k} a_i^2 V(M_i) = 2\sum_{1}^{k} a_i^2 E^2(M_i)/f_i$. Equating these two expressions for $V(M)$, $f = \left[\sum_{1}^{k} a_i E(M_i)\right]^2 / \sum_{1}^{k}\left[a_i^2 E^2(M_i)/f_i\right]$ degrees of freedom. In practice $f$ is obtained by removing the expectation signs in this expression.

# 13

# Survival analysis

## 13.1  Introduction

The survival times of individuals or patients receiving treatments for certain types of serious medical problems are recorded until an event like relapse, remission or death occurs. They can be days, weeks, months or specified lengths of time. They are obtained from the case control, cohort and similar experiments or studies. Section 13.2 presents the definitions of the *Survival function* and the related *Hazard function*.

The survival times for some individuals become *right - censored* if (a) the times of the events do not become available during the study, (b) they withdraw from the study during the experiment, or (c) the events do not occur before the completion of the study. They become *left-censored* if the events had occurred before the study. In some cases, they are *interval-censored*. The nonparametric *Product-Limit Estimation* of the survival function suggested by Kaplan-Meier (1958) is widely used in medical studies. It is presented in Section 13.3 for both the uncensored and right-censored cases. Section 13.4 contains the standard errors of the estimates and confidence limits for the survival function with uncensored observations. They are illustrated in Section 13.5 for the case of the right-censored observations. Section 13.6 presents the *log-rank test* for the equality of two survival functions, for instance, of two treatments or a treatment and a control. The role of the *Proportional Hazard Model* recommended by Cox (1972) for adjusting the responses to the treatments or medical procedures for the confounding variables such as age and length of illness of the patients is described in Section 13.7. The presentation of the different definitions and estimation procedures follow the descriptions of Cox and Oakes (1984), Lee (1992) and others on this topic.

*Statistical Methodologies with Medical Applications*, First Edition. Poduri S.R.S. Rao.
© 2017 John Wiley & Sons, Ltd. Published 2017 by John Wiley & Sons, Ltd.

## 13.2   Survival and hazard functions

With the random variable $T$ representing time of an event, the *Survival probability* or *Survival function*

$$S(t) = P(T \geq t) \quad t \geq 0 \tag{13.1}$$

is the probability of surviving beyond time t. The *hazard function*

$$h(t) = \left[ \frac{S(t) - S(t + \Delta_t)}{\Delta_t} \right] / S(t) \quad \text{as} \quad \Delta_t \to 0 \tag{13.2}$$

is the probability of the event occurring instantaneously after surviving up to time t.

If the time $T$ is continuous $S(t) = [1 - F(t)]$ and $h(t) = f(t)/[1 - F(t)]$, where $f(t)$ and $F(t)$ are the p.d.f and c.d.f of $T$ respectively. If the p.d.f of $T$ is of the exponential form $f(t) = e^{-t/\beta}/\beta$, $t > 0$, the c.d.f becomes $F(t) = 1 - e^{-t/\beta}$ and $S(t) = e^{-t/\beta}$. As a result, the hazard function becomes $h(t) = 1/\beta$, which is a constant and does not depend on the time. In general, it can depend on the shape, scale and other parameters of the p.d.f.

If the above types of parametric distributions are suitable for $T$, $S(t)$ and $h(t)$ can be estimated by substituting the estimators for the parameters. For instance, the mean of the sample times $t_i$, $i = (1, 2, ..., n)$ is $\bar{t} = \sum t_i/n$. For the above exponential distribution $E(T) = \beta$. The survival and hazard functions can be estimated by substituting $\bar{t}$ for $\beta$ in their expressions.

## 13.3   Kaplan-Meir product-limit estimator

In the nonparametric procedure of Kaplan and Meier (1958), the sample times of survival are ranked in increasing order as $(t_1, t_2, ..., t_n)$ with the corresponding ranking $i = (1, 2, ..., n)$ for the sampled patients. Patients with the same survival times are also included in the ranking. Now, the number of patients surviving longer than time $t_i$ is $(n - i)$, and an estimate of $S(t_i)$ is given by $\hat{S}(t_i) = (n - i)/n$. It follows that the estimator of $S(t_1)$ is $(n - 1)/n$, which is the sample proportion of the $n$ patients surviving beyond the first time interval $t_1$, $S(t_2) = (n - 2)/n$ is the proportion surviving beyond the second interval $t_2$, and $S(t_3) = (n - 3)/n$ is the proportion surviving beyond the third interval $t_3$, and so on. Note that $S(t_2) = [(n-2)/(n-1)][(n-1)/n] = \hat{p}_2 \cdot \hat{p}_1$, where $\hat{p}_1$ is the proportion of the $n$ patients surviving beyond $t_1$ and $\hat{p}_2 = (n-2)/(n-1)$ is the proportion of the $(n-2)$ patients surviving beyond $t_2$ among the $(n-1)$ patients surviving beyond $t_1$. Thus, $\hat{p}_2$ is the estimate of the conditional probability of survival, $P(T > t_2 | T > t_1)$. Similarly, $S(t_3) = (n-3)/n = \hat{p}_3 \cdot \hat{p}_2 \cdot \hat{p}_1$, where $\hat{p}_3 = (n-3)/(n-2)$, which is the proportion of the $(n-2)$ patients surviving beyond $t_3$.

Two or more patients may have the same survival time. For instance, if the ranked survival times for the fourth and fifth patients are the same, that is, $t_4 = t_5$, the estimates of both $S(t_4)$ and $S(t_5)$ are equal to $(n-5)/n$ and their conditional probabilities of survival times become $p_4 = p_5 = (n-5)/(n-3)$.

The *Product-Limit Estimator* for the $m$ ($\leq n$) *distinct* survival times can be expressed in general as

$$\hat{S}(t_m) = \hat{p}_1 \cdot \hat{p}_2 \cdot \hat{p}_3 \ldots \hat{p}_m \qquad (13.3a)$$

$$= \frac{(r_1 - d_1)}{r_1} \cdot \frac{(r_2 - d_2)}{r_2} \cdot \frac{(r_3 - d_3)}{r_3} \ldots \ldots \frac{(r_m - d_m)}{r_m}. \qquad (13.3b)$$

In this expression, $r_i$ and $d_i$ respectively are the number of patients alive at the beginning of the $i$th interval and not surviving beyond that interval. As can be seen, $d_i = 1$ if only one patient survives in the $i$th interval, $d_i = 2$ if two patients survive in that interval, and so on.

## 13.4    Standard error of $\hat{S}(t_m)$ and confidence limits for $S(t_m)$

As shown in Appendix A13, the variance of $\hat{S}(t_m)$ and its estimate are obtained by applying – Taylor's series approximation to $\ln\hat{S}(t_m)$. The estimate of this variance is given by

$$v\left[\hat{S}(t_m)\right] = \left[\hat{S}(t_m)\right]^2 \sum_{1}^{m} \frac{d_i}{r_i(r_i - d_i)} \qquad (13.4)$$

and $(1-\alpha)$ percent Confidence limits for $S(t_m)$ are obtained from $\hat{S}(t_m) \pm z_{\alpha/2}\left\{v\left[\hat{S}(t_m)\right]\right\}^{1/2}$, where $z_{\alpha/2}$ is the percentile of the standard normal distribution.

*Example 13.1*    The above estimates, their Standard Errors and confidence limits for $S(t_i)$ obtained from the observed survival times (5, 8, 12, 18, 24, 24, 24, 35, 42, 50) in months for ten individuals obtained from the R-program are presented in Table 13.1 and Figure 13.1.

## 13.5    Confidence limits for $S(t_m)$ with the right-censored observations

In this case, $S(t_i)$ for the uncensored patients are estimated from (13.3a) by setting $p_i$ for the censored patients to be unities or from (13.3b) by setting the corresponding $d_i$ to zeros.

Table 13.1    Uncensored observations of Example 13.1. Survival times $t_i$: (5, 8, 12, 18, 24, 24, 24, 35, 42, 50).

| $t_i$ | $r_i$ | No. of events | $\hat{S}(t_i)$ | S.E. $\hat{S}(t_i)$ | 95% Confidence Limits |
|---|---|---|---|---|---|
| 5 | 10 | 1 | 0.9 | 0.095 | (0.73, 1.0) |
| 8 | 9 | 1 | 0.8 | 0.127 | (0.59. 1.0) |
| 12 | 8 | 1 | 0.7 | 0.145 | (0.47, 1.0) |
| 18 | 7 | 1 | 0.6 | 0.155 | (0.36, 1.0) |
| 24 | 6 | 3 | 0.3 | 0.145 | (0.12, 0.77) |
| 35 | 3 | 1 | 0.2 | 0.137 | (0.06, 0.69) |
| 42 | 2 | 1 | 0.1 | 0.095 | (0.02, 0.64) |
| 50 | 1 | 1 | 0.0 | – | – |

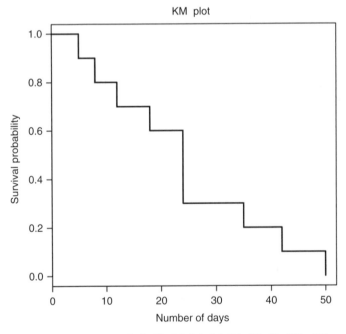

*Figure 13.1    Survival times $t_i$ : (5, 8, 12, 18, 24, 24, 24, 35, 42, 50) of Example 13.1.*

*Example 13.2*    Estimates of $S(t_i)$ along with the standard errors and confidence limits for the observed survival times (5, 8, 12+, 18, 24+, 26, 28, 35, 42, 50) of ten individuals obtained from the R-program are presented in Table 13.2; (12+, 24+) are the censored times.

Table 13.2    Survival times $t_i$: (5, 8, 12+, 18, 24+, 26, 28, 35, 42, 50).

| $t_i$ | $r_i$ | No. of events | $\hat{S}(t_i)$ | S. E. $\hat{S}(t_i)$ | 95 % Confidence limits |
|---|---|---|---|---|---|
| 5  | 10 | 1 | 0.9  | 0.095 | (0.73, 1.0)  |
| 8  | 9  | 1 | 0.8  | 0.127 | (0.59, 1.0)  |
| 18 | 7  | 1 | 0.69 | 0.152 | (0.45, 1.0)  |
| 26 | 5  | 1 | 0.55 | 0.172 | (0.30, 1.0)  |
| 28 | 4  | 1 | 0.41 | 0.176 | (0.18, 0.95) |
| 35 | 3  | 1 | 0.27 | 0.162 | (0.09, 0.87) |
| 42 | 2  | 1 | 0.14 | 0.126 | (0.02, 0.83) |
| 50 | 1  | 1 | 0    | –     | –            |

## 13.6    Log-Rank test for the equality of two survival distributions

For this test, the numbers at risk and of the events like relapse or death $(n_{1i}, o_{1i})$ and $(n_{2i}, o_{2i})$, $i = (1, 2, ..., k)$ for two treatments or a treatment and control are recorded at $k$ independent time intervals. The number of survivals for the two treatments at the $i$th interval are $(n_{1i} - o_{1i})$ and $(n_{2i} - o_{2i})$. As in Section (4.3.5), the number of events $(o_{1i}, o_{2i})$ follow the hypergeometric distribution with the probability

$$P(o_{1i}, o_{2i}) = \frac{n_{1i}Co_{1i}\, n_{2i}\, Co_{2i}}{n_i Co_i}, \quad (0 < o_{1i} < n_{1i}, 0 < o_{2i} < n_{2i}) \tag{13.5}$$

where $n_i = (n_{1i} + n_{2i})$ and $o_i = o_{1i} + o_{2i}$.
The expected value $E(o_{1i})$ and variance $V(o_{1i})$ for the first treatment are

$$e_{1i} = (n_{1i}/n_i)(o_i) \tag{13.6a}$$

and

$$v_{1i} = \left(\frac{n_i - o_i}{n_i - 1}\right)\left(\frac{n_{1i}}{n_i}\right)\left(\frac{n_{2i}}{n_i}\right)(o_i) \tag{13.6b}$$

From these results, $O_1 = (o_{11} + o_{12} + ... + o_{1k})$, $E_1 = (e_{11} + e_{12} + ... + e_{1k})$ and $V_1 = (v_{11} + v_{12} + ... + v_{1k})$. For the equality of the two survival functions, the test statistic is given by

$$U = (O_1 - E_1)^2 / V_1, \tag{13.7}$$

which follows the Chisquare distribution with a single degree of freedom. This statistic is obtained from the procedures of Cochran (1954) and Mantel-Hanszeal (1959) described in Section 9.5.2 for combining observations from a set of contingency tables with two rows and two columns, the (2 × 2) classifications.

*Example 13.3*   The numbers at risk and having the event for two treatments at ten time intervals, the expected numbers $e_{1i}$ and variances $v_{1i}$ are as follows.

| $i$ | $n_{1i}$ | $o_{1i}$ | $n_{2i}$ | $o_{2i}$ | $n_i$ | $o_i$ | $n_i - o_i$ | $e_{1i}$ | $v_{1i}$ |
|-----|------|------|------|------|------|------|--------|--------|--------|
| 1   | 25   | 4    | 30   | 2    | 55   | 6    | 49     | 2.73   | 1.35   |
| 2   | 24   | 2    | 28   | 1    | 52   | 3    | 49     | 1.38   | 0.72   |
| 3   | 22   | 3    | 25   | 0    | 47   | 3    | 44     | 1.40   | 0.71   |
| 4   | 20   | 4    | 24   | 0    | 44   | 4    | 40     | 1.82   | 0.92   |
| 5   | 18   | 1    | 20   | 1    | 38   | 2    | 36     | 0.95   | 0.49   |
| 6   | 15   | 1    | 16   | 2    | 31   | 3    | 28     | 1.45   | 0.70   |
| 7   | 14   | 2    | 12   | 1    | 26   | 3    | 23     | 1.62   | 0.69   |
| 8   | 10   | 0    | 6    | 1    | 16   | 1    | 15     | 0.63   | 0.23   |
| 9   | 6    | 1    | 5    | 0    | 11   | 1    | 10     | 0.55   | 0.25   |
| 10  | 4    | 0    | 2    | 0    | 6    | 0    | 6      | 0.00   | 0.00   |

From these figures, $O_1 = 18$, $E_1 = 12.53$, $V_1 = 6.06$ and $U = (18 - 12.53)^2/6.06 = 4.94$ with the *p*-value of 0.026. The difference between the two survival functions is significant at the five percent level.

## 13.7   Cox's proportional hazard model

The hazard function $h(t)$ in general depends on one or more confounding variables such as age and length of illness. The regression of $h(t)$ on $p$ confounding variables $X' = (x_1, x_2, \ldots x_p)$ may take the linear form

$$lnE[h(t|X)] = \beta_0 + \beta_1 x_1 + \beta_2 x_2 + \ldots + \beta_p x_p = \beta_0 + X'\beta, \qquad (13.8)$$

where $\beta_0$ is the intercept and $\beta' = (\beta_0, \beta_1, \ldots, \beta_p)$ are the regression coefficients.

This model, however, is suitable only if $h(t)$ does not depend on time. For $h(t)$ to depend on time as well as the confounding variables, Cox (1972) recommends the model

$$lnE[h(t|X)] = ln\,E[h_0(t)] + \beta_1 x_1 + \beta_2 x_2 + \ldots + \beta_p x_p = lnE[h_0(t)] + X'\beta, \qquad (13.9)$$

where $h_0(t)$ is not specified. Now, $E[h(t|X)] = E[h_0(t)]\,e^{X'\beta}$. Following this model, for two individuals with confounders $X_1$ and $X_2$,

$$\frac{E[h(t|X_1)]}{E[h(t|X_2)]} = e^{(X'_1 - X'_2)\beta}. \qquad (13.10)$$

Thus, the hazard functions for both the individuals depend on time and the confounders. But, at any point of time, their relative value depends only on the confounders.

## Exercises

**13.1.** The observed survival times $t_i$ in months for 12 individuals receiving a treatment are (8, 10, 10, 12, 13, 14, 14, 16, 18, 19, 20, 24). Estimate the survival probabilities $S(t)$, standard errors of the estimates and confidence limits for $S(t)$.

**13.2.** The observed survival times $t_i$ in months for 12 individuals receiving a treatment are (8, 10, 10, 12, 13+, 14+, 14, 16, 18, 19+, 20, 24). Estimate the survival probabilities $S(t)$, standard errors of the estimates and confidence limits for $S(t)$. The censored survival times for individuals (5, 6, 10) are (13+, 14+, 19+).

**13.3.** The numbers at risk and having the event for two treatments at ten time intervals are as follows. Test for the equality of the two survival functions.

| $i$ | $n_{1i}$ | $o_{1i}$ | $n_{2i}$ | $o_{2i}$ | $i$ | $n_{1i}$ | $o_{1i}$ | $n_{2i}$ | $o_{2i}$ |
|---|---|---|---|---|---|---|---|---|---|
| 1 | 28 | 3 | 35 | 1 | 6 | 15 | 1 | 18 | 2 |
| 2 | 25 | 2 | 30 | 1 | 7 | 14 | 0 | 12 | 1 |
| 3 | 24 | 2 | 25 | 0 | 8 | 10 | 2 | 5 | 1 |
| 4 | 20 | 3 | 24 | 0 | 9 | 5 | 1 | 4 | 0 |
| 5 | 18 | 1 | 22 | 2 | 10 | 2 | 0 | 2 | 0 |

# Appendix A13    Expected value and variance of $\hat{S}(t_m)$ and confidence limits for $S(t_m)$

Consider a function $f(x)$ of a random variable $X$ with $E(X)=\mu$ and $V(X)=\sigma^2$. From Taylor's approximation, $E[f(X)]=f(\mu)$ and $V[f(X)]=[f'(\mu)]^2\sigma^2$.

(1) Expressing $\hat{S}(t_m)$ as $exp\,[ln\,\hat{S}(t_m)]$, following the above approximation,

$$E\left[\hat{S}(t_m)\right] = exp[ln\,S(t_m)] = S(t_m)\ and\ V\left[\hat{S}(t_m)\right] = [S(t_m)]^2 V\left[ln\,\hat{S}(t_m)\right]$$

(2) Since $ln\hat{S}(t_m)=\sum_1^m ln\hat{p}_i$, $E\left[ln\,\hat{S}(t_m)\right]=\sum_1^m ln p_i$ and

$$V\left[ln\,\hat{S}(t_m)\right] = \sum_{i=1}^m (1/p_i^2)[p_i(1-p_i)/r_i] = \sum_{i=1}^m [(1-p_i)/r_i p_i].$$

Substituting $\hat{p}_i = (r_i-d_i)/r_i$ for $p_i$, the estimate of this variance becomes $v\left[ln\hat{S}(t_m)\right]=\sum_1^m d_i/r_i(r_i-d_i)$ and $S.\,E.\,[ln\,\hat{S}(t_m)]$ is obtained from the square root of this expression. Approximate $(1-\alpha)$ percent upper and lower confidence limits $(c_u, c_l)$ for $ln\,\hat{S}(t_m)$ are obtained from

$$ln\,\hat{S}(t_m) \pm S.E.\left[ln\,\hat{S}(t_m)\right].$$

The confidence limits for $S(t_m)$ are given by $(e^{c_l}, e^{c_u})$.

Confidence limits for $S(t_m)$ can be directly obtained as follows. Substituting $\hat{S}(t_m)$ for $S(t_m)$ and $\hat{p}_i = (r_i - d_i)/r_i$ for $p_i$, from (1) and (2), the estimate for $V[\hat{S}(t_m)]$ becomes

$$v\left[\hat{S}(t_m)\right] = \left[\hat{S}(t_m)\right]^2 \sum_1^m d_i/r_i(r_i - d_i)$$ and S. E. $[\hat{S}(t_m)]$ is given by the square root of this

expression. Approximate $(1-\alpha)$ percent confidence limits for $S(t_m)$ are obtained from $\hat{S}(t_m) \pm z_{\alpha/2}S.E.\left[\hat{S}(t_m)\right].$

# 14

# Nonparametric statistics

## 14.1  Introduction

The test for the mean of a population with the assumption of normality for the distribution, the various $t$-tests, the $F$-test for the ANOVA and similar tests considered in the previous chapters are *parametric* tests. The test for a proportion, the Chisquare goodness of fit, Fisher's exact test are *nonparametric*. In certain situations, the assumptions regarding the distributions of the random variables may not be valid. Further, instead of the above type of parameters, the required inference may be related to the differences of the proportions or percentages of an attribute of two groups, the relative ranking of a characteristic and similar factors. The following sections present some of the nonparametric methods of practical interest that are easy to implement. Siegel (1956) presents the early developments on this topic with illustrations.

## 14.2  Spearman's rank correlation coefficient

This correlation coefficient $\rho_s$ is the same as the correlation coefficient $\rho$ of the ranks of $(X, Y)$. Its estimate $r_S$ from the sample is the same as the simple correlation coefficient $r$ of the ranks $(u, v)$ of the observed measurements of $(x, y)$. For the hypothesis $H_0 : \rho_s = 0$, the test statistic

$$t = \frac{r_s \sqrt{n-2}}{\sqrt{1 - r_s^2}} \tag{14.1}$$

approximately follows the $t$-distribution with $(n - 2)$ d.f.

*Statistical Methodologies with Medical Applications*, First Edition. Poduri S.R.S. Rao.
© 2017 John Wiley & Sons, Ltd. Published 2017 by John Wiley & Sons, Ltd.

*Example 14.1*    The ranks $(u, v)$ of the heights and weights $(x, y)$ in Table 1.1 of the sample of $n = 20$ boys are as follows:

| u | v | u | v | u | v | u | v |
|---|---|---|---|---|---|---|---|
| 1 | 1 | 6.5 | 6 | 11 | 11.5 | 16 | 16 |
| 2 | 2 | 6.5 | 7 | 12 | 11.5 | 17.5 | 17 |
| 3 | 3 | 8 | 8 | 13 | 13 | 17.5 | 18 |
| 4 | 4 | 9 | 9 | 14.5 | 14 | 19 | 19 |
| 5 | 5 | 10 | 10 | 14.5 | 15 | 20 | 20 |

If two or more ranks are equal (tied), they are replaced by their average. For these ranks, the means, standard deviations and covariance are $(\bar{u}, \bar{v}) = (10.5, 10.95)$, $(s_u, s_v) = (5.90, 6.21)$ and $s_{uv} = 35.05$. As the simple correlation, the rank correlation coefficient becomes $r_S = s_{uv}/s_u s_v = 0.97$. From (14.1), $t = 16.75$ with 18 d.f, with a very small $p$-value suggesting the rejection of $H_0$.

## 14.3    The Sign test

In several medical applications, it becomes of interest to examine whether a particular treatment is more effective than a second one or a placebo. For instance, consider the decreases $(X_1, X_2)$ of the systolic blood pressures (SBPs) for two treatments. From the observed differences $(x_{1i}, x_{2i})$, $i = (1, 2, \ldots, n)$, of a sample of $n$ pairs of adults, the mean differences can be evaluated through the assumption of normality for $(X_1, X_2)$ and the paired $t$-test.

For the nonparametric evaluation of the two treatments without the normality assumption, the null hypotheses

$$H_0 : P(X_1 > X_2) = P(X_1 < X_2) = (1/2) \tag{14.2}$$

is considered. This hypothesis specifies that the distributions of $X_1$ and $X_2$ are the same. For the alternative hypothesis $H_1$, these two probabilities are not equal, or one is greater than the other. It is also the same as that the median of the distribution of the difference $D = (X_1 - X_2)$ is zero.

For the *Sign test* of (14.2), the difference $d_i = (x_{1i} - x_{2i})$ is replaced by the $(+)$ sign if it is greater than zero and by the $(-)$ sign if it is less than zero. A "tie" with zero for the observed difference $d_i = (x_{1i} - x_{2i})$ for a sample unit is not included in the sample.

To test the above hypothesis, consider $(x_{1i}, x_{2i})$ obtained by administering the two treatments to a sample of n pairs of individuals. Under the null hypothesis in (14.2), the number of $(+)$ or $(-)$ signs follows the binomial distribution with probability $p = 1/2$. For the one-sided alternative, the $p$-value for the test is given by the probability of the smaller of the number of these two signs $Y$ becoming less than the observed value. This probability is doubled for the two-sided alternative.

*Example 14.2*    Decrease in the SBPs of two treatments and the signs of their differences for a sample of $n = 16$ individuals are as follows.

| $x_{1i}$ | $x_{2i}$ | $d_i$ | Sign of $d_i$ | $x_{1i}$ | $x_{2i}$ | $d_i$ | Sign of $d_i$ |
|---|---|---|---|---|---|---|---|
| 16 | 14 | 2 | + | 22 | 15 | 7 | + |
| 12 | 10 | 2 | + | 23 | 15 | 8 | + |
| 7 | 10 | −3 | − | 10 | 5 | 5 | + |
| 10 | 8 | 2 | + | 8 | 8 | 0 | 0 |
| 21 | 15 | 6 | + | 12 | 6 | 6 | + |
| 15 | 10 | 5 | + | 6 | 5 | 1 | + |
| 6 | 8 | −2 | − | 10 | 15 | −5 | − |
| 12 | 10 | 2 | + | 20 | 18 | 2 | + |

Excluding the individual with the "tie," the sample size is 15. Numbers of the ( + ) and ( − ) signs are 12 and 3 respectively. For the smaller number, $P(Y < 3 \,|\, n = 15, p = 0.5) = 0.0176$ from the binomial distribution. The $p$-value for $H_0$ : $P(X_1 > X_2) = P(X_1 < X_2)$ becomes 0.0352 with the two-sided alternative. As a result, the null hypothesis that both the treatments are equally effective in reducing the SBP can be rejected at the 3.52 percent level of significance. The $p$-value for the null hypothesis with the alternative hypothesis $H_1 : P(X_1 > X_2) > P(X_1 < X_2)$ is 0.0176, which leads to the rejection of the null hypothesis at the 1.76 percent level of significance. The first treatment is more effective than the second.

With $(a, b)$ denoting the number of observed ( + , − ) signs, $Z = [|a - np| - (1/2)] / [np(1-p)]^{1/2}$ approximately follows the standard normal distribution. Since $p = 1/2$ under the null hypothesis, this statistic is the same as $Z = [|a - b| - 1] / \sqrt{n}$. From the above observations, $z = 8/(15)^{1/2} = 2.07$ with the $p$-values of 0.0192 and 0.0384 for the one- and two-sided alternative hypotheses.

The square of the above statistic becomes $U = [|a - b| - 1]^2 / n$, which follows the Chisquare distribution with a single degree of freedom. As Snedecor and Cochran (1967, p. 127) pointed out, for the goodness of fit test in Section 9.3,

$$U = \frac{[|a - (n/2)| - 0.5]^2}{n/2} + \frac{[|b - (n/2)| - 0.5]^2}{n/2} = \frac{[|a - b| - 1]^2}{n} \qquad (14.3)$$

follows the Chisquare distribution with a single degree of freedom. For this example, $U = 64/15 = 4.2667$ with the $p$-value of 0.0388, which leads to the rejection of the null hypothesis. The slight difference of this $p$-value from $2(0.0176) = 0.0352$ for the exact test is the result of the Chisquare approximation.

The characteristics of the Sign test are as follows: (1) It is a *nonparametric* test since it is not related to the parameters such as the means of distributions. (2) Assumptions of normality for $X_1$ or $X_2$ or for their difference are not required. (3) The measurements $(X_1, X_2)$ can be ranks of the type (1, 2), (High, Low) and (Yes, No). (4) The individuals in each pair should be similar with respect to age and health-related characteristics. (5) As has been shown in the literature, the $t$-test for the difference of two means with matched observations on $(X_1, X_2)$ and the assumptions of normality will have higher power than the Sign test.

For the 16 sample differences, the mean, standard deviation and S.E. of the mean are 2.375, 3.686 and 0.922. Hence $t_{15} = (2.375 - 0)/(0.922) = 2.58$ with the $p$-value of 0.01 and 0.02 for the one- and two sided-alternatives. The null hypothesis $H_0 : p = 1/2$ can be rejected as above.

## 14.4    Wilcoxon (1945) Matched-pairs Signed-ranks test

This test is an alternative to the $t$-test with paired samples. The absolute values $|d_i|$ of the differences of a sample of $n$ pairs are ranked, and the original signs are returned to the ranks. For more than one value of $|d_i|$, the average of their ranks is considered. The smaller of the sums $W$ of these ranks for the positive and negative $d_i$'s approximately follows the normal distribution with mean $E(W) = n(n + 1)/4$ and variance $V(W) = n(n + 1)(2n + 1)/24$. Since this test uses the actual differences, its inference for the null hypothesis in (14.2) can be different from the Sign test in some situations.

*Example 14.3*    From Example 14.2, the following ranks of $|d_i|$ and the signed ranks are obtained.

| Rank of $|d_i|$ | Signed rank | Rank of $|d_i|$ | Signed rank |
|---|---|---|---|
| 4.5 | 4.5 | 14 | 14 |
| 4.5 | 4.5 | 15 | 15 |
| 8 | −8 | 10 | 10 |
| 4.5 | 4.5 | — | — |
| 12.5 | 12.5 | 12.5 | 12.5 |
| 10 | 10 | 1 | 1 |
| 4.5 | −4.5 | 10 | −10 |
| 4.5 | 4.5 | 4.5 | 4.5 |

The third, seventh and fifteenth ranks (8, 4.5, 10) are for the negative $d_i$'s and the remaining 12 are for the positive differences. The rank for $|d_i| = 2$ is $(2 + 3 + 4 + 5 + 6 + 7)/6 = 4.5$. Similarly, the rank for $|d_i| = 5$ is $(9 + 10 + 11)/3 = 10$, and the rank for $d_i = 6$ is $(12 + 13)/2 = 12.5$. The sum for the smaller number of ranks is $w = (8 + 4.5 + 10) = 22.5$. Since $E(W) = 15(16)/4 = 60$ and $V(W) = 15(16)(31)/24 = 310$, $z = (|22.5 - 60| - 0.5)/(310)^{1/2} = 2.10$. The $p$-values for the test for the null hypothesis with the two-sided and one-sided alternatives are

0.036 and 0.018 respectively. The null hypothesis that both the treatments are equally effective can be rejected at the 3.6 percent level of significance.

For the $t$-test, the average and standard deviation of the actual 16 differences are $\bar{d} = 2.375$ and $s_d = 3.684$ with S.E.$(\bar{d}) = 3.686/4 = 0.922$. Since $t_{15} = (2.375 - 0)/0.922 = 2.58$, the $p$-values for the two-sided and one-sided alternatives are 0.022 and 0.010. As above, the null hypothesis that both the treatments are equally effective can be rejected at the 2.2 percent level of significance. The first treatment is more effective than the second.

## 14.5    Wilcoxon's test for the equality of the distributions of two non-normal populations with unpaired sample observations

This test, also known as Mann-Whitney (1947) test, is the nonparametric alternative to the $t$-test presented in Section (7.6.1) for the equality of the means of two normal populations. The null hypothesis for this test is that the means or the distributions of two non-normal populations are the same.

Consider independent samples of sizes $n_1$ and $n_2$ from two populations. Rank all the $n = (n_1 + n_2)$ observations together and denote the sum of the ranks for the first and second samples by $W_1$ and $W_2$ respectively. Under the null hypothesis of the equality of the two distributions, following Snedecor and Cochran (1967, p. 131), the expected value and variance of $W_1$ are $E(W_1) = n_1(n + 1)/2$ and $V(W_1) = n_1 n_2(n + 1)/12$. Similarly, the expected value of $W_2$ is $n_2(n + 1)/2$ and its variance is the same as $V(W_1)$.

Denote the smaller of $W_1$ and $W_2$ by W. If $W_1$ is smaller than $W_2$, $E(W) = n_1(n + 1)/2$ and $V(W) = n_1 n_2(n + 1)/12$. For large $(n_1, n_2)$, the test statistic for the above null hypothesis is given by $Z = [|W - E(W)| - (1/2)]/\sqrt{V(W)}$. If $W_2$ is smaller than $W_1$, $E(W)$ in this expression is replaced by $n_2(n + 1)/2$. Percentiles of W are available in some of the software programs.

*Example 14.4* Consider the SBPs before the exercise program in Table T11.2 for the first and second groups with $n_1 = n_2 = 10$ observations. Ranking the $n = 20$ observations together, we find that $W_1 = 114$ and $W_2 = 96$. As a result, $W = 96$ with $E(W) = n_2(n + 1)/2 = 105$ and $V(W) = n_2 n_1(n + 1)/12 = 175$. Now, $z = [|96 - 105| - 0.5]/(175)^{1/2} = 0.64$ with a large $p$-value suggesting that the distributions of the SBPs of the two groups before the exercise program are not significantly different.

The sample means and standard deviations of the two groups are (140, 142.40) and (5.5, 9.48) respectively with the pooled variance $s^2 = 60.06$. With the S.E. of $(60.06/5)^{1/2} = 3.47$ for the difference of the two means, and the normality assumption for the two groups, $t_{18} = (140 - 142.4)/3.47 = -0.69$. With a large $p$-value for this statistic, the null hypothesis of equality of the means of the SBPs of the two groups before the exercise program is not rejected.

### 14.5.1    Unequal sample sizes

If $n_1$ and $n_2$ are not equal, an adjustment is made to $W_1$ and $W_2$. If $n_1$ is smaller than $n_2$, $W_1$ remains the same, but sum of the ranks for the second group is obtained from $W_2 = n_1(n + 1) - W_1$. The test statistic is obtained from $W$, the smaller of $(W_1, W_2)$.

*Example 14.5*    Consider the SBPs before the exercise program of the first and second groups in Table 11.4, with sample sizes $n_1 = 9$ and $n_2 = 13$. From the combined sample, $W_1 = 57$. Since $n_1$ is smaller than $n_2$, $W_2 = 9(23) - 57 = 150$. Now, $W = 57$ with $E(W) = n_1(n + 1)/2 = 103.5$ and $V(W) = n_1 n_2 (n + 1)/12 = 224.25$. The test statistic becomes $z = [|57 - 103.5| - 0.5]/14.98 = 3.07$ with a very small $p$-value. The distributions of the SBPs of the two groups differ significantly.

The sample means and standard deviations of the two groups are $(132.22, 142.62)$ and $(6.67, 5.47)$. The pooled estimate of variance becomes $s^2 = 35.75$ with 20 d.f. With the S.E. of 2.59 for the difference of the two sample means and the assumption of normality for the two groups, $t_{20} = (132.22 - 142.62)/2.59 = -4.02$ with a very small $p$-value. The difference between the means of the two groups is highly significant.

## 14.6    McNemer's (1955) matched pair test for two proportions

Each of two treatments can have positive or negative responses. For instance, two experimental diets may increase or decrease high-density lipids (HDL). If $P_1$ is the proportion of the experimental units with positive responses for the first treatment and negative responses for the second treatment, and $P_2$ is the proportion with positive responses for the second treatment and negative response for the first treatment, the null hypothesis $H_0 : P_1 = P_2$ specifies that both the treatments are equally effective. The alternative hypothesis can be $H_1 : P_1 \neq P_2$ or one-sided.

The positive $(+)$ and negative $(-)$ responses to the treatments randomly administered to n pairs of units will be of the form

|  |  | Treatment 2 | |
|---|---|---|---|
|  |  | + | − |
| Treatment 1 | + | $a$ | $b$ |
|  | − | $c$ | $d$ |

The estimates of $P_1$ and $P_2$ respectively are $b/(b + c)$ and $c/(b + c)$. Under $H_0$, the estimate of the common proportion becomes $(b + c)/2$. As in (14.3), the test statistic for the null hypothesis of the equality of $P_1$ and $P_2$ is given by

$$\chi_1^2 = \frac{[|b-c|-1]^2}{b+c} \qquad (14.4)$$

*Example 14.6*   For a sample of 100 pairs of units, $a = 35, b = 25, c = 10$ and $d = 30$. From (14.4), $\chi_1^2 = 5.6$ with the *p*-value of 0.018. There is a significant difference between the effectiveness of the two treatments.

The above test can also be considered to examine the change in the responses before and after administering a diet or treatment.

## 14.7  Cochran's (1950) *Q*-test for the difference of three or more matched proportions

Systolic blood pressure (SBP) is classified as Medium, High and Very High. The reduction of the SBP by 10 percent or more, for instance, with a treatment can be examined for a sample of $n$ groups of $k = 3$ patients with the three levels of the SBP. The $k$ patients are matched in age and other characteristics except for their SBP levels. The null hypothesis of interest is that the $k$ proportions or percentages of the reductions for the three levels of the SBP are the same.

Another kind of common medical interest is whether diet $(T_1)$, diet with exercise $(T_2)$, or diet with exercise and treatment $(T_3)$ reduce SBP by more than 10 percent. In this case, a sample of $n$ patients follow each of the $k = 3$ treatments, for instance, each for six months. The null hypothesis now is that the proportions of the reductions of the SBP by 10 percent or more, for instance, for the $k = 3$ types of treatment are the same.

For both the above two representations, the null hypothesis for the k matched proportions is

$$Ho: P_1 = P_2 = \ldots = P_k \qquad (14.5)$$

For the n groups or patients as described above, denote the reduction of the SBP by (1), which represents success, and the absence of reduction by (0), which represents failure. Consider the totals $R_i, i = (1,2,\ldots,n)$ of the rows and $C_j, j = (1,2,\ldots,k)$ of the columns. This representation may appear as follows:

| Row ($i$) | Column ($j$) | | | | | | | Row total $R_i$ |
|---|---|---|---|---|---|---|---|---|
| | 1 | 2 | 3 | ... | k | | | |
| 1 | 1 | 1 | 0 | 1 | 1 | 0 | | $R_1$ |
| 2 | 1 | 0 | 1 | 1 | 0 | 1 | | $R_2$ |
| . | ........................... | | | | | | | |
| . | ........................... | | | | | | | |
| $n$ | ........................... | | | | | | | $R_n$ |
| Column total $C_j$ | $C_1$ $C_2$ $C_3$ ... $C_k$ | | | | | | | |

For the hypothesis in (14.5), Cochran's test statistic is given by

$$Q = \frac{k(k-1)\sum_{1}^{k}(C_j - \bar{C})^2}{k\sum_{1}^{n}R_i - \sum_{1}^{n}R_i^2} = \frac{(k-1)\left[k\sum_{1}^{k}C_j^2 - \left(\sum_{1}^{k}C_j\right)^2\right]}{k\sum_{1}^{n}R_i - \sum_{1}^{n}R_i^2} \qquad (14.6)$$

which follows the Chisquare distribution with $(k-1)$ d.f.

## 14.8   Kruskal-Wallis one-way ANOVA test by ranks

The one-way unbalanced ANOVA in Section 11.5 considered testing the hypothesis of equality of the means of $k$ normal populations. Kruskal and Wallis (1952) suggest a procedure for examining the hypothesis that $k$ samples of sizes $n_i$, $i = (1,2,...,k)$, have come from the same population or $k$ populations with a common mean. In this approach, all the $n = \sum_{i=1}^{k} n_i$ observations of the $k$ samples are ranked from the lowest to the highest, and the observations in each sample are replaced by the corresponding ranks. With the totals $R_i$ of the ranks of the $k$ groups, the test statistic for the above hypothesis is

$$KW = [12/n(n+1)]\sum_{1}^{k}(R_i^2/n_i) - 3(n+1) \qquad (14.7)$$

which approximately follows the Chisquare distribution with $(k-1)$ d.f., unless $n_i$ are very small.

*Example 14.7*   Age and weight of samples of sizes $n_1 = 9$, $n_2 = 13$ and $n_3 = 8$ from three groups are presented in Table T11.3. Ranking the $n = 30$ observations for age from $(1-30)$, the ranks for the three groups are as follows:

| | Ranks for age | |
|---|---|---|
| Group 1 | Group 2 | Group 3 |
| 1 | 11 | 24 |
| 2.5 | 10 | 24 |
| 7 | 11 | 27.5 |
| 5 | 17 | 24 |
| 8.5 | 20 | 27.5 |
| 8.5 | 14.5 | 29 |
| 4 | 17 | 30 |
| 2.5 | 20 | 26 |
| 6 | 11 | |
| | 14.5 | |
| | 17 | |
| | 22 | |
| | 20 | |

| | Group 1 | Group 2 | Group 3 |
|---|---|---|---|
| Total $R_i$ | 45 | 205 | 212 |
| Mean | 5.0 | 15.77 | 26.5 |
| S.D. | 2.72 | 4.10 | 2.38 |

From the totals $R_i$, $\sum_1^3 R_i^2/n_i = 9075.692$ and from (14.7), $KW = (12/930)$ $(9075.692) = 24.11$. From the Chisquare distribution with 2 d.f., the $p$-value for this statistic becomes $5.82 \times 10^{-6}$, which is very small. The three samples for the age cannot be considered to have come from the same population.

# Exercises

**14.1.** Find the Spearman's correlation coefficient and the simple correlation coefficient for the heights and weights of (a) the 20 sixteen-year-old boys in Table T1.3 and (b) the 20 sixteen-year-old girls in Table T1.4.

**14.2.** From the observations in Table T11.2 for the SBPs before the exercise program of the samples of 10 each, examine the hypothesis of equality of the distributions of the first and third groups through the Wilcoxon test with unpaired samples.

**14.3.** From the observations in Table T11.4 for the SBPs before the exercise program of the samples of sizes $n_1 = 9$ and $n_3 = 8$, examine the hypothesis of equality of the distributions of the first and third groups through the Wilcoxon test with unpaired samples.

**14.4.** In a sample of 100 adults, the number of them with SBP above ($+$) and below ($-$) 140 before and after administering a treatment are $a = 38$, $b = 22$, $c = 12$ and $d = 28$. Test whether the change is significant.

**14.5.** A sample of 20 patients were prescribed a treatment, treatment and a diet, and treatment with diet and exercise for the reduction of low-density lipids (LDL). Each of these three programs was implemented for six months one after the other in turn, and the reduction of LDL by 10 percent was recorded as described in Section (14.7). The column totals were (8, 12, 16). The frequencies for the row totals (0, 1, 2, 3) were (4, 4, 4, 8). Perform Cochran's Q-test to examine whether the proportions for the three types of treatments are the same.

**14.6.** Perform the Kruskal-Wallis one-way ANOVA test for the samples on weight in Table T11.3.

# 15

# Further topics

## 15.1   Introduction

This chapter presents the estimation and inference procedures of general interest in clinical and medical studies. The Joint Confidence Region for a pair of means or treatment effects is described in Section 15.2. Sections 15.3 and 15.4 present procedures for finding confidence limits for the differences of pairs of treatment effects. The simultaneous confidence interval procedure for contrasts of treatment effects is described in Section 15.5. The bootstrap method in Section 15.6 is used for finding the standard error of an estimator and the confidence limits for a population parameter. The variance stabilizing transformations in Section 15.7 are employed when the assumption of equality of the variances in the ANOVA classification cells is not satisfied.

For clinical experiments, samples are considered to be selected randomly from populations of large sizes. In several medical and epidemiological studies, the patients, hospitals and similar *units* are selected randomly *without replacement* from a finite populations. Cochran (1977) and Rao (2000) present stratification, clustering, single and multistage sampling and related topics for the estimation of the means, variances and similar quantities of interest from such populations

## 15.2   Bonferroni inequality and the Joint Confidence Region

Consider the events $(A, B)$, $(A$ or $B)$ and $(AB)$ and their respective compliments $(A', B')$, $(A$ or $B)'$ and $(AB)'$. Now, $P(A \text{ or } B)' = P(A') + P(B') - P(AB)'$. Since the

*Statistical Methodologies with Medical Applications*, First Edition. Poduri S.R.S. Rao.
© 2017 John Wiley & Sons, Ltd. Published 2017 by John Wiley & Sons, Ltd.

left- hand side is nonnegative, $[P(A') + P(B')] \geq P(AB)'$. Hence, $P(AB) = [1-P(AB)'] \geq [1-P(A')-P(B')]$.

Two results follow from this inequality:

(a) Denote by $P(A) = (1-\alpha_1)$ and $P(B) = (1-\alpha_2)$ the probabilities of the confidence limits for two means, and by P(AB) the probability for the joint confidence region for the means enclosed by the two sets of limits. Since $P(A') = \alpha_1$ and $P(B') = \alpha_2$, $P(AB) \geq (1-\alpha_1-\alpha_2)$.

(b) If the significance level for the tests of hypotheses for two means are $P(A') = \alpha_1$ and $P(B') = \alpha_2$, the significance level $P(AB)'$ for the test of hypothesis for the two means together does not exceed $(\alpha_1 + \alpha_2)$.

Consider the $(1-\alpha)$ percent confidence limits for two means. From the Bonferroni inequality, the probability for the joint confidence region for the two means enclosed by the two sets of limits is at least $(1-2\alpha)$. It follows that if the probability for the joint confidence region is required to be at least $(1-\alpha)$, the probabilities for the confidence limits for each of the means enclosing it should be $(1-\alpha/2)$. Similarly, the probability would be at least $(1-\alpha)$ for the region enclosed by the $(1-\alpha/k)$ percent confidence limits of $k \geq 2$ means.

*Example 15.1*    From Table T11.2, for samples of size $m = 10$, the means, standard deviations and standard errors of the systolic blood pressures (SBPs) for three groups before the exercise program respectively are (142.4, 140.0, 148.7), (5.5, 9.45, 7.47) and (1.74, 2.99, 2.36).

Since $t_{9,0.025} = 2.262$, 95 percent confidence limits for the mean of the first group are $142.4 - 2.262(1.74) = 138.46$ and $142.4 + 2.262(1.74) = 146.34$, with the confidence width of 7.88. For the second group, 95 percent confidence limits are $140 - 2.262(2.99) = 133.24$ and $140 + 2.262(2.99) = 146.76$, with the confidence width of 13.52. The probability for the joint region enclosed by these two sets of limits is at least 90 percent.

Since the two means are included in the ANOVA procedure, the confidence limits for each mean should be obtained with the S.E. $\sqrt{\hat{\sigma}^2/m} = \hat{\sigma}/\sqrt{m}$ with $(n-k)$ d.f.

From the ANOVA table of Example 11.1, $\sqrt{\hat{\sigma}^2/m} = (58.61/10)^{1/2} = 2.42$ with 27 d.f. Since $t_{27,0.025} = 2.052$, 95 percent confidence limits for the mean of the first group are $142.4 - 2.052(2.42) = 137.43$ and $142.4 + 2.052(2.42) = 147.37$. For the mean of the second group, they are $140 - 2.052(2.42) = 135.03$ and $140 + 2.052(2.42) = 144.97$. The 90 percent confidence region of the two means is enclosed by (137.43, 147.37) and (135.03, 144.97).

For the unbalanced classification, confidence limits for the $i$th mean are obtained with the S.E. of $\sqrt{\hat{\sigma}^2/n_i} = \hat{\sigma}/\sqrt{n_i}$ with $(n-k)$ d.f.

## 15.3 Least significant difference (LSD) for a pair of treatment effects

In several medical experiments, the difference between the effects of a treatment and control or a pair of treatments is examined. For the one-way balanced classification in Section 11.2, the estimator of $(\alpha_i - \alpha_j)$ of the $i$th and $j$th treatments is $(\bar{y}_i - \bar{y}_j)$ with variance $2\sigma^2/m$. The sample S.E. for this difference becomes $\hat{\sigma}\sqrt{2/m}$ with $(n-k)$ d.f. In the LSD procedure, $(\alpha_i - \alpha_j)$ for any pair of treatments is considered significant at the $\alpha$ level if $|(\bar{y}_i - \bar{y}_j)|$ exceeds $t_{n-k,\alpha/2}\hat{\sigma}\sqrt{2/m}$.

From the ANOVA table of Example 11.1 for the SBPs before the exercise program, $t_{27,0.025}\hat{\sigma}\sqrt{2/m} = 2.052(3.42) = 7.02$. The sample means for the three groups are (142.4, 140.0, 148.7). The differences between the sample means of treatment pairs (1, 2), (3, 1) and (3, 2) respectively are 2.4, 6.3 and 8.7. As a result, only the difference between the means of the third and second treatments is significant at the 5 percent level.

Snedecor and Cochran (1967, p. 272) mention that for the LSD procedure, the probability of $(\alpha_i - \alpha_j)$ becoming significantly different from zero increases with the number of pairs of treatments, and Fisher (1935) recommended using it only if the $F$-test of the ANOVA procedure shows significant difference among the k treatment effects. Note that the alternative hypothesis for the ANOVA procedure is that at least one of the treatment effects differs from the rest.

## 15.4 Tukey's studentized range test

Consider a random sample $(y_1, y_2, \ldots, y_k)$ from a normal distribution with an unbiased estimator $s^2$ of its variance with $f$ degrees of freedom. The range of the sample observations is $r = (y_{max} - y_{min})$, the difference between the largest and smallest values. When $s^2$ is independent of $y_i$, $i = (1, 2, \ldots, k)$,

$$Q = r/s \tag{15.1}$$

follows the *Studentized Range* distribution. The percentiles $q_{k,f;\alpha}$ of this distribution are tabulated.

For the balanced one-way classification for k means in Section 11.2, the estimate of the variance of the sample mean is $\hat{\sigma}^2/m$ with $(n-k)$ d.f. Tukey's (1949) simultaneous $(1-\alpha)$ percent confidence limits for $(\mu_i - \mu_j)$ are obtained from

$$(\bar{y}_i - \bar{y}_j) \pm \frac{q_{(k,n-k),\alpha}}{\sqrt{2}} \sqrt{\frac{2\hat{\sigma}^2}{m}} \tag{15.2}$$

The probability of coverage of these limits for the differences of all the pairs is at least $(1-\alpha)$.

From the samples of sizes $m = 10$ in Table T11.2 for the SBPs before the exercise program, the means for the three groups are (142.4, 140.0, 148.7). From the ANOVA table of Example 11.1, $v(\bar{y}_i) = (\hat{\sigma}^2/m) = 5.861$ and $S.E.(\bar{y}_i) = 2.42$ with 27 d.f. Since $t_{27, 0.025} = 2.052$, 95 percent confidence limits for $(\mu_i - \mu_j)$ are obtained from $(\bar{y}_i - \bar{y}_j) \pm (2.052)[2(5.861)]^{1/2}$, that is, $(\bar{y}_i - \bar{y}_j) \pm 7.02$. With $q_{(3,27),0.05} = 3.51$, the confidence limits become $(\bar{y}_i - \bar{y}_j) \pm 3.51(5.861)^{1/2}$, that is, $(\bar{y}_i - \bar{y}_j) \pm 8.50$.

For the unbalanced one-way classification in Section 11.6 with the sample sizes $n_i$, $i = (1, 2, ..., k)$, the standard error $\sqrt{2\hat{\sigma}^2/m}$ on the right-hand side of (15.2) is replaced by $\hat{\sigma}(1/n_i + 1/n_j)^{1/2}$. This extension is known as the Tukey-Kramer method.

If there are only $k = 2$ means, the confidence limits for $(\mu_1 - \mu_2)$ are obtained form $(\bar{y}_1 - \bar{y}_2) \pm t_{n-k,\alpha/2}\sqrt{2(\hat{\sigma}^2/m)}$, and by replacing the standard error by $\hat{\sigma}(1/n_i + 1/n_j)^{1/2}$ when the sample sizes are unequal. In both cases, they become the same as the limits obtained from the above limits obtained from the Studentized Range distribution.

## 15.5    Scheffe's simultaneous confidence intervals

The Least Significant Difference and the Studentized Range test are employed for examining the differences between pairs of means or treatments and for finding their confidence limits. In the case of $k \geq 2$ treatments, it is frequently of interest to test the hypotheses of the type $H_0 : \mu_1 = \mu_2$ or $H_0 : \mu_2 = (\mu_1 + \mu_3)/2$. In general, each of these hypotheses can be expressed as $H_0 : L = 0$, where

$$\begin{aligned} L &= C_1\mu_1 + C_2\mu_2 + ... + C_k\mu_k \\ &= C_1\alpha_1 + C_2\alpha_2 + ... + C_k\alpha_k \end{aligned} \tag{15.3}$$

is a linear combination of the treatment means or effects. It is a comparison or a *contrast* if $(C_1 + C_2 + ... + C_k) = 0$. For the first hypothesis above, $C_1 = 1$ and $C_2 = -1$. For the second, $C_1 = 1/2$, $C_2 = -1$ and $C_3 = 1/2$. With sample sizes $n_i$, $i = (1, 2, ..., k)$, for the treatments as in the case of the one-way unbalanced classification, an unbiased estimator of $L$ is given by

$$\hat{L} = C_1\bar{y}_1 + C_2\bar{y}_2 + ... C_k\bar{y}_k \tag{15.4}$$

with variance $V(\hat{L}) = \sigma^2 \sum_1^k (C_i^2/n_i)$. The estimator of variance of $\hat{L}$ and its sample S.E. are $v(\hat{L}) = \hat{\sigma}^2 \sum_1^k (C_i^2/n_i)$ and $S.E.(\hat{L}) = \sqrt{v(\hat{L})}$ with $(n-k)$ d.f. The Least Squares procedure provides unique estimates for the contrasts of the treatment effects.

The hypothesis $H_0 : L = 0$ for any of the contrasts can be tested through the statistic $t_{n-k} = \hat{L}/S.E.(\hat{L})$. Even if the $F$-test of the ANOVA procedure does not reject the hypothesis of the equality of the $k$ means, the $t$-test may lead to rejecting the hypothesis $H_0 : L = 0$ for some of the contrasts. From Scheffe's (1959) procedure, this hypothesis for each of the contrasts of interest is rejected if

$$|\hat{L}|/S.E.(\hat{L}). > \sqrt{(k-1)F_\alpha(k-1, n-k)} \tag{15.5}$$

For any $L$, the Confidence coefficient for the limits obtained from

$$\hat{L} \pm S.E.(\hat{L})\sqrt{(k-1)F_\alpha(k-1, n-k)} \tag{15.6}$$

exceeds $(1-\alpha)$.

*Example 15.2* For the SBPs before the exercise program in Table T11.4, the estimate of the contrast $L = (\mu_1 + \mu_3)/2 - \mu_2$ is $\hat{L} = (132.22 + 148.13)/2 - 142.62 = -2.455$. Since $\hat{\sigma}^2 = 37.5$ from the ANOVA table of Example 11.3, $v(\hat{L}) = [(1/4)(1/9) + (1/4)(1/8) + (1/13)](37.5) = 5.10$ and $S.E.(\hat{L}) = 2.26$. Since $k = 3$ and $(n - k) = 27$, $F_{0.05}(2, 27) = 3.35$, and the right-hand side of (15.5) becomes $\sqrt{2(3.35)} = 2.59$. The left-hand side is $(2.455/2.26) = 1.09$, which is smaller than 2.59. Hence, $H_0 : L = 0$ is not rejected at the 5 percent significance level. The 95 percent confidence limits for $L$ are and $-2.455 - 2.26(2.59) = -8.31$ and $-2.455 + 2.26(2.59) = 3.40$.

## 15.6  Bootstrap confidence intervals

As seen throughout the previous chapters, tests of hypothesis and confidence limits for the mean of a population, differences of the population means, regression coefficients and similar parameters are obtained from their sampling distributions. In some cases, the Central Limit Theorem provides the approximations to such distributions. As in the case of the sample correlation coefficient, suitable transformations are employed for the tests of hypotheses and for finding the confidence limits. In the bootstrap method, standard errors for the estimators and confidence limits for the population parameters are obtained from the empirical distribution of the sample estimator.

Consider a parameter $\theta$ like the population correlation coefficient, median of a population distribution or the ratio of the means of two characteristics, and its estimate $\hat{\theta}$ obtained from a sample of n units. In the bootstrap method, a large number ($B$) of estimates $\hat{\theta}_i$, $i = (1, 2, ..., B)$, are obtained by selecting samples of size $(n - 1)$ randomly with replacement from the original $n$ units. The average of these estimates is

$$\hat{\theta}_B = \sum_{i=1}^{B} \hat{\theta}_i/B, \text{ and } S_B^2 = \sum_{i=1}^{B} (\hat{\theta}_i - \hat{\theta})^2/B \text{ is an estimate of } V(\hat{\theta}).$$

Bootstrap procedures for finding the confidence limits for a parameter were developed, for instance, by Davison and Hinkley (1997) and Efron and Tibishirani (1998). For the *percentile* method, the bootstrap estimates are ranked from the lowest to the highest as $\hat{\theta}_{(1)}, \hat{\theta}_{(2)}, \ldots, \hat{\theta}_{(B)}$. With 2.5 percent of the ranked values below $\hat{\theta}_{(l)}$ and above $\hat{\theta}_{(u)}$, 95 percent confidence limits for $\theta$ are obtained from $\left(\hat{\theta}_{(l)}, \hat{\theta}_{(u)}\right)$. For the *Centered bootstrap* method, the empirical distribution of the bootstrap estimates $\hat{\theta}_i$ is considered. With the percentiles $(B_{0.025}, B_{0.975})$ of this distribution, 95 percent confidence limits for $\theta$ are obtained from $\left(2\hat{\theta} - B_{0.975}, 2\hat{\theta} - B_{0.025}\right)$.

For another method, the distribution of $T_B = \left(\hat{\theta}_B - \hat{\theta}\right)/SE_B$ is considered. In this expression, $SE_B$ is the sample estimate of the standard error of $\hat{\theta}_B$ obtained from the bootstrap sample. Denoting the percentiles of $T_B$ by $b_{0.025}$ and $b_{0.975}$, 95 percent confidence limits for $\theta$ are obtained from $\hat{\theta} - SE_B b_{0.975}$, $\hat{\theta} - SE_B b_{0.025}$.

*Example 15.3*    In this illustration, confidence intervals for the correlation of the heights and weights of boys and of girls obtained from Fisher's transformation and the percentile and Centered bootstrap methods are compared.

(a) From the sample observations in Table T1.3 for the sixteen year old boys, the correlation of the heights and weights is $r = 0.755$. From Fisher's (1915) transformation, $z = (1/2)ln[(1 + 0.755)/(1 - 0.755)] = 0.984$. As described in Section 10.10.3, 95 percent confidence limits for the population correlation become (0.469, 0.897). From the R-program the confidence limits obtained from the percentile and bias adjusted BCa bootstrap methods respectively are presented as (0, 446, 0.933) and (0.367, 0.921).

(b) From the sample observations in Table T1.4 for the sixteen-year-old girls, the correlation of the heights and weights is $r = 0.869$. From Fisher's transformation $z = 1.328$ and the 95 percent confidence limits for the population correlation become (0.693, 0.947). For the bootstrap procedure, the R-program presents the limits for the percentile and BCa method as (0.745, 0.948) and (0.697, 0.934) respectively.

## 15.7    Transformations for the ANOVA

As seen throughout Chapter 11, for the ANOVA of one-way, two-way and other classifications, the variance of the observation $y_{ij}$ is assumed to be the same in all the cells. If the observation in each cell is the estimate $\hat{p}_{ij}$ of the proportion $p_{ij}$ of successes in n trials, its variance becomes $p_{ij}(1 - p_{ij})/n$, different for the cells. If the observation in the cell follows the Poisson distribution, its variance becomes the same as the mean. Similarly, in some experiments, the variance of the observation can be proportional to the square of its mean. The transformations for these three cases obtained from Taylor's approximation are presented in Appendix A15.

For the binomial proportion, the transformed variable is obtained from the *arcsin* or *angular* transformation $f\left(\hat{p}_{ij}\right) = sin^{-1}\left(\hat{p}_{ij}\right)$. For the Poisson random variable $X$ with mean $\lambda$, the transformed variable is given by the *square root* transformation $f(X) = \sqrt{X}$. For the random variable $X$ with mean $\mu$ and variance $\mu^2$, the transformed variable is given by the ***log*** transformation $f(X) = \log(X)$.

# Exercises

**15.1.** From the sample observations in Table 11.4 and Example 11.3, find the ninety percent confidence region for the means of first two groups for the SBPs after the exercise program

**15.2.** For the SBPs before the exercise program with the unbalanced data in Table T11.4, consider the contrast corresponding to $H_0 : \mu_2 = \mu_3$. (a) Test for its significance through Scheffe's procedure and the t-test. (b) Compare the 95 percent confidence limits for $(\mu_2 - \mu_3)$ through both the procedures.

**15.3.** Percentages of total fatty acids of foods of five types prepared with partially hydrogenated vegetable oils obtained from the figures presented by Mozaffarian et al. (2006) were presented in Exercise 11.17. Two of the foods in the fifth type with extremely low percentages were ignored. Find 95 percent confidence limits for the difference of (a) the first and fifth and (b) fourth and fifth types of food through the Student's $t$-distribution and the Studentized range distribution.

# Appendix A15

## A15.1   Variance stabilizing transformation

Consider a random variable with expectation $\mu$ and variance $\sigma^2$. For a function $f(X)$ of this random variable, from Taylor's series,

$$f(X) = f(\mu) + (X - \mu)f'(\mu)...,$$

where $f'(\mu)$ is the first derivative of $f(X)$ at $\mu$. Higher order terms are ignored for this expansion of $f(X)$. From this expression, $E[f(X)] = f(\mu)$ and $V[f(X)] = \sigma^2[f'(\mu)]^2$. For this variance to be a constant $C^2$, $f'(\mu) = C/\sigma$. From integrating this derivative, $f(\mu)$ and hence $f(X)$ are obtained.

If $X$ is the proportion $\hat{p}$ of the successes in $n$ trials, $E(X) = p$ and $\sigma = \sqrt{p(1-p)/n}$. If each cell of an ANOVA classification contains $\hat{p}$ from the same number of trials, the transformed variable is obtained from the *arcsin* or *angular* transformation $f(\hat{p}) = sin^{-1}\sqrt{\hat{p}}.$; the variance of this transformed variable becomes $C^2 = 1/4n$. If $\sigma = \sqrt{\mu}$ as in the case of the Poisson variable, $f(X)$ is obtained from $\sqrt{X}$, with the variance $C^2 = 1/4$. If $\sigma$ is proportional to $\mu$, $f(X)$ is obtained from $\log(X)$.

# Solutions to exercises

## Chapter 1

**1.1.**

|  | | Boys | | | Girls | |
|---|---|---|---|---|---|---|
|  | Height | Weight | BMI | Height | Weight | BMI |
| Mean | 142.25 | 34.6 | 17.14 | 136.8 | 33.6 | 17.89 |
| S.d. | 5.12 | 3.0 | 1.76 | 6.78 | 4.94 | 1.69 |
| $m_3$ | −21.73 | 13.81 | 0.35 | −41.2 | 11.53 | −1.67 |
| $m_4$ | 2115.15 | 171.98 | 15.95 | 3518.66 | 990.91 | 20.62 |
| $K_1$ | 0.026 | 0.260 | 0.004 | 0.018 | 0.009 | 0.06 |
| $K_2$ | 3.08 | 2.12 | 1.66 | 1.67 | 1.66 | 2.59 |

**1.2.** (a)

|  | | Boys | | | Girls | |
|---|---|---|---|---|---|---|
|  | Height | Weight | BMI | Height | Weight | BMI |
| Mean | 171.1 | 62.8 | 21.37 | 163.35 | 61.1 | 22.61 |
| S.D. | 7.67 | 9.34 | 2.09 | 6.91 | 12.04 | 2.90 |

(b) Boys: For classes (155–160), ..., (180–185) and mid-values (157.5, 162.5, ..., 182.5) for the heights, the frequencies are (1, 3, 6, 4, 3, 3). Now the mean and S.D. of the heights are 171 and 7.27.

Girls: For classes (150–155),...., (170–175) and mid-values (152.5, 157.5, ..., 172.5) for the heights, the frequencies are (3, 4, 5, 4, 4). The mean and S.D. are 163 and 6.86.

*Statistical Methodologies with Medical Applications*, First Edition. Poduri S.R.S. Rao.
© 2017 John Wiley & Sons, Ltd. Published 2017 by John Wiley & Sons, Ltd.

There is very little change in the means and standard deviations as a result of grouping.

**1.3.**

$$\bar{x} = 154, s_x^2 = 65.33 \text{ and } s_x = 8.08.$$

$$\bar{y} = 142, s_y^2 = 96.48 \text{ and } s_y = 9.82.$$

$$s_{xy} = 4.02 \text{ and } r = 0.05.$$

**1.4.**

$$\bar{x} = 3.09, s_x^2 = 2.17 \text{ and } s_x = 1.47.$$

$$\bar{y} = 1.43, s_y^2 = 0.92 \text{ and } s_y = 0.96.$$

$$s_{xy} = 0.9936 \text{ and } r = 0.70.$$

**1.5.**

|  | Mean, S.D. | | |
|---|---|---|---|
|  | Age | Income | Household size |
| Insured | 40.44, 12.53 | 52.13, 26.42 | 3.05, 1.28 |
| Uninsured | 36.25, 12.29 | 29.35, 19.16 | 3.26, 1.34 |

Age. Mid-values: (23.5, 34.5, 44.5, 57). For the uninsured, percentage for the last class is changed to 17 from 18.

Income. Mid-values: (12.5, 20, 30, 42.5, 62.5, 87.5)

**1.6.**

|  | Measles | DTP 3 | Hep B3 |
|---|---|---|---|
| Mean | 82.92 | 83.91 | 84.65 |
| S.D. | 15.98 | 15.29 | 14.36 |

**1.7.** To convert $x_i$ in kg to $y_i$ in lbs, $y_i = 2.2046 \ x_i$. Now, $\bar{y} = 2.2046 \bar{x}$, $s_y^2 = (2.2046)^2 s_x^2$ and $s_y = (2.2046) s_x$. From the summary figures in Table 1.2, average weight becomes $(2.2046)(73.1) = 161.16 \text{ lbs}$, with variance $(2.2046)^2 (188.09) = 914.17$ and standard deviation $(2.2046)(13.71) = 30.23 \text{ lbs}$.

**1.8.** (a) The mean, variance and standard deviation of $u_i$ are $(-3.5, 14.38, 3.79)$. (b) For $v_i$, they are $(11.33, 21.39, 4.62)$.

**1.9.** The covariance of $(u_i, v_i)$ is $s_{uv} = (1/6)s_x^2 + (1/3)s_y^2 + (1/2)s_{xy} = 17.29$. The correlation of $(u_i, v_i)$ becomes $r_{uv} = (17.29)/(3.79 \times 4.62) = 0.987$.

# Chapter 2

**2.1.** Received and not received the vaccination: $(V_1, V_2)$. Affected and not affected by the flu: $(F_1, F_2)$.

| Prior Probability | Conditional Probability | Joint Probability |
|---|---|---|
| $P(V_1) = 0.80$ | $P(F_1|V_1) = 0.10$ | $P(V_1F_1) = 0.08$ |
| | $P(F_2|V_1) = 0.90$ | $P(V_1F_2) = 0.72$ |
| $P(V_2) = 0.20$ | $P(F_1|V_2) = 0.60$ | $P(V_2F_1) = 0.12$ |
| | $P(F_2|V_2) = 0.40$ | $P(V_2F_2) = 0.08$ |

$$P(F_1) = 0.08 + 0.12 = 0.20 \text{ and } P(F_2) = 0.72 + 0.08 = 0.80.$$
$$P(V_1|F_1) = P(V_1F_1)/P(F_1) = (0.08/0.20) = 2/5 \text{ or } 40 \text{ percent.}$$
$$P(V_2|F_1) = P(V_2F_1)/P(F_1) = (0.12/.20) = 3/5 \text{ or } 60 \text{ percent.}$$

Of those who were affected by Flu, 40 percent received the vaccination but 60 percent did not.

$$P(V_1|F_2) = P(V_1F_2)/P(F_2) = (0.72/0.80) = 0.90 \text{ or } 90 \text{ percent.}$$

$$P(V_2|F_2) = P(V_2F_2)/P(F_2) = (0.08/0.80) = 0.10 \text{ or } 10 \text{ percent.}$$

Of those not affected by flu, 90 percent received the vaccination and 10 percent did not.

**2.2.** (a) P(Overweight or low HDL) $= 0.60 + 0.50 - (0.60)(0.50) = 0.80$ or 80 percent.

(b) P(Overweight or low HDL) $= 0.60 + 0.50 - (0.40)(0.60) = 0.86$ or 80 percent.

**2.3.** (a) $P(AB) = (0.306)(0.274) = 0.084$ or 8.4 percent.

(b) $P(A \text{ or } B) = 0.306 + 0.274 - 0.084 = 0.496$ or 49.6 percent, that is, nearly 50 percent of the adults.

(c) P(An adult is nonhypertensive) $= 1 - 0.306 = 0.694$, and P(both the adults are nonhypertensive) $= (0.694)^2 = 0.482$. Hence P(at least one adult is hypertensive) $= 1 - 0.482 = 0.518$ or 51.8 percent.

(d) P(cholesterol of an adult is less than 240 mg/dL) $= 1 - 0.274 = 0.726$, and P(cholesterol of both the adults is less than 240 mg/dL) $= (0.726)^2 = 0.527$. Hence P(cholesterol of at least one of the adults is 240 mg/dL or higher) $= 1 - 0.527 = 0.473$ or 47.3 percent.

# Chapter 3

**3.1.** (1) The odds that a high LDL person is on a high-fat diet versus he is on a low-fat diet are $(a/c) = (150/70) = (15/7)$.

(2) The odds that a person with the normal LDL is on the high-fat versus the low-fat diet is $(b/d) = (100/80) = (5/4)$.

(3) Odds ratio for the high versus low LDL is $(ad/bc) = (12/7) = 1.71$.

**3.2.** (1) Risk of high LDL from the high-fat diet is $a/(a+b) = (150/250) = (9/15)$.

(2) Risk of high LDL from the low-fat diet is $c/(c + d) = (70/150) = (7/15)$.

(3) Risk of high LDL from the high-fat diet relative to the low-fat diet is $(9/15)/(7/15) = (9/7) = 1.29$.

**3.3.** (1) Sensitivity $= a/(a + c) = (30/70) = (3/7)$.

(2) Specificity $= d/(b + d) = (60/80) = (3/4)$.

**3.4.** (a) Sensitivity $= (10 + 12)/30 = 0.73$ and specificity $= (25/120) = 0.21$.

(b) Sensitivity $= (12/30) = 0.40$ and Specificity $= (25 + 15)/120 = 0.33$.

# Chapter 4

**4.1.** (a) 0.1859, (b) 0.2173, (c) 0.0093, and (d) 0.7765.

**4.2.** (a) 0.1815, (b) 0.2146, (c) 0.0089, and (d) 0.5697.

**4.3.** (a) Denote the probabilities by $(p_1, p_2, p_3)$ and the observed numbers by $(X_1, X_2, X_3)$. Note that $q_1 = 1 - p_1$, $q_2 = 1 - p_2$ and $q_3 = 1 - p_3$.

(a) $E(X_1 - X_2) = E(X_1) - E(X_2) = np_1 - np_2 = 100\,(0.5 - 0.4) = 10$.

$V(X_1 - X_2) = V(X_1) + V(X_2) - 2\,\text{Cov}\,(X_1, X_2) = n\,(p_1q_1 + p_2q_2 + 2p_1p_2) = 100$ $(0.89) = 89$, and the S.D. of $(X_1 - X_2)$ becomes 9.43.

(b) $E[(X_1 - X_2) - (X_2 - X_3)] = E(X_1 - 2X_2 + X_3) = E(X_1) - 2E(X_2) + E(X_3) = n(p_1 - 2p_2 + p_3) = 100[0.5 - 2(0.4) + 0.1] = -20$.

$V(X_1 - 2X_2 + X_3) = n(\ p_1q_1 + 4p_2q_2 + p_3q_3 + 4p_1p_2 - 2p_1p_3 + 4p_2p_3) = 216$, and the s.d of $(X_1 - 2X_2 + X_3)$ becomes 14.70.

**4.4.** (a) $P(X = 5 ; \lambda = 10) = 0.0378$. (b) $P(X \le 5; \lambda = 10) = 0.0671$, and (c) $P(5 \le X \le 10; \lambda = 10) = 0.5538$.

**4.5.** (a) $P[F(6,12 > 3.22] = 0.0402$.

(b) Since $P(F_{12,6} > 4) = 0.05$, $P(F_{6,12} < 0.25) = 0.05$.

# Chapter 5

**5.1.** The standard error for each sample mean are obtained from $s = \sqrt{20}$, and $t_{19, 0.025} = 2.093$. Confidence limits obtained from (5.13) are as follows:

|  | Height | Weight | BMI |
| --- | --- | --- | --- |
| Boys | 139.85, 144.65 | 33.2, 36.0 | 16.32, 17.96 |
| Girls | 133.63, 139.97 | 31.29, 35.91 | 17.10, 18.68 |

**5.2.** The pooled estimate of the variance is found from (5.16), and $t_{38,\,0.025} = 2.02$. Confidence limits for the difference of the population means of boys and girls are as follows:

| Height | Weight | BMI |
|---|---|---|
| 1.61, 9.29 | −1.61, 3.61 | −1.86, 0.36 |

**5.3.** (1) When $(1-\alpha)=0.95$, lower and upper percentiles of the F-distribution with (10, 45) d.f. are (0.31, 2.35). Ratio of the sample variances of Asia and Africa is $(26.25/19.05)^2 = 1.90$. From (5.30), $C_l = (1.9/2.35) = 0.81$ and $C_u = (1.9/0.31) = 6.13$.

(2) For Southeast Asia and Europe, the lower and upper percentiles of the F-distribution with (26, 52) d.f. are (0.49, 1.90). With the ratio of the sample variances $(24.12/6.38)^2 = 14.29$, $C_l = (14.29/1.9) = 7.52$ and $C_u = (14.29/0.49) = 29.16$.

**5.4.** (1) Ratio of the sample variances is $(4.22/2.2)^2 = 3.68$. From (5.30), 95 percent confidence limits are $C_l = (3.68/2.35) = 1.57$ and $C_u = (3.68/0.31) = 11.87$.

(2) Ratio of the sample variances is $(3.72/1.85)^2 = 4.04$. The confidence limits are $Cl = (4.04/1.9) = 2.13$ and $C_u = (4.04/0.49) = 8.24$.

**5.5.** Assuming that the variances of the private expenditures for these two countries are the same, from (5.16), the pooled estimate of the variance is $s_p^2 = \left[10(26.25)^2 + 45(19.05)^2\right]/55 = 422.20$. As a result, $v(d) = 422.2(57/506) = 47.56$ and $S.E.(d) = 6.9$. With $d = (47.48 - 45.93) = 1.55$ and $t_{55,\,0.025} = 2.0$, 95 percent confidence limits for the difference are $[1.55 - 2(6.9)] = -12.25$ and $[1.55 + 2(6.9)] = 15.35$.

**5.6.** Without assuming that the population variances are the same, $v(d) = (4.22^2/11 + 2.2^2/46) = 1.72$ and $S.E.(d) = 1.31$. Since $d = (5.49 - 5.27) = 0.22$, approximate 95 percent confidence limits for the difference are $0.22 - 1.96(1.31) = -2.35$ and $0.22 + 1.96(1.31) = 2.79$.

**5.7.** (a) The sample estimates of the difference of the means, variance of the difference and standard error of the difference are $d = (0.81 - 0.36) = 0.45$, $v(d) = [(0.50)^2/60 + (0.33)^2/10] = 0.0151$ and $S.E.(d) = 0.1227$. Ninety-five percent confidence limits for the difference of the means are $[0.45 - 1.96(0.1227)] = 0.21$ and $[0.45 + 1.96(0.1227)] = 0.69$.

(b) Ratio of the sample variances is $(0.50)^2/(0.33)^2 = 2.30$. For $(1-\alpha) = 0.95$, percentiles of the F-distribution with (59, 9) d.f are (0.428, 3.451). From (5.30), confidence limits for the ratio of the population variances become $(2.3/3.451) = 0.67$ and $(2.3/0.428) = 5.37$.

**5.8.** For the confidence probability $(1-\alpha) = 0.95$, the percentiles of the F-distribution with $(22, 14)$ d.f are $(0.40, 2.81)$. We find the following confidence limits for the ratios of the population variances of the second and first groups. FIM change: $(0.59, 4.18)$. LOS : $(0.16, 1.125)$. ER : $(1.04, 7.3)$.

**5.9.** (a) With the S.E. of $(27.8/\sqrt{45}) = 4.14$, 95 percent confidence limits for the mean of the treated group are $[109.8 - 1.96(4.14)] = 101.69$ and $[109.8 + 1.96(4.14)] = 117.91$.

(b) The variance of the difference of the two sample means is $(46.4^2/60 + 27.8^2/45) = 53.06$ and the S.E. of the difference becomes 7.28. Confidence limits for the difference of the means of the untreated and treated groups are $[119.3 - 1.96(7.28)] = 105.03$ and $[119.3 + 1.96(7.28)] = 133.57$.

# Chapter 6

**6.1.** For the first group, $n_1 = 93$, $\hat{p} = 0.96$ and $S.E.(\hat{p}_1) = [(0.96)(.0.04)/93]^{1/2} = 0.0203$. Ninety-five percent confidence limits for the proportion are $[0.96 - 1.96(0.0203)] = 0.92$ and $[0.96 + 1.96(0.0203)] = 0.9998$; that is, 92 and 100 percent. For the second group, $n_2 = 100$, $\hat{p}_2 = 0.80$ and $S.E.(\hat{p}_2) = [(0.8)(0.2)/100]^{1/2} = 0.04$. Ninety-five percent confidence limits for the proportion are $[0.8 - 1.96(0.04)] = 0.7216$ and $[0.8 + 1.96(0.04)] = 0.8784$, that is 72.16 and 87.84 percent.

The difference of the proportion is $d = (0.96 - 0.80) = 0.16$ with the variance of $[0.96(0.04)/93 + 0.8(0.2)/100] = 0.002$ and S.E. of 0.0447. Ninety-five percent confidence limits for the difference are $[0.16 - 1.96 (0.0447)] = 0.0724$ and $[0.16 + 1.96(0.0447)] = 0.2476$, that is, 7.24 and 24.76 percent.

**6.2.** $\hat{p} = (100/500) = 0.20$ and $S.E.(\hat{p}) = [0.2(0.8)/500]^{1/2} = 0.0179$. Ninety-five percent confidence limits for the combined proportion are $[0.20 - 1.96(0.0179)] = 0.165$ and $[0.20 + 1.96(0.0179)] = 0.235$. They are 16.5 and 23.5 percent for the combined percentage.

**6.3.** (a) Difference of the estimate of the percentage of the second group from the first is $d = (0.50 - 0.15) = 0.35$, with variance $v(d) = [(0.5)(0.5) + (0.15)(0.85) + 2(0.5)(0.15)]/200 = 0.006138$ and $S.E.(d) = 0.0783$. Ninety-five percent confidence limits for the difference of the percentages are $[0.35 - 1.96(0.0783)] = 0.1965$ and $[0.35 + 1.96(0.0783)] = 0.5035$, that is, $(20 - 50)$ percent.

(b) Difference of the estimate of the percentage of the second group from the third is $d = (0.50 - 0.35) = 0.15$, with variance $v(d) = [(0.5)(0.5) + (0.35)(0.65) + 2(0.5)(0.35)]/200 = 0.00414$ and $S.E.(d) = 0.064$. Ninety-five percent confidence limits for the difference of the percentages are $[0.15 - 1.96(0.064)] = 0.025$ and $[0.15 + 1.96(0.064)] = 0.275$;, that is, $(2.5 - 27.5)$ percent.

**6.4.** Since the total percentage of the adults is $(35 + 35 + 15) = 85$, the estimates of observed sample sizes for the three groups can be considered to be $n_1 = 200$ $(35/85) = 82$, $n_2 = 200(35/85) = 82$ and $n_3 = 200(15/85) = 36$ approximately.

(a) Overall : $\hat{p} = [82(0.15) + 82(0.25) + 36(0.50)]/200 = 0.254$, $v(\hat{p}) = (0.254)$ $(0.746)/200 = 0.00095$ and $S.E.(\hat{p}) = 0.0308$. Ninety-five percent confidence limits for the overall proportion are $[0.254 - 1.96(0.0308)] = 0.1936$ and $[0.254 + 1.96(0.0308)] = 0.3144$. Twenty-five percent of the adults have low LDL with the confidence limits of $(19.36, 31.44)$ percent.

(b) Estimate for the difference of the proportions of the first two groups is $(0.25 - 0.15) = 0.10$ with the sample variance $[(0.25)(0.75)/82 + (0.15)(0.85)/82] = (0.315/82) = 0.0038$ and S.E. of $0.062$. Ninety-five percent confidence limits for the difference of the proportions are $[0.10 - 1.96(0.062)] = -0.0215$ and $[0.10 + 1.96(0.062)] = 0.2215$. The estimate of the difference is 10 percent with the confidence interval ranging from negative 2 percent to 22.15 percent.

(c) Estimate of the difference is $(0.50 - 0.40) = 0.10$ with the sample variance $[(0.5)(0.5)/36 + (0.4)(0.6)/164] = 0.0084$ and S.E. of $0.09165$. Ninety-five percent confidence limits for the difference are $[0.10 - 1.96 (0.09165)] = -0.08$ and $[0.10 + 1.96(0.09165)] = 0.28$. The estimate of the difference is 10 percent with the confidence interval ranging from negative 8 percent to 28 percent.

**6.5.** (a) $ln\left(\widehat{OR}\right) = ln\ (9) = 2.1972$, $v\left[ln\left(\widehat{OR}\right)\right] = (1/45 + 1/15 + 1/35 + 1/105) = 0.127$ and S.E. $\left[ln\left(\widehat{OR}\right)\right] = 0.3564$. Ninety-five percent confidence limits for $ln$ (OR) are $[2.1972 - 1.96(0.3564)] = 1.4989$ and $[2.1972 + 1.96(0.3564)] = 2.8957$. Ninety-five percent confidence limits for OR are $(4.48, 18.10)$.

(b) $ln\left(\widehat{RR}\right) = ln(3) = 1.0986$, $v\left[ln\left(\widehat{RR}\right)\right] = [(1/4)/60(3/4) + (3/4)/140(1/4)] = 0.027$ and S.E. $\left[ln\left(\widehat{RR}\right)\right] = 0.1643$. Ninety-five percent confidence limits for $ln$ (RR) are $[1.0986 - 1.96(0.1643)] = 0.7766$ and $[1.0986 + 1.96(0.1643)] = 1.4206$. Ninety-five percent confidence limits for RR are $(2.17, 4.14)$.

# Chapter 7

**7.1.** The hypotheses are $H_0 : \mu = 100$ and $H_1 : \mu \geq 100$. With the known value of 25 for the standard deviation, $S.E.(\bar{X}) = 25/5$ and $z = (108 - 100)/5 = 1.6$. Since it does not exceed $z_{0.05} = 1.645$, the null hypothesis is not rejected at the 5 percent level of significance. The $p$ – value becomes $P(Z > 1.6) = 0.055$.

(a) At the significance level of 5 percent, the power of the test at the alternative value of 110 becomes $P[Z > (100 - 110)/5 + 1.645] = P[Z > -0.355] = 0.74$.

(b) For the power of 95 percent at the value of 110 for the alternative value of the mean, $[(100 - 110)/(5/\sqrt{n}) + 1.645] = -1.645$ from (7.6), and $n \geq 68$ from (7.7).

(c) With estimate of 30 for the standard deviation, $S.E.(\bar{X}) = 30/5 = 6$ and $t = (8/6) = 1.33$. Since it does not exceed $t_{24, 0.05} = 2.06$, the null hypothesis is not rejected at the 5 percent level of significance. The $p$-value becomes, $P(t_{24} > 1.33) = 0.098$.

**7.2.** $H_0 : \mu = 45$ and $H_1 : \mu \leq 45$.

(a) With the known standard deviation, $S.E.(\bar{X}) = 25/5 = 5$, and $z = [(35 - 45)/5] = -2$. Since it is smaller than $-z_{0.05} = -1.645$, reject the null hypothesis at the 5 percent level of significance. The $p$-value is $P(Z < -2) = 0.023$, which is small suggesting the rejection of the null hypothesis.

(b) Power of the test at the alternative value of 35 for the mean becomes 0.639.

(c) For the power of 95 percent at the alternative value of 35 for the mean, the required sample size is n = 68.

(d) With the estimate of 30 for the standard deviation, $S.E.(\bar{X}) = 30/5 = 6$ and $t = [(35 - 45)/6] = -1.67$. Since this value is larger than $-t_{24, .05} = -2.06$, the null hypothesis is not rejected at the 5 percent level of significance. The $p$-value becomes $P(t_{24} < -1.67) = 0.054$, suggesting that a level of significance of at least 5.4 percent is needed to reject the null hypothesis.

**7.3.** The null and alternative hypotheses are $H_0 : \mu = 100$ and $H_1 : \mu \neq 100$.

(a) With the known standard deviation, $S.E.(\bar{X}) = 35/5 = 7$ and $z = (110 - 100)/7 = 1.43$. Since it does not exceed $z_{0.025} = 1.96$, the null hypothesis is not rejected at the 5 percent significance level. Since $P(Z > 1.43) = 0.076$, the $p$-value becomes $2(0.076) = 0.152$, which is large and suggests not rejecting the null hypothesis.

(b) The power at the alternative value of 105 for the mean is given by $P[Z > [(100 - 105)/7 + 1.96] = P(Z > 1.25) = 0.106$ or close to 11 percent.

(c) For the power of 20 percent at the alternative value of 105 for the mean, the required sample size becomes $n = 61$.

(d) With the estimated standard deviation, $S.E.(\bar{X}) = 40/5 = 8$ and $t = (110 - 100)/8 = 1.25$. Since it does not exceed $t_{24, 0.025} = 2.39$, the null hypothesis is not rejected at the 5 percent significance level. The $p$-value for the test becomes 0.223.

**7.4.** Following Section 7.4.2, the pooled estimates of the variances, S.E.s of the differences of the means for the two groups, and the t-statistics with 403 d.f for the difference of the means of High fat – high protein and low fat – average protein diets, and the one-sided $p$-values are as follows:

|  | Pooled variance | S.E. | $t_{403}$ | $p$-value |
| --- | --- | --- | --- | --- |
| Total cholesterol | 773.47 | 2.76 | 3.62 | 0.0002 |
| SBP | 169.81 | 1.295 | 2.32 | 0.0224 |
| DBP | 81.00 | 0.8944 | 2.24 | 0.0250 |

These results suggest that the Low fat-low protein diet is preferable to the High fat-high protein diet for reducing the risk factors associated with high levels of total cholesterol, SBP and DBP.

**7.5.** Following Section 5.4, the pooled sample variances $s^2$, S.E. for the difference of the sample means and the $t$-statistics are as follows:

|        | Pooled $s^2$ | S.E.(diff.) | $t_{38}$ |
|--------|--------------|-------------|----------|
| Height | 53.29        | 2.31        | 3.35     |
| Weight | 116.1        | 3.41        | 0.50     |
| BMI    | 6.39         | 0.80        | −1.55    |

The $p$-values for the differences of the means of the weights as well as the BMIs are very large, suggesting that the population means of these characteristics of the boys and girls do not differ significantly. However, the $p$-value for the difference of the means of the heights is very small indicating that the population mean of the heights of the boys is significantly larger than that of the girls.

**7.6.** From (7.20), $u = 15(5.6)^2/(5.2)^2 = 17.4$, which does not exceed $\chi^2_{15,0.05} = 25.0$. The null hypothesis is not rejected at the 5 percent significance level. The $p$-value becomes $P(\chi^2_{15} > 17.4) = 0.30$

**7.7.** (a) $s_p^2 = 45.44$, $\ln s_p^2 = 3.82$, $\ln \Sigma s_i^2 = 11.278$. From (7.25), $u = 3.38$ which is smaller than $\chi^2_{2,0.05} = 5.99$. The null hypothesis of the equality of the three population variances of the heights is not rejected at the 5 percent level of significance. The $p$-value is 0.185.

(b) $s_p^2 = 4.67$, $\ln s_p^2 = 1.541$, $\ln \Sigma s_i^2 = 4.485$. From (7.25), $u = 2.56$ which is smaller than $\chi^2_{2,.0.05} = 5.99$. The null hypothesis of the equality of the three population variances of the BMIs is not rejected at the 5 percent level of significance. The $p$-value is 0.28.

**7.8.** The variance of the sample mean and S.E. are $(27.8^2/45) = 17.17$ and 4.14. Since $Z = [(109.8 - 94.7)/4.14] = 3.65$ with the $p$-value of 0.0001, the null hypothesis can be rejected.

# Chapter 8

**8.1.** From the binomial distribution with $p = 0.3$ and $n = 30$, $P(X \geq 15) = 0.017$ which is smaller than 5 percent. For the normal approximation, $\mu = 30(0.3) = 9$, $\sigma = [30(0.3)(0.7)]^{1/2} = 2.51$ and $z = [(14.5 - 9)/2.51] = 2.19$, which exceeds $z_{0.05} = 1.645$. The null hypothesis is rejected at the 5 percent significance level.

(a) The p-value of the test statistic becomes $P(Z > 2.19) = 0.0143$, which is small.

(b) From (8.5), the required power at $p = 0.5$ becomes, $P(Z > -0.6832) = 0.753$.

(c) When $(1 - \beta) = 0.80$, $z_{0.80} = -0.85$. From (8.7), the required sample size becomes

$$n \geq \left[ -0.85(0.5) - 1.645(0.21)^{1/2} \right]^2 / (0.3 - 0.5)^2 = 35 \text{ approximately.}$$

**8.2.** (a) $P(X \leq 7 \mid n = 20, p = 0.6) = 0.021$, and for the normal approximation, the p-value was 0.0202. (b) $P(X \leq 8 \mid n = 20, p = 0.4) = 0.596$, and from the normal approximation, the power at $p = 0.4$ was 0.571.

**8.3.** (a) The critical values are $X \geq 15$ and $X \leq 5$ since the probability for these events together is $2(0.021) = 0.042$, which is less than 5 percent.

(b) Since $P(X \geq 14 \mid n = 20, p = 0.5) = 0.058$, the p-value becomes $2(0.058) = 0.116$. With the normal approximation, the p-value becomes 0.1164.

(c) The power at $p_1 = 0.8$ is given by the probability of $(X \geq 15)$ or $(X \leq 5)$ of the binomial distribution with $n = 20$ trials and probability of success $p_1 = 0.8$. The probability for $(X \leq 5)$ is very small, and the power becomes 0.804. It was 0.8159 for the normal approximation with the 5 percent significance level.

**8.4.** The estimate of the difference of the proportions is $(\hat{p}_1 - \hat{p}_2) = (0.4 - 0.3) = 0.1$. Under $H_0$, estimate of the common proportion is $\hat{p} = (120 + 600)/500 = 0.36$. Now, the estimates of the variance and S.E. of $(\hat{p}_1 - \hat{p}_2)$ are $(0.36)(0.64)$ $(1/300 + 1/200) = 0.00192$ and 0.0438. Since $z = [(0.4 - 0.3) - 0]/0.0438 = 2.28$ exceeds $z_{0.05} = 1.645$, the null hypothesis of the equality of the proportions is rejected at the 5 percent significance level. The p-value of the test statistic becomes $P(Z > 2.28) = 0.0113$.

**8.5.** The estimates of the proportions $p_1$ and $p_2$ for the first two ranges are $\hat{p}_1 = 250/500 = 0.5$ and $\hat{p}_2 = 150/500 = 0.3$. The estimate of the variance of $(\hat{p}_1 - \hat{p}_2)$ is $[(0.5)(0.5) + (0.3)(0.7) + 2(0.5)(0.3)]/500 = 0.00152$ and the estimate of the S.E. of $(\hat{p}_1 - \hat{p}_2)$ becomes 0.039. The test statistic for $H_0 : (p_1 - p_2) = 0$ becomes $z = [(0.5 - 0.3) - 0]/0.039 = 5.13$. The difference between the percentages for the first two ranges of the SBP is highly significant.

**8.6.** (a) Estimates of the proportions of the males and females controlled are $\hat{p}_1 = (156/224) = 0.696$ and $\hat{p}_2 = (174/219) = 0.795$. Under the null hypothesis of equality of the proportions, the estimate of the common proportion is $\hat{p}_1 = (330/443) = 0.745$. The estimate of $V(\hat{p}_1 - \hat{p}_2)$ becomes $\hat{p}\hat{q}(1/n_1 + 1/n_2) = 0.0017$. Now, $S.E.(\hat{p}_1 - \hat{p}_2) = 0.0412$ and $z = (0.795 - 0.696)/0.0412 = 2.40$, which exceeds $z_{0.025} = 1.96$. The difference between the proportions controlled is different at the 5 percent level of significance.

With the continuity correction, $\hat{p}_1 = 156.5/224 = 0.6987$, $\hat{p}_2 = 173.5/219 = 0.7922$, and $z = (0.7922 - 0.6987)/0.0412 = 2.27$.

(b) The estimates of the proportions of the controlled for the persons 65 years and under 65 years are $\hat{p}_1 = (104/151) = 0.689$ and $\hat{p}_2 = (226/292) = 0.774$. Under the null hypothesis of equality of the proportions, the estimate of the common proportion becomes $\hat{p} = (104 + 226) / 443 = 0.745$. The estimate of $V(\hat{p}_1 - \hat{p}_2)$ is $\hat{p}\hat{q}$ $(1/n_1 + 1/n_2) = 0.0019$. Now, $S.E.(\hat{p}_1 - \hat{p}_2) = 0.0436$ and $z = 0.085/0.0436 = 1.95$. The difference of the proportions of the two age groups controlled is significant just about the 5 percent level.

With the continuity correction, $\hat{p}_1 = 104.5/151 = 0.6921$, $\hat{p}_2 = 225.5/292 = 0.7723$, and $z = (0.7723 - 0.6921)/0.0436 = 1.84$.

(c) The estimates of the proportions of the diabetic (1) and non-diabetic (2) patients controlled are $\hat{p}_1 = (65/138) = 0.471$ and $\hat{p}_2 = (265/305) = 0.8689$. Under the null hypothesis of equality of the proportions, the estimate of the common pro-portion becomes $\hat{p} = (65 + 265)/443 = 0.7449$. The estimate of $V(\hat{p}_1 - \hat{p}_2)$ is $\hat{p}\hat{q}(1/n_1 + 1/n_2) = 0.002$. Now, $S.E.$ $(\hat{p}_1 - \hat{p}_2) = 0.0447$ and $z = 0.3979/0.0447 = 8.90$. The difference of the proportions of the two groups controlled is highly significant.

With the continuity correction, $\hat{p}_1 = 65.5/138 = 0.4746$, $\hat{p}_2 = 264.5/305 = 0.8672$, and $z = (0.8672 - 0.4746) / 0.0447 = 8.78$.

**8.7.** $\hat{p} = [30(0.4) + 30(0.7) + 40(0.7)]/100 = 0.61$, $\hat{p}\hat{q} = 0.2379$ and $\sum n_i$ $(\hat{p}_i - \hat{p})^2 = 1.89$. From (8.39), $U = (1.89/0.2379) = 7.9445$ which exceeds $\chi^2_{2,0.05} = 5.99$. The hypothesis that the percentage of effectiveness is the same for the three age groups is rejected at the 5 percent significance level; the p-value is 0.0188.

**8.8.** From (8.40), $z = \{[|0.61 - 0.5| - 0.005]/0.05\} = 2.1$, which exceeds $z_{0.05} = 1.96$. Equivalently, $U = 4.41$ exceeds $\chi^2_{1,0.05} = 3.84$. The hypothesis that the treatment is effective for 50 percent of each of the groups is rejected at the 5 percent significance level.

# Chapter 9

**9.1.** The expected numbers are (40, 30, 20, 10, 10, 20, 30, 40). From (9.1a), $U = 6.0375$ from, which is smaller than $\chi^2_7(0.05) = 14.067$. Do not reject the hypothesis that the observed numbers support the hypothesized expected numbers.

**9.2.** (a) From (9.1a), $U = \left(5.5^2/54 + 7.5^2/42 + 13.5^2/104\right) = 3.65$, which does not exceed $\chi^2_{2,0.05} = 5.99$. At the 5 percent level of significance, do not reject the hypothesis that the percentages for the three reasons are the same as the national averages.

(b) The estimate for the difference is $(\hat{p}_1 - \hat{p}_2) = (0.30 - 0.25) = 0.05$ with the estimated variance $v(\hat{p}_1 - \hat{p}_2) = [0.3(0.7) + 0.25(0.75) + 2(0.30)(0.25)]/200 = 0.00274$ and $S.E.$ $(\hat{p}_1 - \hat{p}_2) = 0.0523$. The test statistic becomes $z = (0.30 - 0.25)/0.0523 = 0.96$, which does not exceed $z_{0.05} = 1.645$. The hypothesis that the percentages for the cold symptoms and injuries do not differ is not rejected at the 5 percent significant level.

**9.3.** The expected numbers are presented in the parentheses.

|  | Age | | | |
| --- | --- | --- | --- | --- |
| Vaccination | 22 | 22–60 | $\geq 60$ | Total |
| Yes | 60(81) | 70(67.5) | 140(121.5) | 270 |
| No | 60(39) | 30(32.5) | 40(58.5) | 130 |
| Total | 120 | 100 | 180 | 400 |

From (9.3a), $U = 24.38$ with $(2 - 1)(3 - 1) = 2$ d.f. which is much larger than $\chi^2_{2,0.05} = 5.99$ with a very small p-value. There is a significant difference between age and receiving the vaccination.

**9.4.** From (9.3a), $U = 19.50$ with $(3 - 1)(3 - 1) = 4$ d.f. which is larger than $\chi^2_{4,0.05} = 9.49$ with the $p$-value of 0.0006. The hypothesis that age and hypertension levels are not related can be rejected at a very small significant level.

**9.5.** The Chisquare statistic U is obtained from 9.5(a) for all the three parts. (a) $U = 5.10$ with the $p$-value of 0.024. At a significance level of 2.4 percent or smaller, the proportions for the males and females are significantly different. (b) $U = 3.37$ is smaller than $\chi^2_{1,0.05} = 3.84$ with the $p$-value of 0.066. The proportions for the two age groups are not different at the 5 percent level of significance. (c) $U = 77.06$ with a very small $p$-value. The proportions are significantly different for the two types of patients.

**9.6.** For both (a) and (b), the test statistic U follows the Chisquare with a single degree of freedom degree. (a) The row and column totals respectively are (1334, 1830) and (1844, 1320) with the total sample size of $n = 3164$. From (9.5a), $U = 5.79$ with the $p$-value of 0.016. Medical care significantly differs for the full-year and part-year insured.

(b) The row and column totals respectively are (483, 993) and (944, 532) with the total sample size of 1476. From (9.5a), $U = 9.31$ with the $p$-value of 0.002. Medical care differs significantly for the full year public and private insurance.

**9.7.** For these observations, following Section 9.5.2, $A = 54$, $E = (7.5 + 12.0 + 25) = 44.5$, $V = (3.56 + 5.09 + 7.35) = 16.0$. From (9.7), $\chi^2_{MH} = (9.5 - 0.5)^2/16 = 5.06$ with the $p$-value of 0.024. The null hypothesis that the two treatments are equally effective is rejected at a small level of significance. Equivalently, the two SBP levels differ significantly for each of the treatments.

# Chapter 10

**10.1.** Estimate of $E(Y|X)$ is 154.35 with S.E = 6.42. Ninety-five percent confidence and prediction limits are (140.86, 167.84) and (106.77, 201.93).

**10.2.** (a) $t_{19} = (2.23 - 2)/(0.3326) = 0.69$ with the $p$-value of 0.4986. Do not reject $H_0 : \beta_1 = 2$.

(b) $t_{19} = (2.23 - 3)/(0.3326) = -2.32$ with the $p$-value of 0.032. Reject $H_0$: $\beta_1 = 3$ at the 3.2 percent significance level.

**10.3.** $\hat{\beta}_1 = (328.82/126.2) = 2.61$ and $\hat{\beta}_0 = 126.7 - 2.61(42.75) = 15.31$.

(a) The regression estimate for $E(Y/X_{1i})$ is $\hat{Y}_i = 15.31 + 2.61X_{1i}$.

| Coefficient | Estimate | S.E. | t | p-value |
|---|---|---|---|---|
| Intercept | 15.31 | 24.66 | 0.62 | 0.54 |
| Slope | 2.61 | 0.559 | 4.67 | 0.00017 |

(b) ANOVA for the significance of the regression.

| Source | d.f | SS | MS | F | p-value |
|---|---|---|---|---|---|
| Regression | 1 | 16278.36 | 16278.36 | 21.74 | 0.00017 |
| Residual | 18 | 13475.83 | 748.66 | | |
| Total | 19 | 29754.19 | | | |

For $H_0 : \beta_1 = 0$, $t_{18} = 2.61/0.559 = 4.67$ with the $p$-value of 0.00017. The regression of LDL on age is significant at the $p$-value of 0.00017. Same conclusion is obtained from the F-ratio of 21.74. The slight difference of this value from $(4.67)^2 = 21.81$ is due to the rounding-off error.

(c) Since $t_{18, 0.025} = 2.101$, confidence limits for the slope coefficient are $2.61 - 2.101(0.56) = 1.43$ and $2.61 + 2.101(0.56) = 3.79$. Confidence limits for the intercept are $15.31 - 2.101(24.66) = -36.50$ and $15.31 + 2.101(24.66) = 67.12$.

At $X_1 = 75$, $\hat{Y} = 15.31 + 2.61(75) = 211.06$. Further, $v(\hat{Y}) = 748.66[1/20 + (75 - 42.75)^2/2397.8] = 362.17$, and S.E. $(\hat{Y}) = 19.03$. Confidence limits for the mean of the LDL at age 75 are $211.06 - 2.101(19.03) = 171.08$ and $211.06 + 2.101(19.03) = 251.04$. The 95 percent prediction limits at $X_1 = 75$ are (140.71, 280.75).

At $X_1 = 65$, $\hat{Y} = 15.31 + 2.61(65) = 184.96$. Further, $v(\hat{Y}_{new} - Y_{new}) = 748.66$ $\left[1 + 1/20 + (65 - 42.75)^2/2397.75\right] = 940.67$  and  $\left[v(\hat{Y}_{new} - Y_{new})\right]^{1/2} = 30.67$.

Prediction intervals for LDL at the age of 65 are $184.96 - 2.101(30.67) = 120.52$ and $184.96 + 2.101(30.67) = 249.40$.

**10.4.** Estimate of $E(Y|X_{1i})$: $\hat{Y}_i = 56.9 - 0.334X_{1i}$.

ANOVA for the significance of the regression.

| Source | d.f. | SS | MS | F | p-value |
|---|---|---|---|---|---|
| Regression | 1 | 267.58 | 267.58 | 8.64 | 0.009 |
| Residual | 18 | 557.22 | 30.96 | | |
| Total | 19 | 824.80 | | | |

Estimates of the coefficients and S.E.s.

| Coefficient | Estimate | S.E. | t | p-value |
|---|---|---|---|---|
| Intercept | 56.88 | 5.01 | 11.34 | 0.000 |
| Age | -0.334 | .1136 | -2.94 | 0.009 |

HDL significantly decreases with age.

At age $X_1 = 75$, $\hat{Y} = 31.38$, $S.E.\left(\hat{Y}\right) = 3.87$. Ninety-five percent confidence and prediction limits respectively are (23.70, 39.96) and (17.59, 46.07).

**10.5.** Estimate of $E(Y|X_{2i})$ : $Y_i = 89.8 - 0.31X_{2i}$.

ANOVA for the significance of the regression.

| Source | d.f. | SS | MS | F | p-value |
|---|---|---|---|---|---|
| Regression | 1 | 408.89 | 408.89 | 17.7 | 0.001 |
| Residual | 18 | 415.91 | 23.11 | | |
| Total | 19 | 824.80 | | | |

| Coefficient | Estimate | S.E. | t | p-value |
|---|---|---|---|---|
| Intercept | 89.79 | 11.27 | 7.97 | 0.000 |
| Weight | -0.31 | 0.074 | -4.21 | 0.001 |

At weight $X_{2i} = 150$, $\hat{Y} = 43.28$ and $S.E.\left(\hat{Y}\right) = 1.09$. Ninety-five percent confidence and prediction limits respectively are (40.99, 45.56) and (32.92, 53.63).

At weight $X_{2i} = 165$, $\hat{Y} = 38.68$ and $S.E.\left(\hat{Y}\right) = 1.42$ Ninety-five percent confidence and prediction limits respectively are (35.69, 41.67) and (28.15, 49.21).

**10.6.** $\hat{Y} = 76.3 + 0.23X_1 - 0.35X_2 + 0.11X_3$.

(1) ANOVA.

| Source | d.f. | SS | MS | F | p-value |
|---|---|---|---|---|---|
| Regression | 3 | 455.23 | 151.74 | 6.57 | 0.004 |
| Residual | 16 | 369.57 | 23.10 | | |
| Total | 19 | 824.80 | | | |

(2) Estimates and S.E.s.

| Coefficient | Estimate | S.E. | $t$ | p-value |
|---|---|---|---|---|
| Intercept | 76.33 | 15.10 | 5.05 | |
| Age | 0.23 | 0.26 | 0.87 | 0.40 |
| Weight | −0.35 | 0.12 | −2.85 | 0.01 |
| Fitness | 0.11 | 0.08 | 1.35 | 0.20 |

At $X_1 = 70$, $X_2 = 170$ and $X_3 = 90$, $\hat{Y} = 41.74$ with $S.E.(\hat{Y}) = 5.23$; 95 percent Confidence intervals are (30.66, 52.83) and Prediction intervals are (26.69, 56.80).

**10.7.**
Males.

| Coefficient | Estimate | S.E. | $t_8$ | p-value |
|---|---|---|---|---|
| Intercept | 48.13 | 1.402 | 34.33 | $3.57 \times 10^{-9}$ |
| Slope | 0.505 | 0.043 | 11.67 | $3.88 \times 10^{-6}$ |

Females.

| Coefficient | Estimate | S.E. | $t_8$ | p-value |
|---|---|---|---|---|
| Intercept | 36.92 | 1.835 | 20.12 | $1.13 \times 10^{-7}$ |
| Slope | 0.541 | 0.057 | 9.56 | $1.11 \times 10^{-5}$ |

The increase of the overweight percentages over the years for both males and females has been highly significant.

**10.8.** The model is $E(Y/X) = \beta_0 + \beta_1 X + \beta_2 X^2$.

Period (X) and Percapita Expenditure (Y$).

| Coefficient | Estimate | S.E. | $t_6$ | p-value |
|---|---|---|---|---|
| $\beta_0$ | 175.8 | 120.60 | 1.46 | 0.195 |
| $\beta_1$ | −28.5 | 11.0 | −2.58 | 0.042 |
| $\beta_2$ | 3.35 | 0.20 | 16.71 | $0.29 \times 10^{-5}$ |

The second degree polynomial trend is highly significant. From the ANOVA Table, $F(2, 6) = 1900.35$ with a very small p-value. The per capita expenditure has increased significantly over the 50 years.

Period (X) and Private insurance (Y$).

| Coefficient | Estimate | S.E. | $t_6$ | p-value |
|---|---|---|---|---|
| $\beta_0$ | 53.29 | 52.95 | 1.01 | 0.353 |
| $\beta_1$ | −18.63 | 4.84 | −3.85 | 0.008 |
| $\beta_2$ | 1.026 | 0.088 | 11.66 | $0.24 \times 10^{-4}$ |

From the ANOVA Table, $F(2, 6) = 595.47$ with a very small p-value. The private insurance for health has increased significantly over the 50 years.

**10.9.** (a) Estimates of the intercept and slope are (5.12, 0.211) with S.E.s (0.155, 0.017) and $t_{13}$ of (33.0, 12.36). The p-values for both the coefficients are very small and the trend is highly significant. The annual rate of increase is $(0.211)(1000) = 211$ or 2.11 percent.

For the above regression, with $X_i = (1, 2,...,15)$, $\bar{X}=8$, $\sum_1^n (X_i-\bar{X})^2 = 280$

and $\hat{\sigma}^2 = 0.081$.

(b) The year 2020 corresponds to $X = 29$, and the estimate of the average expenditure for that year becomes $\hat{Y} = 5.12 + (0.211)(29) = 11.239$. From (10.10), $v(\hat{Y}) = (0.081)\left[(1/15) + (29-8)^2/280)\right] = 0.133$ and $S.E.(\hat{Y}) = 0.3647$. With $t_{13,0.025} = 2.16$, ninety-five percent confidence limits at $X = 29$ are $11.239 \pm 2.16 (0.3647)$, that is, (10.45, 12.03). For the year $2020, 95 percent. confidence limits for the average expenditure are $\$(10,450 - 12,030)$.

For the prediction at $X = 29$, $v(\hat{Y}_{new} - Y_{new}) = (0.081 + 0.133) = 0.214$ and $[v(\hat{Y}_{new} - Y_{new})]^{1/2} = 0.462$.

The 95 percent prediction intervals are $11.239 \pm 2.16(0.462)$, that is (10.24, 12.24). The prediction interval for 2020 are $\$(10,240 - 12,240)$.

**10.10.** (a)

| Coefficient | Estimate | S.E. | $z$ | p-value | OR | 95% Conf. lts for (OR) |
|---|---|---|---|---|---|---|
| Intercept | −5.43 | 2.578 | −2.11 | 0.035 | | |
| Age | 0.135 | 0.062 | 2.18 | 0.029 | 1.14 | 1.01, 1.29 |

(b)

| Coefficient | Estimate | S.E. | $z$ | p-value | OR | 95% Conf. lts for (OR) |
|---|---|---|---|---|---|---|
| Intercept | −33.82 | 14.574 | −2.32 | 0.02 | | |
| Weight | 0.224 | 0.096 | 2.34 | 0.019 | 1.25 | 1.04, 1.51 |

(c)

| Coefficient | Estimate | S.E. | z | p-value | OR | 95% Conf. lts for (OR) |
|---|---|---|---|---|---|---|
| Intercept | −54.80 | −27.04 | −2.03 | 0.043 | | |
| Age | 0.192 | −0.169 | −1.14 | 0.256 | 0.83 | 0.59, 1.15 |
| Weight | 0.413 | 0.216 | 1.92 | 0.055 | 1.51 | 0.99, 2.30 |

**10.11.** To test the null hypothesis $H_0 : \rho_{23} = 0$ *versus* $H_1 : \rho_{23} \neq 0$, from Table T10.1 (c), $t_{18} = (-0.42 - 0)/(0.0458)^{1/2} = -1.96$ with the $p$-value of 0.066. Hence $H_0$ is not rejected with a significance level of 6.6 percent or higher.

**10.12.** (a) $z = (1/2)ln[(1 + 0.74)/(1 - 0.74)] = 0.9505$ and $E(z) = (1/2)ln[(1 + 0.3)/(1 - 0.3)] = 0.3095$. As a result $Z = (0.9505 - 0.3095)(17)^{1/2} = 2.64$ with the $p$-value of 0.0082.

(b) $z = (1/2)ln[(1 - 0.82)/(1 + 0.82)] = -1.1568$ and $E(z) = (1/2)ln[(1 - 0.4)/(1 + 0.4)] = -0.4236$ Now, $Z = (-1.1568 + 0.4236)(17)^{1/2} = -3.02$ with the $p$-value of 0.0026.

(c) $z = (1/2)ln[(1 - 0.82)/(1 + 0.82)] = -1.1568$ and $E(z) = (1/2)ln[(1-0.6)/(1+0.6)] = -0.6931$ Now, $Z = (-1.1568 + 0.6931)(17)^{1/2} = -1.91$ with the $p$-value of 0.0562.

**10.13.** $C_l = (1/2)ln[(1 -0.82)/(1 + 0.82)] - 1.96/(17)^{1/2} = -1.6322$ and $C_u = (1/2)ln[(1 -0.82)/(1 + 0.82)] + 1.96/(17)^{1/2} = -0.6814$.

From the expressions in Section 10.10.3 or *Fisherinv*, confidence limits for $\rho_{13}$ become $(-0.93, -0.59)$.

**10.14.** $C_l = (1/2)ln[(1 + 0.26)/(1 - 0.26)] - 1.96/(17)^{1/2} = -0.2093$ and $C_u = (1/2)ln[(1 + 0.26)/(1 - 0.26)] + 1.96/(17)^{1/2} = 0.7415$.

Confidence limits for $\rho_{12}$ are $(-0.21, 0.63)$.

# Chapter 11

**11.1.**

ANOVA for the weights.

| Source | d.f. | SS | MS | F | p-value |
|---|---|---|---|---|---|
| Between groups | 2 | 1192.47 | 596.24 | 48.63 | 0.000 |
| Within groups | 27 | 331.0 | 12.26 | | |
| Total | 29 | 1523.47 | | | |

The difference among the means of the weights of the three groups is highly significant.

**11.2.**
ANOVA for the SBPs after the exercise program.

| Source | d.f. | SS | MS | F | p-value |
|---|---|---|---|---|---|
| Between groups | 2 | 1184.87 | 592.44 | 10.76 | 0.000 |
| Within groups | 27 | 1486.60 | 55.06 | | |
| Total | 29 | 2671.47 | | | |

The difference among the means of the SBPs of the three groups after the exercise program is highly significant.

**11.3.** For the weights in Exercise 11.1, $\hat{\sigma}_\alpha^2 = (119247-331)/10 = 86.15$. The 95 percent confidence limits for $R$ are $(48.63 - 4.242)/(10 \times 4.242) = 1.046$ and $(48.63 - 0.025)/(10 \times 0.025) = 194.42$.

**11.4.** For the SBPs after the exercise program in Exercise 11.2, $\hat{\sigma}_\alpha^2 = (592.44-55.06)/10 = 53.738$. The 95 percent confidence limits for R are $(10.76 - 4.242)/(10 \times 4.242) = 0.154$ and $(10.76 - 0.025)/(10 \times 0.025) = 42.94$.

**11.5.**

| Source | d.f | SS | MS | F | p-value |
|---|---|---|---|---|---|
| Between | 2 | 536.4 | 268.2 | 7.91 | 0.002 |
| Within | 27 | 915.8 | 33.9 | | |
| Total | 29 | 1452.2 | | | |

The estimate of $\sigma^2$ is $\hat{\sigma}^2 = 33.9$. The difference between the means of SBPs of the three groups is highly significant.

**11.6.** With $m_0 = 10$ as in Example 11.4, $\hat{\sigma}_\alpha^2 = (268.2 - 33.90/10) = 23.43$ from (11.25) and Exercise 11.5. The estimates of $V_i$ are $v_1 = 27.20$, $v_2 = 26.04$ and $v_3 = 27.67$. Now, the estimates of $W_i$ and $W$ are $w_1 = 1/27.20 = 0.0368$, $w_2 = 0.0384$, $w_3 = 0.0361$ and $w = 0.1113$. The estimate of $\mu$ becomes $\bar{y}_w = 129.56$, with $v(\bar{y}_w) = 1/w = 8.98$ and $S.E.(\bar{y}_w) = 2.997$.

**11.7.**
SS and SP for weight (x) and SBP after (y).

| Source | d.f. | x | y | xy |
|---|---|---|---|---|
| Between | 2 | 1192.47 | 1184.87 | 828.03 |
| Within | 27 | 331.00 | 1486.60 | 353.10 |
| Total | 29 | 1523.47 | 2671.47 | 1181.13 |

From these figures, $\hat{\beta} = 353.1/331 = 1.0668$, Regression $SS = 353.1^2/331 = 376.68$, $W_{y.x} = (1486.6 - 376.68) = 1109.92$ and $\hat{\sigma}^2 = 1109.92/26 = 42.69$ with 26 d.f. The test statistic for $H_0 : \beta = 0$ becomes $F(1, 26) = 376.68/42.69 = 8.82$ with the $p$-value of 0.0063. The SBPs significantly depend on the weights. To test the difference among the means, $T_{y.x} = 2671.47 - 1181.13^2/1523.47 = 1755.75$, and the test statistic becomes $F(2, 26) = [(1755.75 - 1109.92)/2]/42.69 = 7.56$ with the $p$-value of 0.0026. The difference among the means of the SBPs of the three groups after the exercise program is highly significant. From Exercise 11.2, the means of the SBPs of the three groups after the exercise program were found to be significantly different.

**11.8.** From Exercise 11.7, $Wxx = 331$, $\hat{\beta} = 1.0668$ and $\hat{\sigma}^2 = 42.69$ with 26 d.f. The S.E.s and ranks of the estimates appear in the parentheses.

| $\bar{y}_i$ | $\hat{\mu}_i$ | Confidence limits for $\mu_i$ |
|---|---|---|
| 131.2 (3) | 140.62 (1) (3.79) | 132.84, 148.40 |
| 132.9 (2) | 129.30 (3) (2.39) | 124.39, 134.21 |
| 145.3 (1) | 139.46 (2) (2.85) | 133.60, 145.32 |

Adjustment for the weight has altered the rank of the mean of the first group from the lowest to the highest. For the first two groups, $(\hat{\mu}_1 - \hat{\mu}_2) = (140.62 - 129.30) = 11.32$, $v(\hat{\mu}_1 - \hat{\mu}_2) = 42.69\left[(2/10) + (158.3 - 170.5)^2/331\right] = 27.73$, and S.E.$(\hat{\mu}_1 - \hat{\mu}_2) =$ 5.27. With $t_{26,0.025} = 2.056$, Ninety-five percent confidence limits for the difference of the two adjusted means become $(11.32 - 10.84) = 0.48$ and $(11.32 + 10.84) = 22.16$.

**11.9.**

| Source | d.f. | $x$ | $y$ | $xy$ |
|---|---|---|---|---|
| Between | 2 | 518.05 | 536.26 | 381.19 |
| Within | 26 | 865.54 | 915.91 | 306.48 |
| Total | 29 | 1383.59 | 1452.17 | 687.67 |

1. $\hat{\beta} = 306.48/865.54 = 0.3541$.

2. Regression SS $= (308.77 - 306.48)^2/865.54 = 108.18$.
   Error SS $W_{y.x} = (915.91 - 108.18) = 807.73$
   $\hat{\sigma}^2 = 807.73/26 = 31.07$.
   Test for $H_0 : \beta = 0$.
   $F_{1, 26} = (108.18/31.07) = 3.48$ with the p-value of 0.073 suggesting that the SBP does not depend highly on weight.
   Test for $H_0 : \mu_1 = \mu_2 = \ldots = \mu_k$
   $T_{y.x} = 1452.17 - (687.67^2/1383.59) = 1110.39$

$F_{2,26} = [(1110.39 - 797.11)/2]/30.66 = 4.87$ with the p-value of 0.016 suggesting that after adjusting for weight the difference among the means of the SBPs for the three age groups is significantly different.

**11.10.** From Exercise 11.9, $Wxx = 865.54$, $\hat{\beta} = 0.3541$ and $\hat{\sigma}^2 = 31.07$. The estimates of the means and confidence limits are as follows. S.E.s of the estimates are presented in the parentheses.

| Sample size: $n_i$ | $\bar{y}_i$ | $\hat{\mu}_i$ | Confidence limits |
|---|---|---|---|
| 9 | 125.00 (3) | 127.23 (2) (2.21) | 122.69, 131.77 |
| 13 | 127.92 (2) | 127.11 (3) (1.61) | 123.80, 130.42 |
| 8 | 135.90 (1) | 134.68 (1) (2.07) | 130.42, 138.94 |

There is only a very slight change for the adjusted means of the first two groups.

The difference of the adjusted means for the third and first groups is $(134.68 - 127.23) = 7.45$ with the estimate of the variance $31.07[(1/9 + 1/8) + (174.25 - 164.56)^2/865.54] = 10.71$ and S.E. of 3.27. With $t_{26,0.025} = 2.056$, 95 percent confidence limits for the difference of these two adjusted means become $(0.73, 14.17)$.

**11.11.**
ANOVA for the HDLs.

| Source | d.f. | SS | MS | F | p-value |
|---|---|---|---|---|---|
| Age groups | 3 | 299.8 | 99.93 | 4.08 | 0.033 |
| Treatments | 4 | 153.5 | 38.38 | 1.57 | 0.245 |
| Error | 12 | 293.7 | 24.48 | | |
| Total | 19 | 747.0 | | | |

Estimate of $\sigma^2$ is $\hat{\sigma}^2 = 24.48$. The difference of the means of the age groups is significant at the 3.3 percent level, and the difference between the treatment effects is not significant.

**11.12.**
ANOVA for the DBPs.

| Source | d.f | SS | MS | F | p-value |
|---|---|---|---|---|---|
| Patients | 2 | 52.67 | 26.34 | 2.03 | 0.212 |
| Treatments | 3 | 248.12 | 82.71 | 6.38 | 0.027 |
| Error | 6 | 77.83 | 12.97 | | |
| Total | 11 | 378.62 | | | |

$\hat{\sigma}^2 = 12.99$.
The difference between the treatment effects is highly significant. The difference between the patient effects is not significant.

**11.13.**
ANOVA for the decrease of the SBPs.

| Source | d.f. | SS | MS | F | $p$-value |
|---|---|---|---|---|---|
| Rows | 3 | 237.5 | 79.17 | 6.33 | 0.027 |
| Columns | 3 | 50 | 16.67 | 1.33 | 0.35 |
| Treatments | 3 | 112.5 | 37.5 | 3 | 0.117 |
| Residual | 6 | 75 | 12.5 | | |
| Total | 15 | 475 | | | |

The difference between the means of the three age groups is significant at the 2.7 level, but the difference between the treatment effects is not significant.

**11.14.** Row means: (8.83, 8.0, 11.33). Column means: (10.33, 9.67, 8.17). Grand mean = 9.39

ANOVA for the DBPs.

| Source | d.f. | SS | MS | F | $p$-value |
|---|---|---|---|---|---|
| Weight | 2 | 36.11 | 18.06 | 3.95 | 0.046 |
| Fitness | 2 | 14.78 | 7.39 | 1.62 | 0.236 |
| Error | 13 | 59.39 | 4.57 | | |
| Total | 17 | 110.28 | | | |

At the 5 percent level, the difference among the effects of the weights on the DBPs is significant, but not the difference among the exercise programs.

**11.15.**

| Source | d.f. | SS | MS | F | $p$-value |
|---|---|---|---|---|---|
| Weight | 2 | 36.11 | 18.06 | 15.48 | 0.001 |
| Fitness | 2 | 14.78 | 7.39 | 6.33 | 0.019 |
| Interaction | 4 | 48.89 | 12.22 | 10.48 | 0.002 |
| Error | 9 | 10.50 | 1.17 | | |
| Total | 17 | 110.28 | | | |

For this model, $\hat{\sigma}^2 = 1.17$. The difference between the effects of the weights and between the effects of the fitness classifications is highly significant. The interaction between weight and fitness is also highly significant.

**11.16.** For the observations in Exercise 11.15, Total = 232, Total SS 132.8, $S_R$ (unadj.) 51.37, $S_C$ (unadj.) = 38.13 and $S_B$ = 112.13. The adjusted row totals are

$$Q_1 = 88 - [2(58/6) + 2(70/6) + 3(104/8)] = 38/6$$
$$Q_2 = 66 - [2(58/6) + 2(70/6) + 3(104/8)] = -94/6,$$

and

$$Q_3 = 78 - [2(58/6) + 2(70/6) + 2(104/8)] = 56/6.$$

From (11.77), the estimating equations for the row effects are

$$109\alpha_1 - 59\alpha_2 - 50\alpha_3 = 152,$$

$$-59\alpha_1 + 109\alpha_2 - 50\alpha_3 = -376,$$

and

$$-50\alpha_1 - 50\alpha_2 + 100\alpha_3 = 224.$$

Setting $\alpha_1 = 0$ in these equations, $\hat{\alpha}_2 = -22/7$ and $\hat{\alpha}_3 = 234/350$. With these estimates, $S_R(\text{adj.}) = (22/7)(94/6) + (234/350)(56/6) = 55.48$. The adjusted column sum of squares becomes $S_C(\text{adj.}) = S_R(\text{adj.}) + S_C(\text{unadj.}) - S_R(\text{unadj.}) = 55.48 + 38.13 - 51.37 = 42.24$. The Error SS becomes $S_E = \text{Total } SS - S_R(\text{adj.}) - S_C(\text{unadj.}) = 132.8 - 55.48 - 38.13 = 39.19$, which is the same as $\text{Total } SS - S_C(\text{adj.}) - S_R(\text{unadj.}) = 132.8 - 42.24 - 51.37 = 39.19$.

ANOVA for the effects of the weights and fitness without interaction.

| Source | d.f. | SS(adj.) | MS | F | $p$-value |
|--------|------|----------|-----|-----|---------|
| Weight | 2 | 55.48 | 27.74 | 10.63 | 0.0019 |
| Fitness | 2 | 42.24 | 21.12 | 8.09 | 0.0041 |
| Error | 15 | 39.19 | 2.61 | | |
| Total | 19 | 132.80 | | | |

The estimate of $\sigma^2$ is $\hat{\sigma}^2 = 2.61$. For the DBPs, the effects of weight and fitness are highly significant.

With the interaction, $S_I = S_B - S_R(\text{adj.}) - S_C(\text{unadj.}) = 112.13 - 55.48 - 38.13 = 18.52$ with $(r-1)(c-1) = 4$ d.f. and $SE = \text{Total } SS - S_B = 132.8 - 112.13 = 20.67$ with $(n - rc) = 11$ d.f. The ANOVA with the interaction is as follows:

ANOVA for the effects of weight, fitness and interaction.

| Source | d.f. | SS | MS | F | $p$-value |
|--------|------|-----|-----|-----|---------|
| Weight (adj.) | 2 | 55.48 | 27.74 | 14.76 | 0.0008 |
| Fitness (adj.) | 2 | 42.24 | 21.12 | 11.23 | 0.0022 |
| Interaction | 4 | 18.52 | 4.63 | 2.46 | 0.107 |
| Error | 11 | 20.67 | 1.88 | | |
| Total | 19 | 132.8 | | | |

of $\sigma^2$ is $\hat{\sigma}^2 = 1.88$. The effects of weight and fitness are highly significant, but not their interaction.

**11.17.**
ANOVA for the percent of fatty acids.

| Source | d.f. | SS | MS | F | p-value |
|---|---|---|---|---|---|
| Between | 4 | 269.3 | 67.3 | 1.33 | 0.296 |
| Within | 19 | 964.0 | 50.7 | | |
| Total | 23 | 1233.3 | | | |

There is no significant difference among the averages of the fatty acids of the five types of foods.

**11.18.**
1. Private expenditure. $n = 172$. $\bar{x} = [35(42.76) + 53(32.75) + \ldots + 27(31.00)]/172 = 39.29$.

Between $SS = \left[35(42.76 - 39.29)^2 + 53(32.75 - 39.29)^2 + \ldots + 27(31.00 - 39.29)^2\right] = 8114.36$ with 4 d.f.

$\hat{\sigma}^2 = \left[34(13.91)^2 + 52(16.38)^2 + \ldots + 26(24.12)^2\right]/167 = 352.56$ with 167 d.f.

$F(4, 167) = (8114.36/4)/352.56 = 5.73$ with the $p$-value of 0.00024. The difference between the means of the private expenditures for the five regions is highly significant.

Total expenditure. $\bar{x} = 6.51$ and $\hat{\sigma}^2 = 6.41$ with 167 d.f. Between $SS = 129.12$.

$F(4, 167) = (129.12/4)/6.41 = 5.04$ with the $p$-value of 0.00074. The difference between the means of the total expenditure for the five regions is highly significant.

2. Africa and Asia. Private expenditures. Difference of the means is $(47.48 - 45.93) = 1.55$ with the S.E. of $[352.56(1/46 + 1/11)]^{1/2} = 6.3$, $t_{167} = (1.55/6.3) = 0.25$. The difference of the means of the private expenditures of the two regions is not significant.

3. Europe and Americas. Total expenditure. Difference of the means is $(7.35 - 6.83) = 0.52$ with the S.E. of $[6.41(1/35 + 1/53)]^{1/2} = 0.55$, $t_{167} = (0.52/0.55) = 0.95$. The difference between the means of the total expenditures of these two regions is not significant.

# Chapter 12

**12.1.** For the procedure in Section 12.4, $\hat{\sigma}_\alpha^2 = 27.47$, $w = 0.4289$, $\bar{y}_w = 17.53$, and $S.E.(\bar{y}_w) = 1.53$. For the alternative procedure in Section 12.5, $\hat{\sigma}_{\alpha 0}^2 = 32.41$, $r_0 = 0.3755$, $\bar{y}_w = 17.55$ and $S.E.(\bar{y}_w) = 1.63$.

**12.2.** The approximate degrees of freedom for $s_b^2$ and $s^2$ are $f_1 = 13$ and $f_2 = 234$. The test statistic in (12.8) for $H_0 : \sigma_\alpha^2 = 0$ becomes $F = (35.24/7.77) = 4.54$ with (13, 234) d.f. with a very small p-value. The variance component $\sigma_\alpha^2$ is significantly larger than zero.

When $(1 - \alpha) = 0.95$, the lower and upper limits for the $F$-distribution with (13, 234) d.f. are $(F_l, F_u) = (0.38, 1.96)$. The 95 percent confidence limits for $R$ are $(4.54/1.96) - 1 = 1.32$ and $(4.54/0.38) - 1 = 10.95$.

**12.3.**

|  | Before | After |
|---|---|---|
| $y_i$ | 132.22, 142.62, 148.13 | 125, 127.92, 135.88 |
| $s_i^2$ | 4.94, 2.3, 5.3 | 3.47, 1.75, 7.02 |
| $s_b^2$ | 65.28 | 31.75 |
| $s^2$ | 4.18 | 4.08 |
| $\hat{\sigma}_\alpha^2$ | 61.1 | 27.63 |
| $\bar{y}_w$ | 141.0 | 129.35 |
| S.E.$(\bar{y}_w)$ | 4.66 | 3.24 |
| $\bar{y}$ | 140.99 | 129.6 |
| S.E.$(\bar{y})$ | 4.66 | 3.25 |

For both the before and after cases, $\hat{\sigma}_\alpha^2$ is much larger than $s_i^2$ of each group. As a result, there is very little difference between $\bar{y}_w$ and $\bar{y}$ and their standard errors.

**12.4.** Since $y_i$ is the difference of the effects of the treatment and placebo, $s_i^2 = v = (2\hat{\sigma}^2/b)$. For the six institutions, $s_i^2 = (24, 26, 29, 30, 26, 34)$ and $s^2 = \sum_1^6 s_i^2/6 = 28.17$.

From the six values of $y_i$, $s_b^2 = 65.2$. Now $\hat{\sigma}_\alpha^2 = (65.2 - 28.17) = 37.03$. With $w_i = 1/(\hat{\sigma}_\alpha^2 + s_i^2)$, $w = 0.0923$. The estimate of $\mu$ in (12.1) becomes $\bar{y}_w = 5.31$ with its standard error of $1/\sqrt{w} = 3.29$. The unweighted mean is $\bar{y} = 5$ with its sample variance of $(65.2/6) = 10.87$ and standard error of 3.30. The difference between the standard errors of $\bar{y}_w$ and $\bar{y}$ is negligible.

# Chapter 13

**13.1.**
Solution from the *R*-program.

| $t_i$ | $r_i$ | No. of events | $\hat{S}(t_i)$ | S.E. $[\hat{S}(t_i)]$ | 95% Confidence limits |
|---|---|---|---|---|---|
| 8 | 12 | 1 | 0.92 | 0.079 | (0.76, 1.00) |
| 10 | 11 | 2 | 0.75 | 0.125 | (0.51, 1.00) |
| 12 | 9 | 1 | 0.67 | 0.136 | (0.40, 0.93) |
| 13 | 8 | 1 | 0.58 | 0.142 | (0.30, 0.86) |
| 14 | 7 | 2 | 0.42 | 0.142 | (0.14, 0.70) |
| 16 | 5 | 1 | 0.33 | 0.136 | (0.07, 0.60) |
| 18 | 4 | 1 | 0.25 | 0.125 | (0.01, 0.50) |
| 19 | 3 | 1 | 0.17 | 0.108 | (0.00, 0.38) |
| 20 | 2 | 1 | 0.08 | 0.080 | (0.00, 0.24) |
| 24 | 1 | 1 | 0.00 | 0.000 | (0.00, 0.00) |

**13.2.**

From the *R*-program.

| $t_i$ | $r_i$ | No. of events | $\hat{S}(t_i)$ | S.E. $[\hat{S}(t_i)]$ | 95% Confidence limits |
|---|---|---|---|---|---|
| 8 | 12 | 1 | 0.92 | 0.079 | (0.76, 1.00) |
| 10 | 11 | 2 | 0.75 | 0.125 | (0.51, 1.00) |
| 12 | 9 | 1 | 0.67 | 0.136 | (0.40, 0.93) |
| 14 | 7 | 1 | 0.57 | 0.146 | (0.28, 0.86) |
| 16 | 5 | 1 | 0.46 | 0.155 | (0.15, 0.76) |
| 18 | 4 | 1 | 0.34 | 0.153 | (0.04, 0.64) |
| 20 | 2 | 1 | 0.17 | 0.143 | (0.00, 0.45) |
| 24 | 1 | 1 | 0.00 | 0.000 | (0.00, 0.00) |

**13.3.** $O_1 = 15$, $E_1 = 11.29$, $V_1 = 5.32$ and $U = (15 - 11.29)^2/5.32 = 2.59$ with the *p*-value of 0.11. The difference between the two survival distributions is not significant.

# Chapter 14

**14.1.** (a) Boys: $r_S = 0.70$ and $r = 0.76$. (b) Girls: $r_S = 0.90$ and $r = 0.87$.

**14.2.** From the combined sample of the $n = 20$ observations, $W_1 = 80.5$ and $W_3 = 129.5$, with $E(W_1) = 10(21)/2 = 105$ and $V(W_1) = 10(10)21/12 = 175$. Now, $z = [|80.5 - 105| - 0.5]/(175)^{1/2} = 1.81$ with the *p*-values of 0.04 and 0.08 for the one and two-sided alternatives. The difference between the distributions of the two groups is not significant at the 5 percent level.

The sample means and standard deviations for these two groups are (142.4, 148.7) and (5.50, 7.47) respectively. The pooled variance is $s^2 = 43.025$ with 18 d.f. and S.E. for the difference of the sample means becomes 2.93. The test statistic is $t_{18} = -6.3/2.93 = -2.15$ with the *p*-values of 0.023 and 0.046 for the one and two-sided alternatives, suggesting significant difference between the two means at about the 5 percent level.

**14.3.** From the ranks of the combined sample of size $n = (n_1 + n_3) = (9 + 8) = 17$, $W_1 = 48.5$ and $W_3 = 104.5$. Since $n_3$ is smaller than $n_1$, $W_3$ remains the same, but sum of the ranks for the first group is adjusted to $W_1 = n_3(n-1) - W_3 = 8(18) - 104.5 = 39.5$. Now, $W = 39.5$ with $E(W) = n_1(n+1)/2 = 81$ and $V(W) = n_1 n_3(n+1)/12 = 108$. The test statistic becomes $z = [|39.5 - 81| - 0.5]/(108)^{1/2} = 3.95$ with a very small *p*-value for both the one and two-sided alternatives. There is a significant difference between the distributions of the SBPs before the exercise for the first and third groups.

The means and standard deviations of the first and third group are (132.22, 148.13) and (6.67, 6.51). With the pooled variance of $s^2 = 43.5$, the S.E. of the difference of the means becomes 3.20. With the normality assumption for the two groups, $t_{15} = -(15.91/3.2) = 4.97$ with a very small $p$-value for both the one and two-sided alternatives. The difference between the means of the SBPs of the first and third groups is significantly different.

**14.4.** From (14.3), $\chi_1^2 = [(22-12)-0.5]^2/34 = 2.65$ with the p-value of 0.1035. The change of the SBP from 140 is not significant at the 10 percent level.

**14.5.** From (14.6), $Q = 12$ with 2.d.f. and the $p$-value of 0.0025. The difference of the proportions of the patients with the reduction of the LDL by ten is significantly different.

**14.6.** Ranking the thirty observations in Table T11.3 from $(1 - 30)$, the ranks for the three samples are as follows:

|  | Ranks for weights | | |
|---|---|---|---|
|  | Group 1 | Group2 | Group 3 |
|  | 1 | 13 | 21 |
|  | 2 | 21 | 6.5 |
|  | 6.5 | 13 | 21 |
|  | 10.5 | 16.5 | 28.5 |
|  | 3 | 16.5 | 25 |
|  | 6.5 | 28.5 | 6.5 |
|  | 13 | 26.5 | 30 |
|  | 6.5 | 6.5 | 16.5 |
|  | 21 | 24 |  |
|  | 21 |  |  |
|  | 16.5 |  |  |
|  | 10.5 |  |  |
|  | 26.5 |  |  |
| Total $R_i$ | 70 | 240 | 155 |
| Mean | 7.78 | 18.46 | 19.38 |
| S.D. | 6.29 | 6.78 | 9.05 |

From the totals $R_i$, $\sum_1^3 R_i^2/n_i = 7978.339$, and from (14.7), $KW = (12/930)(7978.339) - 93 = 9.95$. From the Chisquare distribution with 2 d.f., the $p$-value becomes 0.0069. The three samples of weights can be considered to have come from populations with significantly different average weights.

# Chapter 15

**15.1.** From Table T11.4, the means of the SBPs after the exercise program for the first two groups are (125, 127.92). From the ANOVA Table of Example 11.3, $\hat{\sigma}^2 = 37.5$ with 27 d.f. The S.E.s of these two means are $\hat{\sigma}/3 = 2.04$ and

$\hat{\sigma}/\sqrt{13} = 1.70$ respectively. Since $t_{27,0.025} = 2.052$, 95 percent confidence limits for the mean of the first group are $125 - 2.052(2.04) = 120.81$ and $125 + 2.052(2.04) = 129.19$. Similarly, 95 percent confidence limits for the mean of the second group are $127.92 - 2.052(1.70) = 124.43$ and $127.92 + 2.052(1.70) = 131.41$. The 90 percent confidence region for the two means is enclosed by the limits (120.81, 129.19) and (124.43, 131.41).

**15.2.** The contrast and its estimate are $L = \mu_2 - \mu_3$ and $\hat{L} = 142.62 - 148.13 = -5.51$.

Since $v(\hat{L}) = [(1/13) + (1/8)](37.5) = 7.57$, S.E.$(\hat{L}) = 2.75$. The right-hand side of (15.5) becomes $\sqrt{2(3.35)} = 2.59$. Since $|\hat{L}|/S.E.(\hat{L}) = 2.004$ does not exceed 2.59, $H_0: L = 0$ is not rejected at the 5 percent significance level. For the $t$-test, $|\hat{L}|/S.E.(\hat{L})$ does not exceed $t_{0.025,27} = 2.052$, and hence this hypothesis is not rejected at the 5 percent significance level.

For Scheffe's approach, 95 percent confidence limits for $L$ from (12.6) are $-5.51 - 7.12 = -12.63$ and $-5.51 + 7.12 = 1.61$, with the confidence width of 14.24. From the $t$-statistic, the 95 percent confidence limits become $-5.51 - 2.052(2.75) = -11.153$ and $-5.51 + 2.502(2.75) = 0.133$ with the confidence width of 11.02.

**15.3.**
ANOVA for the percent of fatty acids.

| Source | d.f. | SS | MS | F | p-value |
| --- | --- | --- | --- | --- | --- |
| Between | 4 | 269.3 | 67.3 | 1.33 | 0.296 |
| Within | 19 | 964.0 | 50.7 | | |
| Total | 23 | 1233.3 | | | |

The difference in the fatty acids of the five types of foods is not significant.

(a) With $t_{19,0.025} = 2.093$, confidence limits for $(\mu_5 - \mu_1)$ are $5.5. \pm 2.093[50.7(1/7+1/3)]^{1/2}$, that is $(-4.75, 16.81)$. Since $\hat{\sigma} = 7.12$, with $q_{(5,19),0.05} = 4.26$, confidence limits for the difference of these two means are $5.53 \pm (4.26/\sqrt{2})(7.12)(1/7+1/3)^{1/2}$, that is, $(-9.27, -20.33)$.

(b) With $t_{19,0.025} = 2.093$, confidence limits for $(\mu_5 - \mu_4)$ are $11 \pm 2.093[50.7(2/3)]^{1/2}$, that is, $(-1.17, 23.17)$. With $q_{(5,9),0.05} = 4.26$, confidence limits for the difference of the two means are $11 \pm (4.26/\sqrt{2})(7.12)(2/3)^{1/2}$, that is, $(-6.51, 28.51)$.

# Appendix tables

Table T1.1   Heights (cm), Weights (kg) and BMI of 20 *ten*-year-old boys.

|        | Height | Weight | BMI   |
|--------|--------|--------|-------|
|        | 140    | 30     | 15.3  |
|        | 142    | 40     | 19.8  |
|        | 142    | 40     | 19.8  |
|        | 140    | 32     | 16.3  |
|        | 145    | 32     | 15.2  |
|        | 143    | 35     | 17.1  |
|        | 130    | 31     | 18.3  |
|        | 150    | 37     | 16.4  |
|        | 152    | 33     | 14.3  |
|        | 139    | 34     | 17.6  |
|        | 142    | 36     | 17.9  |
|        | 142    | 40     | 19.8  |
|        | 135    | 35     | 19.2  |
|        | 140    | 32     | 16.3  |
|        | 145    | 37     | 17.6  |
|        | 150    | 33     | 14.7  |
|        | 145    | 33     | 15.7  |
|        | 138    | 35     | 18.4  |
|        | 145    | 32     | 15.2  |
|        | 140    | 35     | 17.9  |
| Mean   | 142.25 | 34.60  | 17.14 |
| St.dev.| 5.12   | 3.00   | 1.76  |

*Source*: Adapted from "Stature for age and weight for age percentiles", Center for Disease Control, National Center for Health Statistics, May 30, 2000.

*Statistical Methodologies with Medical Applications*, First Edition. Poduri S.R.S. Rao.
© 2017 John Wiley & Sons, Ltd. Published 2017 by John Wiley & Sons, Ltd.

Table T1.2    Heights (cm), Weights (kg) and BMI's of 20 *ten*-year-old girls.

|        | Height | Weight | BMI   |
|--------|--------|--------|-------|
|        | 136    | 35     | 18.92 |
|        | 147    | 38     | 17.58 |
|        | 137    | 33     | 17.58 |
|        | 135    | 28     | 15.36 |
|        | 145    | 40     | 19.02 |
|        | 130    | 25     | 14.79 |
|        | 145    | 40     | 19.03 |
|        | 140    | 34     | 17.35 |
|        | 140    | 42     | 21.43 |
|        | 127    | 31     | 19.22 |
|        | 140    | 36     | 18.37 |
|        | 145    | 38     | 18.07 |
|        | 128    | 30     | 18.31 |
|        | 145    | 40     | 19.03 |
|        | 125    | 31     | 19.84 |
|        | 140    | 35     | 17.86 |
|        | 130    | 30     | 17.75 |
|        | 136    | 28     | 15.14 |
|        | 130    | 30     | 17.75 |
|        | 135    | 28     | 15.36 |
| Mean   | 136.80 | 33.60  | 17.89 |
| St.dev | 6.78   | 4.94   | 1.66  |

*Source*: Adapted from "Stature for age and weight for age percentiles," Center for Disease Control, National Center for Health Statistics, May 30, 2000.

Table T1.3    Heights (cm), Weights (kg) and BMI's of 20 *sixteen* year old boys.

|         | Height | Weight | BMI   |
|---------|--------|--------|-------|
|         | 173    | 60     | 20.05 |
|         | 180    | 72     | 22.22 |
|         | 160    | 52     | 20.31 |
|         | 184    | 80     | 23.63 |
|         | 179    | 55     | 17.17 |
|         | 165    | 55     | 20.20 |
|         | 167    | 58     | 20.80 |
|         | 172    | 60     | 20.28 |
|         | 176    | 65     | 20.98 |
|         | 182    | 78     | 23.55 |
|         | 170    | 75     | 25.95 |
|         | 162    | 63     | 24.01 |
|         | 165    | 48     | 17.63 |
|         | 160    | 57     | 22.27 |
|         | 168    | 61     | 21.61 |
|         | 185    | 80     | 23.37 |
|         | 168    | 57     | 20.20 |
|         | 170    | 62     | 21.45 |
|         | 166    | 58     | 21.05 |
|         | 170    | 60     | 20.76 |
| Mean    | 171.10 | 62.80  | 21.37 |
| St.dev. | 7.67   | 9.34   | 2.09  |

*Source*: Adapted from "Stature for age and weight for age percentiles", Center for Disease Control, National Center for Health Statistics, May 30, 2000.

Table T1.4    Heights (cm), Weights (kg) and BMI's of 20 *sixteen*-year-old girls.

|  | Height | Weight | BMI |
|---|---|---|---|
|  | 168 | 58 | 20.55 |
|  | 170 | 75 | 25.95 |
|  | 172 | 65 | 21.97 |
|  | 160 | 50 | 19.53 |
|  | 155 | 45 | 18.73 |
|  | 170 | 78 | 26.06 |
|  | 173 | 75 | 24.22 |
|  | 165 | 68 | 24.98 |
|  | 162 | 64 | 24.39 |
|  | 160 | 48 | 18.75 |
|  | 173 | 79 | 26.40 |
|  | 155 | 53 | 22.06 |
|  | 153 | 55 | 23.50 |
|  | 162 | 56 | 21.34 |
|  | 151 | 44 | 19.30 |
|  | 170 | 76 | 26.30 |
|  | 168 | 72 | 25.51 |
|  | 162 | 65 | 24.77 |
|  | 160 | 50 | 19.53 |
|  | 158 | 46 | 18.43 |
| Mean | 163.35 | 61.10 | 22.61 |
| St.dev. | 6.91 | 12.04 | 2.90 |

Table T1.5    Immunization Coverage (percentage) among 1-year olds in 2004 in the countries of the world.

| Percentage | Frequency | | |
|---|---|---|---|
|  | Measles | DTP3 | HepB3 |
| 20–30 | 1 | 1 | 1 |
| 30–40 | 4 | 4 | 1 |
| 40–50 | 5 | 5 | 4 |
| 50–60 | 11 | 6 | 5 |
| 60–70 | 15 | 14 | 8 |
| 70–80 | 26 | 26 | 19 |
| 80–90 | 35 | 39 | 33 |
| 90–100 | 95 | 97 | 72 |
| Number of countries: n | 192 | 192 | 143 |

*Source*: World Health Organization (WHO)- Health Service Coverage 2006, pp 34–40. For HepB3, one country has only eight percent, and the figures for 48 countries are not available in the WHO tables.

Table T4.1    US Population in 2006 in millions.

| Age (yrs) | Total | Males | Females |
|---|---|---|---|
| <1 | 4.13 | 2.11 | 2.02 |
| 1–4 | 16.29 | 8.33 | 7.96 |
| 5–14 | 40.34 | 20.64 | 19.70 |
| 15–24 | 42.44 | 21.85 | 20.59 |
| 25–34 | 40.42 | 20.57 | 19.85 |
| 35–44 | 43.67 | 21.85 | 21.82 |
| 45–54 | 43.28 | 21.29 | 21.99 |
| 55–64 | 31.59 | 15.22 | 16.36 |
| 65–74 | 18.92 | 8.67 | 10.25 |
| 75–84 | 13.05 | 5.30 | 7.75 |
| >85 | 5.30 | 1.69 | 3.61 |
| Total | 299.40 | 147.51 | 151.89 |
| Average of Age | 36.81 | 35.58 | 35.86 |
| St.dev. of Age | 22.51 | 21.85 | 23.19 |

*Source*: Health US, 2008, Table 1.

Table T4.2    Number of physicians in the U.S. per 10,000 civilian population.

| Number of Physicians | Frequency |
|---|---|
| 16.5–19.5 | 4 |
| 19.5–22.5 | 9 |
| 22.5–25.5 | 12 |
| 25.5–28.5 | 15 |
| 28.5–31.5 | 2 |
| 31.5–34.5 | 2 |
| 34.5–37.5 | 3 |
| 37.5–40.5 | 3 |
| 40.5–43.5 | 1 |

$n = 51$    $E(X) = 26.41$    $V(X) = 33.89$
$\mu_3 = 178.78$    $\mu_4 = 3765.72$    $k_1 = 0.82$
$k_2 = 0.12$

Table T4.3    Lowest per capita healthcare expenditures in 2006 at the average exchange rate (US$); 150 countries.

| Expenditure | Frequency |
| --- | --- |
| 0–50 | 52 |
| 50–100 | 21 |
| 100–150 | 12 |
| 150–200 | 9 |
| 200–250 | 10 |
| 250–300 | 11 |
| 300–350 | 7 |
| 350–400 | 5 |
| 400–450 | 3 |
| 450–500 | 5 |

*Source*: WHO

| Range ($) | Number of Countries | Average | Standard deviation |
| --- | --- | --- | --- |
| 4–500 | 135 | 140.79 | 133.29 |
| 500–1000 | 21 | 672.57 | 150.48 |
| 1000–6714 | 35 | 3325.54 | 1645.66 |

Table T5    Expenditure on health in 2006. Averages (top) and standard deviations (bottom).

| Region | Number of Countries | (a) | (b) | (c) | (d) |
| --- | --- | --- | --- | --- | --- |
| Americas | 35 | 345.09 | 619.03 | 42.76 | 6.83 |
| | | 657.20 | 1244.75 | 13.91 | 2.01 |
| Europe | 53 | 1424.25 | 1874.38 | 32.75 | 7.35 |
| | | 1585.61 | 1963.71 | 6.38 | 1.85 |
| Africa | 46 | 50.15 | 79.43 | 47.48 | 5.27 |
| | | 86.79 | 124.42 | 19.05 | 2.20 |
| Asia | 11 | 44.18 | 63.91 | 45.93 | 5.49 |
| | | 74.33 | 86.69 | 26.25 | 4.22 |
| South East Asia | 27 | 437.67 | 597.30 | 31.00 | 6.98 |
| | | 655.05 | 876.18 | 24.12 | 3.72 |

(a) Per capita government expenditure on health at average exchange rate (US$)

(b) Per capita total expenditure on health at average exchange rate (US$).

(c) Private expenditure on health as percentage of total expenditure on health

(d) Total expenditure on health as percentage of gross domestic product

*Source*: World Health Organization. http//:www.who.int

Table T10.1 (a)    Physical and diagnostic measurements of $n = 20$ adults.

| Age | Weight | Fitness | LDL | HDL |
|---|---|---|---|---|
| 35 | 136 | 120 | 85 | 46 |
| 26 | 140 | 120 | 90 | 49 |
| 29 | 134 | 120 | 75 | 49 |
| 39 | 159 | 120 | 174 | 37 |
| 53 | 156 | 60 | 150 | 40 |
| 45 | 156 | 90 | 130 | 35 |
| 32 | 150 | 120 | 100 | 36 |
| 41 | 154 | 90 | 169 | 38 |
| 33 | 140 | 120 | 129 | 55 |
| 46 | 120 | 60 | 80 | 48 |
| 41 | 159 | 120 | 150 | 40 |
| 53 | 163 | 60 | 155 | 35 |
| 64 | 171 | 60 | 175 | 38 |
| 37 | 144 | 120 | 80 | 50 |
| 50 | 166 | 120 | 160 | 38 |
| 35 | 148 | 120 | 75 | 54 |
| 27 | 137 | 120 | 72 | 46 |
| 56 | 164 | 90 | 150 | 45 |
| 59 | 180 | 60 | 170 | 35 |
| 54 | 170 | 60 | 165 | 38 |
| 42.75 | 152.35 | 97.50 | 126.7 | 42.6 |
| 11.23 | 14.98 | 27.31 | 39.57 | 6.59 |
| 126.2 | 224.35 | 746.05 | 1566.01 | 43.41 |
| 2397.75 | 4262.55 | 14174.95 | 29754.2 | 824.8 |

Means, standard deviations, variances and sums of squares of deviations from the mean are presented in the last four rows.

Table T10.1 (b)    Variances and Covariances of the measurements.

|        | Age     | Weight  | Fit     | LDL     | HDL   |
|--------|---------|---------|---------|---------|-------|
| Age    | 126.20  |         |         |         |       |
| Weight | 124.36  | 224.35  |         |         |       |
| Fit    | −250.66 | −171.71 | 746.05  |         |       |
| LDL    | 328.82  | 501.11  | −534.47 | 1566.01 |       |
| HDL    | −42.16  | −69.48  | 83.68   | −185.34 | 43.41 |

Table T10.1 (c)    Correlations of the measurements.

|        | Age   | Weight | Fit   | LDL   | HDL |
|--------|-------|--------|-------|-------|-----|
| Age    | 1     |        |       |       |     |
| Weight | 0.74  | 1      |       |       |     |
| Fit    | −0.82 | −0.42  | 1     |       |     |
| LDL    | 0.74  | 0.85   | −0.49 | 1     |     |
| HDL    | −0.57 | −0.70  | 0.47  | −0.71 | 1   |

Table T10.1 (d)    Corrected Sums of squares (SS) and Sums of Products (SP) of the measurements.

|        | Age      | Weight   | Fit       | LDL      | HDL    |
|--------|----------|----------|-----------|----------|--------|
| Age    | 2397.80  |          |           |          |        |
| Weight | 2362.84  | 4262.65  |           |          |        |
| Fit    | −4762.54 | −3262.49 | 14174.95  |          |        |
| LDL    | 6247.58  | 9521.09  | −10154.93 | 29754.19 |        |
| HDL    | −801.04  | −1320.12 | 1589.92   | −3521.46 | 824.79 |

Table T10.2   Weight and LDL of two groups of adults ($n_1 = 9$, $n_2 = 11$); first group followed by the second.

| Weight | LDL |
|--------|-----|
| 140 | 125 |
| 140 | 110 |
| 137 | 100 |
| 134 | 110 |
| 130 | 110 |
| 140 | 135 |
| 148 | 130 |
| 144 | 130 |
| 144 | 125 |
| 154 | 120 |
| 159 | 130 |
| 156 | 125 |
| 150 | 122 |
| 166 | 130 |
| 156 | 135 |
| 163 | 140 |
| 170 | 145 |
| 164 | 135 |
| 175 | 140 |
| 170 | 135 |

Table T10.3   Percent of the overweight (includes obesity, $BMI \geq 25$) 20–74 years old persons.

| Years | X | Males and females | Males | Females |
|-------|---|-------------------|-------|---------|
| 1960–1962 | 0 | 44.8 | 49.5 | 40.2 |
| 1971–1974 | 10 | 47.7 | 54.7 | 41.1 |
| 1976–1980 | 15 | 47.4 | 52.9 | 42.0 |
| 1988–1994 | 30 | 56.0 | 61.0 | 51.2 |
| 1999–2002 | 40 | 65.2 | 68.8 | 61.7 |
| 2003–2006 | 45 | 66.9 | 72.6 | 61.2 |
| 2007–2010 | 50 | 68.5 | 73.3 | 63.9 |

Source: Health United States, 2012.
Table 68 Healthy weight, overweight and obesity among adults 20 years and over.

Table T10.4    Personal Healthcare Expenditure.

| Year | Time period | Per capita expenditure ($) | All persons (billions $) | Private insurance ($) |
|------|-------------|----------------------------|--------------------------|-----------------------|
| 1960 | 0  | 125  | 23.4   | 6.6    |
| 1970 | 10 | 300  | 63.1   | 29.6   |
| 1980 | 20 | 943  | 217.2  | 132.0  |
| 1990 | 30 | 2430 | 616.8  | 403.3  |
| 2000 | 40 | 4128 | 1165.4 | 844.8  |
| 2005 | 45 | 5745 | 1697.2 | 1281.1 |
| 2008 | 48 | 6615 | 2010.2 | 1544.9 |
| 2009 | 49 | 6886 | 2109.0 | 1637.1 |
| 2010 | 50 | 7082 | 2186.0 | 1703.0 |

*Source*: *Health Statistics United States, 2012.*

Table T11.1    Age and weight of three groups of size $m = 10$ adults each. (for balanced one-way).

|        | Group 1 | | Group 2 | | Group 3 | |
|--------|---------|--------|---------|--------|---------|--------|
|        | Age | Weight | Age | Weight | Age | Weight |
|        | 45 | 155 | 55 | 170 | 75 | 175 |
|        | 40 | 165 | 50 | 168 | 75 | 170 |
|        | 36 | 160 | 56 | 172 | 72 | 170 |
|        | 35 | 155 | 58 | 170 | 70 | 172 |
|        | 30 | 150 | 60 | 175 | 74 | 170 |
|        | 42 | 160 | 58 | 170 | 72 | 175 |
|        | 36 | 156 | 60 | 175 | 75 | 175 |
|        | 35 | 160 | 60 | 172 | 70 | 168 |
|        | 40 | 162 | 56 | 168 | 78 | 175 |
|        | 42 | 160 | 55 | 165 | 78 | 176 |
| Mean   | 38.1 | 158.3 | 56.8 | 170.5 | 73.9 | 172.6 |
| S.D.   | 4.46 | 4.30  | 3.12 | 3.14  | 2.89 | 2.91  |

Table T11.2   Systolic blood pressures (mmHg) of the three groups of the adults in Table 11 before and after an exercise program; balanced case.

|        | Group 1 | | Group 2 | | Group 3 | |
|--------|---------|-------|---------|-------|---------|-------|
|        | Before | After | Before | After | Before | After |
|        | 145 | 130 | 150 | 140 | 155 | 150 |
|        | 150 | 135 | 138 | 130 | 140 | 142 |
|        | 148 | 130 | 135 | 125 | 140 | 138 |
|        | 140 | 120 | 135 | 120 | 146 | 144 |
|        | 140 | 135 | 140 | 138 | 140 | 138 |
|        | 140 | 132 | 155 | 148 | 158 | 152 |
|        | 136 | 130 | 150 | 145 | 158 | 148 |
|        | 150 | 132 | 142 | 138 | 145 | 140 |
|        | 135 | 130 | 130 | 125 | 150 | 145 |
|        | 140 | 138 | 125 | 120 | 155 | 156 |
| Mean   | 142.4 | 131.2 | 140.0 | 132.9 | 148.7 | 145.3 |
| S.D    | 5.5 | 4.8 | 9.45 | 10.25 | 7.47 | 6.11 |

Table T11.3   Age (years) and weight (lbs) of $n = 30$ adults in three age groups of sizes $n_1 = 9$, $n_2 = 13$ and $n_3 = 8$.

|        | Group1 | | Group 2 | | Group 3 | |
|--------|--------|--------|---------|--------|---------|--------|
|        | Age | Weight | Age | Weight | Age | Weight |
|        | 30 | 155 | 56 | 170 | 70 | 175 |
|        | 35 | 158 | 55 | 175 | 10 | 165 |
|        | 46 | 165 | 56 | 170 | 75 | 175 |
|        | 44 | 168 | 60 | 172 | 70 | 180 |
|        | 48 | 160 | 65 | 172 | 75 | 177 |
|        | 48 | 165 | 58 | 180 | 77 | 165 |
|        | 38 | 170 | 60 | 178 | 78 | 185 |
|        | 35 | 165 | 65 | 165 | 74 | 172 |
|        | 45 | 175 | 56 | 176 |    |    |
|        |    |    | 58 | 175 |    |    |
|        |    |    | 60 | 172 |    |    |
|        |    |    | 66 | 168 |    |    |
|        |    |    | 65 | 178 |    |    |
| Mean   | 41 | 164.556 | 60 | 173.154 | 73.63 | 174.25 |
| S.D.   | 6.61 | 6.187 | 4 | 4.337 | 3.25 | 6.902 |

Table T11.4    Systolic Blood Pressures (mmHg) for the adults in Table T11.3 before and after an exercise program.

| | Group 1 | | Group 2 | | Group 3 | |
|---|---|---|---|---|---|---|
| | Before | After | Before | After | Before | After |
| | 120 | 120 | 140 | 140 | 155 | 150 |
| | 125 | 120 | 135 | 130 | 145 | 130 |
| | 135 | 130 | 135 | 125 | 155 | 135 |
| | 135 | 130 | 140 | 130 | 150 | 135 |
| | 130 | 120 | 145 | 128 | 135 | 125 |
| | 130 | 120 | 150 | 130 | 145 | 135 |
| | 140 | 135 | 150 | 130 | 150 | 142 |
| | 135 | 125 | 140 | 125 | 150 | 135 |
| | 140 | 125 | 145 | 125 | | |
| | | | 140 | 120 | | |
| | | | 142 | 125 | | |
| | | | 140 | 125 | | |
| | | | 152 | 130 | | |
| Mean | 132.22 | 125 | 142.62 | 127.92 | 148.13 | 135.90 |
| S.D. | 6.67 | 5.59 | 5.47 | 4.77 | 6.51 | 7.49 |

# References

Allan, F. G., and Wishart, J. (1930). A method of estimating the yield of a missing plot in field experiments. *J. Agri. Sci.* 20, 399–406.

Baignet, C., Blackwell, L., Emberson, J., et al. (2010). Efficacy and safety of more intensive lowering of LDL cholesterol: a meta-analysis of data from 170,000 participants in 26 randomized trials. *Lancet* 376(9753), 1670–1681.

Bartlett, M. S. (1937). Properties of sufficiency and statistical tests. *Proc. Roy. Statist. Soc.*, Series A., 160, 268–282.

Beherens, W. V. (1964). The comparison of means of independent normal distributions with different variances. *Biometrics* 20, 16–27.

Chrysant, S. G., Neutel, J. M., and Ferdinand, K. C. (2009). Irbersartan/hydrochlorothiazide for the treatment of isolated systolic hypertension: a subgroup analysis of the inclusive trial. *J. Natl. Med. Assoc.* 101, 300–307.

Cochran, W. G. (1937). Problems arising in the analysis of a series of experiments. *J. Roy. Statist. Soc.*, Suppl. 4, 102–118.

Cochran, W. G. (1938). Long-term agricultural experiments. *J. Roy. Stat. Soc. Suppl.* 6, 104–148.

Cochran, W. G. (1950). The comparison of percentages in matched samples. *Biometrika* 37, 255–266.

Cochran, W. G. (1954a). The combination of estimates from different experiments. *Biometrics* 10, 101–129.

Cochran, W. G. (1954b). Some methods of strengthening the common $\chi^2$ tests. *Biometrics*, 10, 417–451.

Cochran, W. G. (1964). Approximate significance levels of the Behrens-Fisher test. *Biometrics* 20, 191–195.

Cochran, W. G. (1977). *Sampling Techniques*. Third ed. New York: Wiley.

Colson, E. R., Rybin, D., Smith, L. A., Colton, T., et al. (2009). Trends and factors associated with infant sleeping position; the National Infant Sleeping Position study, 1993–2007. *Arch. Pediatr. Adolesc. Med.*, 163(120), 1122–1128.

Colton, T., Gosselin, R. E., and Smith, R. P. (1968). The tolerance of coffee drinkers to caffeine. *Clin. Pharmacol. Ther.* 9, 31.

Cox, D. R. (1972). Regression models and life-tables. *J. Roy. Statist. Soc.* B34(2), 187–220.

Cox, D. R., and Oakes, D. (1984). *Analysis of Survival Data*. Chapman & Hall.

*Statistical Methodologies with Medical Applications*, First Edition. Poduri S.R.S. Rao.
© 2017 John Wiley & Sons, Ltd. Published 2017 by John Wiley & Sons, Ltd.

Cushman, L. A., Poduri, K. R., and Palenski, C. (1995). Predicting discharge functional status and rehabilitation efficiency from preadmission functional assessments. *J. Stroke Cerebrovasc. Dis.* 5(1), 33–38.

Davison, A. C., and Hinkley, D. V. (1997). *Bootstrap Methods and Their Applications*. Cambridge Series in Statistics and Probabilistic Methods. Cambridge: Cambridge University Press.

DerSimonian, R., and Laird, N. (1986). Meta-analysis in clinical trials. *Controlled Clinical Trials* 7, 177–188.

Efron, B., and Tibishirani, R. J. (1998). *An Introduction to Bootstrap*. Chapman & Hall/CRC Press.

Fisher, R. A. (1915). Frequency distribution of the values of the correlation coefficient in samples from an indefinitely large population. *Biometrika* 10, 507–521.

Fisher, R. A. (1921). On the probable error of a coefficient of correlation deduced from a small sample. *Metron* 1, 3–32.

Fisher, R. A. (1925). *Statistical Methods for Research Workers*. Hafner Publishing Company.

Fisher, R. A. (1935). *The Design of Experiments*. Oliver and Boyd.

Fisher, R. A. (1941). The asymptotic approach to Beheren's integral, with further tables for the *d* test of significance. *Ann. Eugen.* 11, 141–172.

Fisher, E. S., Bynum, J. P., and Skinner, J. S. (2009). Slowing the growth of health care costs – lessons from regional variation. *N. Engl. J. Med.*, 360(9), 849–852.

Flegal, K. M., Graubard, B. I., Williamson, D. F., and Gail, M. H. (2005). Excess deaths associated with underweight, overweight, and obesity. *J. Am. Med. Assoc.* 293(15), 1861–1867.

Galton, F. (1885). Regression towards mediocrity in hereditary stature. *J. Anthropological Institute* 15, 246–263.

Josyula, S., Lin, J., Xue, X., et al. (2015). Household air pollution and cancers other than lung: a meta-analysis. *Environmental Health* 14, 24.

Kaplan, E. L., and Meier, P. (1958). Nonparametric estimation from incomplete observations. *J. Am. Statist. Assoc.* 53 (282), 457–481.

Kruskal, W. H., and Wallis, W. A. (1952). Use of ranks in one-criterion variance analysis. *J. Am. Statist. Assoc.*, 47, 583–621.

Lee, E. T. (1992). *Statistical Methods for Survival Data*. Second ed. New York: Wiley.

Little, R. J. A., and Rubin, D. B. (1987). Statistical analysis with missing data. New York: John Wiley and Sons.

Louis, T. A., Lavori, P. W., Bailar, J. C., and Polansky, M. (1992). Crossover and self-controlled designs in clinical research. In *Medical Uses of Statistics*, Bailar, J. C. and Mosteller, M. (Eds.), 83–103. Second ed. Boston, MA: NEJM Books.

Mann, H. B., and Whitney, D. R. (1947). On a test of whether one of two random variables is stochastically larger than the other. *Ann. Math. Statist.* 18, 50–60.

Mantel, N., and Haenszel, W. (1959). Statistical aspects of the analysis of data from retrospective studies of disease. *J. Nat. Cancer Inst.* 22, 719.

McNemar, Q. (1947). Note on the sampling error of the difference between correlated proportions or percentages. *Psychometrika* 12, 153–157.

Mosselli, G. et al. (2010). Celiac disease: evaluation with dynamic contrast-enhanced MR imaging. *Radiology* 256(3), 783–790.

Mozaffarian, D., Katan, M. B., Ascherio, A. et al. (2006). Trans fatty acids and cardiovascular disease. *N. Engl. J. Med.* 354(15), 1601–1612.

Muhm, J. M., Rock, P. B., McMullin, D. L. et al. (2007). Effect of aircraft-cabin altitude on passenger discomfort. *N. Engl. J. Med.* 357, 18–27.

Neyman, J., and Pearson, E. S. (1933). On the problem of the most efficient tests of statistical hypotheses. *Phil. Trans. Roy. Soc. A : Math. Phy. and En. Sci.* 231, 694–706.

Ogden, C. L., and Carroll, M. (2010). Prevalence of obesity among children and adolescents: United States, trends 1963–1965 through 2007–2008. *Health E-stat.* Available at http://www.cdc.gov/nchs/data/hestat/obesity_child_07_08/obesity_child_07_08.htm.

Ogden, C. L., Carroll, M.D., Curtin, L. R. et al. (2006). Prevalence of overweight and obesity in the United States, 1999–2004, *J. Am. Med. Assoc.* 295, 1549–1555.

Olson, L. M., Tang, S. S., and Newacheck, P. W. (2005). Children in the United States with discontinuous health insurance coverage. *N. Engl. J. Med.* 353(4), 382–391.

Poduri, K. R., Cushman, L. A., and Gibson, C. J. (1996). Inpatient rehabilitation: the correlation between functional gains and appropriateness of admissions. *Int. J. Rehab. Res.* 19, 327–332.

Poduri, K. R., Palenski, C., and Gibson, C. J. (1996). Inpatient rehabilitation: Physiatristic and nurse practitioner admission assessment of stroke patients and their rehabilitation outcomes. *Int. J. Rehab. Res.* 19, 111–121.

Rao, Poduri S. R. S. (1997). *Variance Components estimation: Mixed models, Methodologies and Applications.* London: Chapman & Hall.

Rao, Poduri S. R. S. (2000). *Sampling Methodologies with Applications.* Boca Raton, FL; New York: Chapman & Hall/CRC.

Rao, Poduri S. R. S., Kaplan, J., and Cochran, W. G. (1981). Estimators for the One-way Random Effects Model With Unequal Error Variances. *J. Am. Stat. Assoc.* 76, 89–97.

Ross, J. S., Bradley, E. H., and Busch, S. H. (2006). Use of health care services by lower-income and higher-income uninsured adults. *J. Am. Med. Assoc.* 295(17), 2027–2036.

Rothwell, P. M., Fowkes F. G., Belch J. F. et al. (2011). *Lancet* 377(9759), 31–41.

Satterthwaite, F.E. (1946). An Approximate Distribution of Estimates of Variance Components. *Biometrical Bulletin* 2, 110–114.

Sachs, F. M., Bray, G. A., Carey V. J. et al. (2009). Comparison of weight-loss diets with different compositions of fat, protein, and carbohydrates. *N. Engl. J. Med.* 360 (9), 859–873.

Scheffe, H. (1959). *The Analysis of Variance.* New York: John Wiley and Sons.

Siegel, S. (1956). *Nonparametric Statistics for the Behavioral Sciences.* McGraw-Hill Series in Psychology. New York: McGraw-Hill.

Snedecor, G. W., and Cochran, W. G. (1967). *Statistical Methods.* Sixth ed. Ames: Iowa State University Press.

Tukey, J. W. (1949). One Degree of Freedom for Non-Additivity. *Biometrics* 5, 232–242.

Wilcoxon, F. (1945). Individual comparisons by ranking methods. *Biometrics Bull.* 1, 80–83.

Yates, F., and Cochran, W. G. (1938). The analysis of groups of experiments. *J. Agri. Sci.* 28(4), 556–280.

Zanobetti, A., Bind, M. A., and Schwartz, J. (2008). Particulate air pollution and survival in COPD cohort. *Environ Health* 7, 48.

Smoking and Health: Report of the Advisory Committee to the Surgeon General of the Public Health Service (1964) U. S. Department of Health, Education and Welfare. Jan 11.

Chart Tables of the CDC. (2008). Health Statistics.

Health United States. 2012. Figure 23. Patients, primary reason for emergency department visit, by age and reason. United States, average annual 2009–2010.

National Health and Nutrition Examination Survey (NHANES), 1999–2002.

World Health Organization (WHO) Reports.

# Index